ABJECTLY BOUNDLESS

Dedicated to Elza Rudge 1908–2009

Abjectly Boundless
Boundaries, Bodies and Health Work

Edited by
TRUDY RUDGE
University of Sydney, Australia
and
DAVE HOLMES
University of Ottawa, Canada

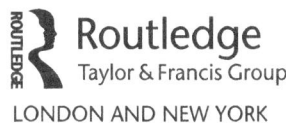

LONDON AND NEW YORK

First published 2010 by Ashgate Publishing

2 Park Square, Milton Park, Abingdon, Oxforshire OX14 4RN
711 Third Avenue, New York, NY 10017

Routledge is an imprint of the Taylor & Francis Group, an informa business

First issued in paperback 2018

British Library Cataloguing in Publication Data
Abjectly boundless : boundaries, bodies and health work.
   1. Human body--Social aspects. 2. Medical care--
   Psychological aspects. 3. Medical personnel--Attitudes.
   4. Medical personnel and patient. 5. Aversion. 6. Kristeva,
   Julia, 1941-
   I. Rudge, Trudy. II. Holmes, Dave, 1967-
   362.1'019-dc22

Library of Congress Cataloging-in-Publication Data
bjectly boundless : boundaries, bodies, and health work / [edited by] by Trudy Rudge and Dave Holmes.
      p.cm.
   Includes bibliographical references and index.
   ISBN 978-0-7546-7910-3 (hardback) 1. Medical personnel and patient. 2. Medical personnel--Attitudes. 3. Social medicine. 4. Medical anthropology. I. Rudge, Trudy. II. Holmes, Dave, 1967-
   [DNLM: 1. Attitude of Health Personnel. 2. Attitude to Health. 3. Burnout, Profes-sional. 4. Human Body. 5. Patient Care--psychology. W 21 A149 2009]
   R727.3.A247 2009
   610.69'6--dc22

                                                                          2009037624
ISBN 978-0-7546-7910-3 (hbk)
ISBN 978-1-138-36702-9 (pbk)

Contents

List of Figures

List of Tables

Notes on Contributors

Jackie Cook is a Senior Lecturer in the School of Communications Studies at the University of South Australia, Australia. Her PhD explored community and talk back radio's place in the capitalist enterprise. Her work has considered masculinity and sport, comedy and sports reporting, cultural and textual analysis of talk back radio, the development of innovative cross disciplinary educational innovations in local communities and Aboriginal communities in Central Australia. Her work is published in cultural and communications studies journals and she is a founding organizer of the international conference *Consoling Passions: Feminism, Soaps and Media Studies*.

Alicia Evans practises clinical psychoanalysis and is a member of The Freudian School of Melbourne (a school of Lacanian psychoanalysis). She is also a Senior Lecturer (Mental Health) in the School of Nursing and Midwifery at the Australian Catholic University in Melbourne.

Cary Federman is the author of *The Body and the State: Habeas Corpus and American Jurisprudence* (SUNY Press, 2006). He has a PhD from the Department of Government, the University of Virginia. Professor Federman has been a Fulbright Scholar at the Faculty of Political Science, the University of Zagreb, Croatia, and at the Institute of Criminology, Faculty of Law, University of Ljubljana, Slovenia. Currently, he is Assistant Professor of Justice Studies in the Department of Justice Studies, Montclair State University, New Jersey, United States.

Marilou Gagnon is Assistant Professor of Nursing in the School of Nursing, Faculty of Health Sciences, University of Ottawa (Canada). Her field of study addresses the experience of HIV positive women living with lipodystrophy.

Audrey Giles completed her doctoral dissertation in the Faculty of Physical Education and Recreation at the University of Alberta. She is Assistant Professor in the School of Human Kinetics at the University of Ottawa (Canada). Her SSHRC-funded program of research focuses on the intersections of gender, culture and physical practices, primarily in Canada's North.

Dave Holmes is Professor of Nursing and Vice-Dean (Academic) in the Faculty of Health Sciences, University of Ottawa (Canada). He is also University Research Chair in Forensic Nursing. His scholarly interests lie in the critique of prevailing orthodoxies and regimes of truth that influence the operations of the health care apparatus (*dispositif*). His work has been, and continues to be, strongly influenced by those of Canguilhem, Deleuze & Guattari, Foucault, Nietzsche and other writings from a postmodernist/poststructuralist perspective. He is the Editor-in-Chief of *Aporia*, an international peer-reviewed nursing journal and co-editor (with SJ Murray) of the book titled *Critical Interventions in the Ethics of Healthcare* (Ashgate, 2009).

Katrina Jaworski has recently completed her doctoral thesis which examined gender and gendering in suicide in suicidology, and sites of practice including sociology, law, medicine, psy-knowledge and newsprint media. She currently works as a Post Doctoral Research Associate at the School of Health Sciences, University of South Australia.

David Kissane is Professor of Psychiatry and Attending Psychiatrist, Memorial Sloan-Kettering Cancer Centre. He has a medical degree and M.D. from University of Melbourne, Faculty of Medicine (Australia). He is the Alfred P. Sloan Chair of and Chairman, Department of Psychiatry and Behavioural Sciences at the MSK Cancer Center. He has, across a 30-year medical career, trained in family medicine, psychiatry of the medically ill and palliative medicine. His research has focussed on group therapy in cases of breast cancer and family therapy during palliative care and bereavement. He has published widely in this area and in 2002, published *Family Focused Group Therapy.*

Deborah Lupton Freelance writer and profressional researcher. Former Professor of Sociology and Cultural Studies at Charles Sturt University, Australia. She has authored/co-authored over 100 journal articles and book chapters, and eleven books on topics primarily relating to the sociocultural aspects of health, medicine and risk, including *Risk* (Routledge, 1999), *Medicine as Culture* (2nd edition, Sage, 2003) and *Risk and Everyday Life* (with J. Tulloch, Sage, 2003).

Marc Lafrance is Assistant Professor in the Department of Sociology and Anthropology at Concordia University, Montreal (Canada). Winner of two Commonwealth Scholarships, Lafrance earned his Master's and Doctoral degrees at the University of Oxford. Lafrance's research relates to questions of subjectivity, embodiment and culture and has been published in refeered journals like *Body and Society* and edited collections like *Reading Nip/Tuck* (Palgrave-MacMillan, 2008).

Joanna Latimer is Reader in Social Science at Cardiff University, United Kingdom. She has published widely in medical and cultural sociology, particularly in relation to power and participation. Joanna is chair of the Ageing, Science and Older People network and the Medicine and Society Research Interest Group at Cardiff, and is currently working on a number of research projects that investigate the relation between science, medicine, culture and conceptions of personhood, including a new book *The Gene, the Clinic & the Family: Diagnosing Dysmorphology, Reviving medical dominance.* Joanna is associate editor of *Gender, Work and Organization*, and a member of the editorial board of *The Sociological Review*.

Sylvie Lauzon is Associate Vice-President Academic at the University of Ottawa and also Associate Professor of Nursing in the School of Nursing, Faculty of Health Sciences, University of Ottawa (Canada). Her work involves nursing epistemology and care of older adults. Her research focused on the experience of family caregivers living with people suffering from dementia and chronic mental disorders.

Janet McCabe is Assistant Professor of Nursing at the College of Nursing, University of Saskatchewan (Canada) and PhD candidate in the School of Nursing, Faculty of Health Sciences at the University of Ottawa (Canada). She received her Masters in Education from the University of Toronto. She has worked as a pediatric nurse (in both acute care and outpatient settings) for several years. Her research interests lie in the areas of disability studies, Foucauldian analysis of nursing work, and sexual health.

Patrick O'Byrne is currently Assistant Professor of Nursing in the School of Nursing at the University of Ottawa (Canada). His field of study addresses the intersection of desire, drugs, and unsafe sexual practices from a critical public health perspective. He works as a Registered Nurse in the fields of harm reduction and sexual health at the City of Ottawa.

Beverleigh Quested is a registered nurse who has worked in the specialization of Haematology and Bone Marrow Transplantation for more than 25 years. She is currently the Transfusion Nurse Educator, Transfusion Medicine Services, Australian Red Cross Blood Service as well as continuing in a clinical role on a Haematology Bone Marrow Transplant Unit. She has a Master of Nursing (Advanced Practice) and this chapter is a part of her unpublished PhD thesis exploring blood stem cell transplantation.

Jeanne Randolph is a retired psychiatrist and also an independent intellectual whose most recent book is titled *Ethics of Luxury: Materialism and Imagination.* Dr Randolph is noted for her performances and writing about psychoanalytic theory, visual arts, the technological ethos, mass spectator sports, and occasional allegories about the lives of bugs.

Allison Roderick is a registered nurse with extensive experience in Critical Care nursing in Australia and the United Kingdom. Her academic career combined her love of clinical work and education, teaching undergraduate patho-physiology, sociology and research. Allison is currently enrolled in the Doctoral program at

Flinders University (Australia) and her thesis explores nurses' infection control practices. In particular her research interests are risky and abject bodies in nursing and health.

Trudy Rudge is a Professor of Nursing at the University of Sydney, Australia. She is a nurse with specializations in trauma and mental health. She has an honours degree in Anthropology and a PhD in nursing from LaTrobe University, Melbourne. Her continuing project is to bring a critical perspective such as Foucault and Kristeva to nursing and health care research by applying theoretical perspectives from the humanities and social sciences to enquiry. She publishes analyses of embodiment, nursing and spatial analysis, technology studies in nursing and cultures of care in acute and primary health care environments.

Virginia Schmied is an Associate Professor (Midwifery/Child and Family Health) in the School of Nursing at the University of Western Sydney, Australia. Dr Schmied has over twenty-five years experience in clinical practice, education, research and consultancy. She has built a program of nursing and midwifery research using both qualitative and quantitative methodologies. Dr Schmied has conducted funded research on the transition to parenthood, women's experiences of pregnancy, childbirth and parenting education, breastfeeding, models of midwifery care and postnatal care and the role of child and family health nurse in Australia.

Annette Street Professor of Nursing at LaTrobe University (Australia) has an international reputation in health care and nursing research. She has a track record of bringing research projects to a timely conclusion and to publication. She has received grant support from major funding bodies in Australia, New Zealand, and Thailand. Annette has conducted research consultancies throughout Australia, New Zealand, Sweden, Canada, Thailand, the UK and in the USA. Her research books *Inside Nursing* and *Nursing Replay*, along with other published monographs, are used in graduate programs in nursing and education in Asian and English-speaking countries.

Roanne Thomas-MacLean is Associate Professor in the Department of Sociology at the University of Saskatchewan (Canada). Prior to her appointment there, she completed a postdoctoral fellowship in interdisciplinary primary health care research. Her interests focus on the exploration of chronic illness, particularly cancer, and its implications for people's everyday lives. She holds a Canadian Institutes of Health Research/Saskatchewan Health Research Foundation New Investigator Award.

Foreword

The education of nurses has always been under the authority of a society's dominant values. The most iconic example is Florence Nightingale, whose diaries express and explain a Christian interpretation of the dedication intrinsic to nursing. As this volume's authors explore, however, another paradigm – Kristeva's theory of abjection – offers an interpretation that extends the experience of nursing beyond society's dominant values. This is significant and relevant to all caregivers, and particularly to nurses, who must contend with aspects of nursing that cannot be articulated by our currently dominant values: the methods and language of science. Quite simply, the extremes of both religious and scientific interpretations of damaged, dirty, leaking, decaying bodies and body parts, ignore the experience of two of the most engaged parties – the nurses themselves and their patients. Extreme Christian dualism valorizes the patient's soul and demeans 'the flesh' as transient; yet nurses are called to tend, comfort and help restore this highly suspect vessel. Extreme scientism positions both the nurses' practice and the patients' bodies as objects; yet nurses are called to tend, comfort and help restore people who scream, moan, bleed, stink and ooze. As the authors of these chapters emphasize, the position of the nurses is paradoxical to be sure. Trudy Rudge and Dave Holmes, the Editors, propose that the experience of nursing exceeds the dominant language's depiction. And, most importantly, this collection illustrates the many possibilities available when the interpretation of nursing praxis is translated into Kristeva's language of the abject. The position and the experience of abjection, the concepts of disgust, pollution and chaos, return nursing to its foundational elements, maternal compassion, for example, which occupies and is a fine embodiment of abjection. Breastfeeding itself has been translated over the past century from the language of 'Natural' to the language of technology (bottle feeding is more convenient, efficient and sanitary) and now into the language of science (breast-fed babies are more intelligent, less allergic, more immune, etc.). The concept of abjection reveals the enchantment of materials that are both inside and outside the body. For example semen is of the body yet leaves the body to enter another body. In fact, some essays develop the necessary re-evaluation of the social connotations of semen since the AIDS epidemic, when previously semen was rarely a relevant aspect of nursing consciousness. As this book demonstrates, dominant value systems are in place to eliminate confusion, ambiguity and indeed ambivalence. Yet abjection floridly asserts the reality of the confusion between sanitary and unsanitary, the ambiguity of healing and decaying, the ambivalence of nurses' response to mutilation, to spillage, to deterioration of mind and body, to another person's corpse. If nurses are to be educated humanely, their function as humans caught between polarities of clean and unclean, whole and fragmented, strong and weak, autonomous and dependent, order and chaos, between life and death, has to be acknowledged and navigated. The concept of abjection reveals the plenitude of understanding that is necessary for the practice of nursing to meet the ethical dilemmas of a changing world.

Jeanne Randolph MD, F.R.C.P.(C)
Winnipeg, Manitoba, CANADA

Acknowledgements

Trudy Rudge and Dave Holmes would like to acknowledge the financial support of the Faculty of Health Sciences at the University of Ottawa. Thanks to Sébastien Dunn, whose patient work at various stages of the manuscript has been indispensable. Special thanks to Diana Thorneycroft for authorising the use of her work for the book cover.

Introduction
Abjectly Boundless: Boundaries, Bodies and Health Work

Trudy Rudge and Dave Holmes

Introduction

From the seeming chaos of war zones and emergency rooms to the ritualized order of forensic psychiatric settings and many other practice environments, nurses often experience feelings of disgust and repulsion in their practice. For these intense feelings to occur, an abject object must exist. Cadaverous, sick, disabled bodies, troubled minds, wounds, vomit, faeces, and so forth are all part of nursing work and threaten the clean and proper bodies of nurses. The unclean side of nursing is rarely accounted for in academic literature: it is silenced (Holmes, Perron, and O'Byrne 2006).

The objective of this edited collection is to demonstrate to what extent the concept of abjection have been used in nursing, health and social sciences to look at boundary work. This proposed book is an edited collection of authors who use the work of Julia Kristeva, usually the psychoanalytical defence mechanism of abjection, to analyse bodies and boundary work in health-related situations. The editors have noted a continuing return to her work with its particular salience to all that disgusts, horrifies and renders the certain, uncertain. While there is a constant use of her work in film and cultural studies, there is a less obvious, but equally constant, use of her work in health care research. This use of Kristeva arises out of the relevance of the emotional defence of the abject to explanations about lack of boundaries, sullying of subjectivities, and when various attempts to regain certainty are mobilized. Much of what occurs in these situations is challenging to describe let alone provide accounts representing the range and extent of human reactions. Kristeva's theorization of the psychical defence of abjection affords the possibility of voicing the incomprehensible in bodies that leak, in the chaos of illness and disease, and in the monstrosity of illnesses such as cancer, as well as much that is deemed 'out of place' in health care.

Therefore, all contributors are committed to engage the reader in a philosophical/psychoanalytical (thus theoretical) analysis of abjection and disgust in the health care domain. To achieve this goal, authors have drawn on ideas gleaned from the works of renowned theorists such as Mary Douglas (2002), Julia Kristeva

(1982), and William Miller (1998) to illustrate major concepts such as abjection, disgust, and pollution in order to provide sufficient theoretical insight to allow for the application of these works to a broad range of day-to-day health-related experiences. As pointed out lucidly by Parker (2004) and Lawler (1991), nursing and health care practices are caught within a matrix where subjectivities, systems, and order are intertwined but can easily be disrupted by the breakdown of bodies (or parts of bodies), persons, and places. For example, nurses and other health care professionals are exposed to and confronted by many forms of disruptive health issues and practices that challenge the order of the clean and proper and engage them at a personal level of anxiety and perhaps even fear. The very nature of abjection is to bring about a retreat from the abject even in the face of extensive socialization to do otherwise. Our challenge is to bring into the open the important impact of the concept of abjection, which historically has been silenced in the health sciences.

Abjection and the Abject Body

Late postmodern psychoanalyst Julia Kristeva is a prominent figure in the literature on abjection (Sim 2002). According to her, the feeling of abjection is first developed during infancy when the young child (between 6 and 18 months of age), as part of the process of self-identification, begins to reject certain parts of his being. The rejected elements may be such things as faeces and sour milk, but they may also include symbolic representations of the child's relationship with their mother (Kristeva 1982). This process is necessary for any child who strives to construct his own identity and become a person; in doing so, the child begins to enter the realm of the symbolic. Following Lacan, and against the primacy of the patricide in the Oedipal myth of Freud, Kristeva argues for the defence of abjection as emotional primer for all other defence mechanisms that follow. Located in the pre-linguistic psychical structures, she asserts that abjection and the abject body drive the infant to the symbolic order and language – to the paternal function. This rejection of the maternal function and its authority (as a part of the incest taboo) lies under many of the ambiguities that follow.

The rejected matter may be under voluntary control or not. It includes what one excretes or spits but also what leaves the body unaided through the mouth, nose, or genitals. What is rejected is never completely dissociated from the body, however, because it remains attached to it at an unconscious level (McAfee 2004). In other words, although it leaves the body, rejected matter is still bound to the body through the unconscious, and the threat it poses to the immaculate manifests itself at the conscious and the unconscious level; the semiotic and symbolic levels (McAfee 2004). Therefore, that which is rejected is both manifest (concrete), a physical product of the subject (excrement, secretions, and so on), and imaginary (symbolic), existing metaphorically because of the cognitive process taking place in which the abject evokes filth and is associated with pollution of the body and mind.

The mapping of what counts as proper and improper, clean and unclean, possible and impossible is accomplished through the work and authority of the maternal function (Kristeva 1982). The maternal function forever is associated with civilizing of the infant body, just as abjection places this function outside of the control of the symbolic order and signifies the maternal function as 'lack'. Paradoxically, such exclusion constitutes the basis of the maternal power – a power that both repels and pleasures. It is this duality of the abject that signifies why nurses and their work are a challenge to present in the symbolic order of language. Nurses, who civilize and contain, are doubly implicated in the feminine. As a part of this, feminist analyses or interest in nurses' work is rare, and some reasons for this may be that nurses (male and female) are too abject, too feminine and too defiled. Kristeva's psychoanalytic concept offers nurses (and other health researchers) a way to bring this incomprehensibility to our understanding. She makes it obvious why nurses also run to religious symbolism such as 'vocation' to understand their work and their pleasure in it; or on the other hand, to science, to contain and disavow the horror of the work they do.

The abject is considered to be abject because it threatens the non-abject that is, the clean and proper (Kristeva 1982). Its threat derives from its promise of unwanted outcomes (faeces or fluids secreted because of a disease). For example, food, an absolute necessity for keeping the body alive, inevitably breaks down into digested waste material and in this way mirrors the reality that the body will eventually die and decompose. Kristeva (1982) maintains that a corpse constitutes the utmost portrayal of the abject. In this case, the abject is real; it takes on a physical and visible shape. The corpse embodies the unbreakable interrelationship between life and death, and the observer is forced to recognize that one cannot exist without the other. The dead body functions as the intermediate between these states; it is the inescapable outcome of having lived. The proximity of a cadaver to a living body emphasizes the frailness of the latter, whose physical boundaries are thus violated by the former (Kristeva 1982).

The abject constitutes a threat only insofar as it makes its demarcating lines illusory. In constructing the self, the 'separateness of our individual bodies' (Mansfield 2000: 82) is perceived as essential in defining one's subjectivity. Kristeva argues, however, that this separateness is tenuous because it is born within our idealism and ideology (Mansfield 2000). This process of alienation is necessary in order to get a sense of one's separateness: 'I give birth to myself amid the violence of sobs, of vomit' (Kristeva 1982: 3). However it challenges and questions one's sense of integrity: is the expelled matter still part of me because it comes from me? Do I own it? Because of this uncertainty, the lines that differentiate the inside from the outside of the body shift and fluctuate, thus destabilizing the sense of subjectivity because the abject belongs to both sides. An individual needs to reject subhuman matter in order to strengthen his or her subjectivity and preserve a *Self propre* (clean, proper, self-controlled body) but in doing so is continuously facing doubt about personal integrity and autonomy: 'The subject remains in process, forever trying to establish itself, forever pushing away at those things that relentlessly challenge its limits' (Mansfield 2000: 83).

Shildrick (2002) echoes some of Kristeva's ideas, but she uses the metaphor of the monster to illustrate the demarcation between the self and the nonself. Like the abject, the monstrous helps individuals define their identity through their corporeality because monsters have a 'confused and essentially fluid corporeality' (Shildrick 2002: 48). The monstrous forces itself into one's consciousness, thus defining the subjectivity of the majority by comparison (and opposition). Securing one's subjectivity, according to this author, revolves around an inviolable, distinct, and autonomous self/body. The monstrous thus gives meaning to the self by serving as a nonself against which comparisons may be made. For instance, representations of 'nurse' have been influenced by the monstrous, and the self-sacrificing maternal function where the person is subject of and subject to, abjection (Kristeva 1982). The defence of abjection constitutes nurses in many of popular culture's icons as monstrous and improper, as much as divine and angelic. While the symbolic order is set to control for abjection's effects and affect – *jouissance* in sublimation and disavowal in law and science, yet its power to horrify remains installed in our psyche always already a threat to our hard-won singularity. In such a situation, the monstrous and angelic nurse may well be one and the same thing, as each simultaneously signals and disavows the abject/abjected body and its correlate emotion (Kristeva 1982).

The abject is both disgusting and irresistible, outraging and fascinating (Kristeva 1982). As such, the person experiences what Kristeva describes as a loss of meaning, a breakdown of the distinction between the subject and the object, a collapse of symbolic order. The abject represents instability and ambiguity because it is neither subject nor object (Mansfield 2000). Abjection goes beyond the perception of one's body. It even goes beyond fluid subjectivity: the abject challenges established 'systems of order, meaning, truth and law … and laws that produce a controlled and manageable subject' (Mansfield 2000: 85). The abject, therefore, brings forth the uncertainty or chaos that systems of order attempt to govern through structures of truth: Thus the meaning of the abjection of the individual subject and its clean and proper body is entangled in the abstract and general sphere of truth and power. Put simply, the stability of both the dominant symbolic and the political order relies on individual subject's commitment to the desperate self-discipline of the clean and proper body (Mansfield 2000: 85).

A Cautionary Word

Much of Kristeva's work is contentious and in contention. As with all uses of theories or concepts, there are many difficulties and challenges put forward as to the effectiveness of abjection as an explanatory device. Some of these issues come from the sheer difficulty of her writing – the style of exegesis, the difficult language and the use of many terms from literary theories, philosophy and psychoanalysis that are unfamiliar to an audience not *au fait* with the refinements of the Freudian and Lacanian debates, or Kristeva's philosophical roots. Many of the critiques of her work focus on her debates with feminism (later French feminists and the Anglo-American feminists), their charges against her seeming unqualified acceptance of Freudian and Lacanian psycho-sexual development and with what they term, Kristeva's essentialist arguments about femininity, motherhood and the body. Such debates are more indicative of the concerns (perhaps horrors) of Anglo-American feminists such as Judith Butler, Nancy Fraser and Toril Moi and their fears that writings such as Kristeva's on abjection, return to an essentialism that they had fought against to obtain equalities for women (Oliver 1993, Beardsworth 2004, McAfee 2004). Kristeva has not always bothered to repudiate such attacks, instead offering a view that some feminist authors in their rush to separate themselves from the oppression and female embodiment, have not done anything for women or their embodiment as women, mothers and so on.

Issues such as this also feed into the difficulties many have with her use of psychoanalytic theories to work through deeper philosophical issues around embodiment, and ontological concerns about life, death and the connectedness of people. In this case, Kristeva, while having a bias towards Lacanian psychoanalytical models of the psyche, still uses Freudian psychoanalytical insights to generate and ground her arguments. For instance, in the developing the notion of the abject, her arguments use the notion of phobia and the uncanny to develop where this affective realm emerges, its affects and effects. In working out the inner life of abjection, she reworks the Oedipal drama, asking how Freud discounted or lessened the role of maternal incest in his use of the mythical story. Such reworkings have laid her open to critiques from Lacanian and Freudian analysts alike, and continues her debates with feminists who are wary of their use. Moreover, others such as Frosh (1987) and Lechte (1990) wonder why she has not explored or challenged the powers that are embedded in psychoanalysis in relation to the authority of the figure of the analyst. This in particular relates to the unquestioning rights of analysts to diagnose and label the normalities or abnormalities of the psyche against the rights of the analysand.

Many would assert that there is more to this than the power of psychoanalysts to define abnormality in the psyche. Others find the very idea of psychical structures such as the conscious and unconscious problematic, let alone the figures of ego, id and superego, and their defence mechanisms. The entire façade of contemporary psychology is built around a focus on the empirical view of the mind (what is available for analysis made evident in psychometric tests, reviews of visible behaviours and now with brain imaging, what the areas of the brain light up, when…) and debates as to the 'scientific' validity of psychoanalysis – as either treatment or model of human understanding. In this respect, the figuring of abjection comes into question as explanatory of anything at all.

Located as this is at the edges of consciousness, like a movement half seen at the periphery of our field of vision, abjection seems a most flimsy explanation for these elements of great moment. Yet as we hope to show in this collection, Kristeva opens up for exploration the singularities of the experiences of the body, health and illness and what counts as significant in such events. Her development of the idea of the subject in process/on trial following from Heidegger, Nietzsche and Deleuze, affords the writers in this collection a way into the various issues about what lies inside or outside, the transgressive and sacred, the self and Other. The idea of abjection provides a view of embodiment that overcomes the scientized medical view of illness and the flattening of experiences that flow from this. Moreover, this idea also affords a view of the apparatus (*dispositif*) that raises science, empirical evidence and biopower above the symbolic and expressive realms in health and illness. As many authors show, it is in the fold of the process between body and other, inside and outside where abjection hovers and where the great systems we raise to keep it 'in place' so often fail. It is these systems – health care priorities, managerialism, scientific explanations and professional agendas – that so often impede or reduce such experiences to their orderings and priorities, and in setting each ordering and re-ordering, are doomed to fail. The abject locates the paradoxes of working with and for people with spoiled identities and whose bodies have the potential to defile. It is the hope, too, in what follows to show that abjection is not a singular or essentialized affective realm, but rather 'an unfolding' that expresses the ambiguities and contingencies that the sciences of health care set out to disavow. In this respect, the analyses explore the politics and ethics of the processes of health and body work – from the perspective of patient and health workers. It also explores nurses and their work in particular – a group of health workers that many feminists perceive as too traditionally female to study. The concept of the abject also affords nurses a positive and affirming view of their work with patients, confirming the power and attraction of nurturance, forbearance and tolerance. It is the hope that this collection affords a resistance to the rejection of nurses' relational work, and its diminishment in the rush to efficiencies offered in the 'management' of health care and the nursing workforce.

Part I: Fluids and Transgression of Boundaries

This book is constituted of three distinct, yet interdependent sections. Part I deals with bodily fluids and the transgression of bodily boundaries that occur when these fluids leak, cross its orifices or otherwise are not containable. Kristeva identifies two key types of defiling substances. These are excremental and menstrual. 'Excrement and its equivalents (decay, infection, disease, corpse, etc.) stand for the danger to identity that comes from without… Menstrual blood, on the contrary, stands for the danger issuing from within the identity (social or sexual)' (Kristeva 1982: 71). However Kelly Oliver (1993), in her analysis of Kristeva, highlights how the substances that defile change. A recent focus on the toxicity and effects of the toxins in current environments has changed how semen is coded. Moreover, all blood, not just menstrual blood has been destabilized through its association with

HIV/AIDS and other viral pollutants, particularly in Western society. In the case of blood it can be coded in the two main categories as a threat from the outside and a threat to identity when it is menstrual.

In this first section of the book, our contributors highlight how fluids are viewed in contemporary society. Through explorations of bodily fluids such as, semen, breast milk, or menstruation or through analysis of the toxicity of bodies, or representations of the suicide corpse each shows how the abject positions us and creates emotions that horrify and transfix, as they simultaneously fascinates us. In a traditional analysis of fluids, semen and breast milk would not have made the list as a fluid that transgresses, whereas menstrual blood in 'tradition' has always been considered polluting and dangerous (see Giles below). Schmied and Lupton (in this collection) outline how, when women's relation to maternity changed, they also developed a different relationship with breastfeeding. While some of their participants viewed their breastfeeding from within the discourses of 'breast is best', many others found the leakiness of their bodies and the chaos of breastfeeding at odds with the picture of present day womanhood as autonomous and in control.

Similarly by association, the transgressive in homosexual sexuality (Holmes and Federman this volume) has been amplified by the addition of a body viewed as having the potential to pollute others. As this body is represented in public health messages as 'risky', such messages contain within them the seeds of horror and also fascination and excitement. The structural components of gender and sex combine to promote alternative messages from those that the public health discourses seek to promote. Such an exploration indicates how the abject plays out in the discourse of health, and renders those who are its target, subject of and subject to its discursive effects. A psychoanalytical reading of these messages using Kristeva promotes an understanding of the hidden implications in such messages and provides reasons why these messages stigmatize and 'other', and also shows how, from within the group, these influences may promote less than helpful practices against safe sex (O'Byrne in this collection).

A further theme in this part of the book is on the abject and abjected body. In the case of the representations of lethal suicide in forensic textbooks, the lethality of the act promulgates the view of the gendering of suicide as intrinsically a masculine practice. As an indicator, lethality and its re-presentations present the abject body as corpse where that corpse has resulted from an act of taking one's life. Like the homosexual body, the corpse resulting from suicide signifies an act of self-destruction that is surrounded by medical assemblages that want us to read them as mere neutral, objective records of the events leading to the death (see Jaworski in this volume). However, the results of such records are to present a corpse, one that science considers stabilized but one that nevertheless escapes, signifying chaos and disorder – the abject. Bodies, not only their fluids, transgress the boundaries that surround them, and escape our futile efforts at control and objectification (Holmes and Federman, Jaworski, Schmied and Lupton in this collection).

Part II: Abject Positioning

In this section of the book, we turn to an exploration of how bodies and identity are inextricably linked as what affects one, invariably affects one's certainty in identity. The body/self registers its abject positioning says Kristeva because bodies always already escape our best efforts to obtain their civilization. Our *self propre* has the germs of its decay within it, as chaos waits on the other side of order to challenge all of the rules, strategies, dictums and ordering we use to bind and control our bodies. Moreover, abject positioning relates to order/chaos beyond the body itself, reaching into the systems (discursive and extra-discursive) where structures are mobilized to contain the abject and abject bodies. In this section our contributors explore in various ways how bodies, and the systems which contain them, fail to take account of how abject positioning and the abject body resist systemic effort.

In cancer care Thomas-MacLean and Quested identify how loss of identity, bodily mutilations and annihilation of body systems are where abjection resides. Thomas-MacLean shows how in the process of breast cancer diagnosis, the body itself becomes the danger; whereas with the treatment for blood cancers, equally life threatening, the preparation for the treatment of grafting drives stem cell transplant recipients into the abject spaces of betwixt and between (Quested in this collection). An exploration of abject positioning discloses much about cancer survivorship and its narratives, where the body becomes a source of chaos, the position of survivor signals a return to containment; a containment nevertheless underpinned by a heightened awareness of the certainty of our future deaths.

In this section we consider how acts such as euthanasia and the development of care models may work to overcome some of the effects of abjection on the dying and those with chronic, stigmatized conditions such as HIV/AIDS. In exploring the act of euthanasia, we more deeply understand how the dying seek to control for abjection's effects, even as these acts remain outside the parameters of end of life care. It is clear too, why practitioners of end of life care would invalidate the dying who enact euthanasia as a solution to the insolubility of their dying process (see Street and Kissane below). Similarly, Marilou Gagnon argues that an ethical response to the care of people with HIV/AIDS is possible when we take account of the symbols of their illness and the social and personal experience of abjection, and when this is done we will further our understanding of corporeality in such a stigmatizing condition.

In the case of a person who loses their face, to reclaim a face that will not be considered horrific, Marc Lafrance explores the challenge mounted by such restorative surgery to our understandings about the stability of identity. Simultaneously as this surgery is trumpeted as heroic restitution of a person to normality, the operation also speaks of ambivalence we feel for the work of such surgeons. Clearly, the transformations made possible through cosmetic surgery trouble as much as they excite, but in the case of this surgery, an identity is re-constituted by a process of normalizing that which was made abnormal through trauma. Can an identity be re-made in such a fashion or is identity destabilized, made abject, hence causing our ambivalence despite cosmetic surgery's heroic stance?

The corpse signifies the abject body without parallel. We have many rules and regulations around its containment and disposal (religious, health and governmental). The bodies represented above, all escape social structures during life, but in death, the abject body can disappear and destabilize all our best endeavours to contain it. As the *News Hour with Jim Lehrer* reports the death of US army soldiers in the face of the silencing and hiding the toll of US dead in Iraq, the loss of an Australian soldier's body *en route* to his home from Iraq indicates how such a body slips through the processes and rules for its safe conduct. In an avalanche of chaos, the loss of the body reverberated throughout the media disclosing military (dis)order, possible soldierly (mis)conduct and failures of masculinity. The case of losing the dead body of Private Kovko came to frame much of Australian discontent with the war in Iraq, its military imperatives and the values underpinning the politics of Australia at the time. Moreover, it is a case without boundaries as it continues to enthral with detail from a continuing judicial case destabilizing the image of military discipline, supposed military order and the particular brand of masculinity on which it relies.

Part III: Containment of Bodies

In this final section, our contributors focus on the containment of the abject body through nursing and health care practices. The civilizing of the abject body and its products, both material and emotional, require an analysis that recognizes all of the ways that abjection affects those who encounter and work closely with those who are experiencing it. Abjection is a psychical defence mechanism, but as we show throughout this collection, its effects reverberate and challenge 'identity, system, order' (Kristeva 1982: 4). Many health care and nursing practices do not take account of these emotional conditions of nursing and health care work. Instead nursing practices continue the tradition of ignoring the patient as a body (see McCabe below). These same practices deny the impact witnessing the body's abjection has on the health workers and nurses who are in intimate contact, to the detriment of developing a constructive ethics of care. The civilizing of the abject body resides in the maternal function that is excluded from the realm of the symbolic order, yet the maternal function is given social authority to contain it. Nurses and other health workers work in such a location, and are reviled/valorized for the part they play in abjection's containment (see Alicia Evans this volume).

As Holmes, Lauzon and Gagnon (this collection) illustrate, care of the person with dementia is a challenge for all involved, in watching its long slow decline to abjection in a body completely disengaged from its previous 'holding' identity. Once again, the body contains the condition; a condition that destroys its former inhabitant, as well as the relationships which connected the person to a social world. Dementia and the care of its sufferers faces nurses with challenges to sustain relationships that would be considered chaotic by society, to comfort the discomforted, and civilize a body that is decaying while seeming to be normal, as it forgets all that previously systematizes and regulates. The body in the dementing person fails to remember how it is contained, becoming other to those who care for them as well as, tragically, for their kin. Holding such a body becomes, in the end: an impossibility.

The chapters in the final section focus on nurses and their practices – as these attempt to deal with abjection – theirs and their patients. Residing in the maternal function, the containment of abjection through their work with patients goes beyond the mere materiality of nursing practice into a realm of an ethics of care which takes account of patient and nurse as they are positioned by abjection (Roderick, Rudge, McCabe in this collection). Rippling out from the pebble of abjection, are a collection of nursing responses requiring a framework for analysis beyond viewing the work they do as merely clinical. Sure, nurses have a matter of fact response to all that they see in their work (much like a mother cleaning a baby's bottom), but they also have stresses and anxieties that are difficult to articulate and comprehend, let alone communicate to others outside of nursing or health care work (Evans in this collection). It is to this situation our contributors turn to explicate some of what makes nursing work difficult for the long term, and the affects it has on nurses' health and work satisfaction. Each contributor suggests that abjection, and the maternal function requires to be taken seriously and their presence acknowledged in the workplace and education of nurses, patients and other health workers. A mere surface response to the conditions of work will not suffice as such an action silences. Instead, suggesting that a nurse learns to work with their response, acknowledge the disappointments that attend abjection, and wait for the feeling to pass does not obtain much traction in the science of nursing management or the economic imperatives of the health care system. It is clear we need to rethink the power and nurturance of the maternal function in nursing, to progress nurses' part in the provision of health care. Disavowing abjection and its social and emotional sequels will not work. It is the hope that this volume will begin the necessary wider debate.

References

Beardsworth, S. 2004. *Julia Kristeva: Psychoanalysis and Modernity.* Albany: SUNY Press.

Douglas, M. 2002. *Purity and Danger: An Analysis of the Concepts of Pollution and Taboo.* New York: Routledge.

Frosh, S. 1987. *The Politics of Psychoanalysis.* London: MacMillan.

Holmes, D., Perron, A. and O'Byrne, P. 2006. Understanding disgust in nursing: abjection, self, and the 'other'. *Research and Theory for Nursing Practice: An International Journal*, 20(4), 305–315.

Kristeva, J. 1982. *Powers of Horror: An Essay on Abjection*. New York: Columbia University Press.

Lawler, J. 1991. *Behind the Screens*. Melbourne: Churchill Livingstone.

Lechte, J. 1990. *Kristeva.* London: Routledge.

Mansfield, N. 2000. *Subjectivity: Theories of the Self from Freud to Haraway*. New York: New York University Press.

McAfee, N. 2004. *Julia Kristeva.* New York: Routledge.

Miller. W. 1998. *The Anatomy of Disgust.* Cambridge, MA: Harvard University Press.

Oliver, K. 1993. *Reading Kristeva: Unraveling the Double-bind*. Bloomington and Indianapolis: Indiana University Press.

Parker, J. 2004. Nursing on the medical ward. *Nursing Inquiry,* 11(4), 210–217.

PART I
Fluids and Transgression of Boundaries

Chapter 1

Blurring the Boundaries: Breastfeeding and Maternal Subjectivity

Virginia Schmied and Deborah Lupton

Introduction

The majority of writings about breastfeeding, whether academic or lay, are profoundly in favour of the practice. The professional accounts of medicine, nursing, midwifery, public health and public policy continually emphasize that 'breast is best' for infants, the environment and global economy (Meershoek 1993, Smith and Ingham 1997)[1]. It is claimed that breastfeeding is essential for bonding or securing the relationship between a mother and child (Virden 1988, Dettwyler 1995) and that it promotes the health, development and psychological wellbeing of the infant (Walker 1993, Riordan 1997).

In these accounts, the decision to breastfeed is largely considered a matter of individual choice and rational decision making. There is also a focus on the biological aspects of breastfeeding to the exclusion of insights into how the practice contributes to a woman's sense of self and embodiment. Medical and nursing accounts, while claiming the significance of the intimate contact between a mother and infant, predominantly frame this connection around a biological or 'natural' account of symbiosis, emphasizing anatomical functioning of the breasts and the production of breast milk, particularly the action of hormones (see Henschel and Inch 1996, Royal College of Midwives 1996). Even in anthropological accounts, a strong link is often drawn between biology and breastfeeding (see, for example, the edited volume by Stuart-Macadam and Dettwyler 1995).

---

1   There is considerable support for breastfeeding in Australia at the level of public policy. The Australian Government has rated breastfeeding first in the 'Dietary Guidelines for Children and Adolescents' and since 1996 has made a strong commitment to breastfeeding through the allocation of two million dollars for a National Breastfeeding Strategy. The Australian government policy – Health Throughout Life – encourages breastfeeding awareness, with the aim of increasing Australia's rate of breastfeeding, particularly for babies up to six months of age. Australia's target for breastfeeding for the year 2000 is to have 80 per cent of babies at least partially breastfed up to six months of age (Commonwealth Government of Australia 1993). Rates of breastfeeding in Australia (at time of first publication) are approximately 84 per cent at birth, 60 per cent at three months of age and 40 per cent at six months of age (ABS 1996).

Nor has this dimension of breastfeeding been addressed adequately in other disciplines. Indeed, some commentators are puzzled by the lack of critical debate from sociologists and feminists in the topic of breastfeeding (Blum 1993, Carter 1995, Maher 1992). Where this debate has occurred, writers have mainly articulated the possibility for breastfeeding to be seen as an expression of women's power, providing new, positive ways to view the unique features and capacities of women's bodies and subjectivities. Van Esterik (1989: 107), for example, insisted that 'the vague murmurings or submerged discourse about the power to nurture' should be seized by women to reassert feminine values. Sichtermann (1983) stressed the potential to recapture the lost eroticism of the breasts and celebrate breastfeeding as a form of female sexuality and sensual pleasure. More recently, Blum (1993: 300) argued that, as a unique experience of the female body, breastfeeding can provide a deeply satisfying interlude of intense engagement with and delight in one's child.

The present chapter contributes to a sociological and feminist understanding of breastfeeding in three ways. First, we overview some of the sociological and related anthropological and feminist literature that moves understandings of infant feeding decisions and practices away from the biomedical and health promotional discourses that dominate current debates on infant feeding. Second, the discussion draws upon our own Australian research using qualitative methods to explore women's lived experiences of breastfeeding and the discourses upon which they draw when articulating and making sense of these experiences. Third, we argue that understandings of the breastfeeding experience can be strengthened by incorporating phenomenological and symbolic perspectives on women's embodiment, particularly those offered in the work of feminist philosophers such as Julia Kristeva, Iris Marion Young and Elizabeth Grosz.

The Sociocultural and Economic Context of Breastfeeding

There are few accounts in the literature on breastfeeding that canvas the diversity of the breastfeeding experience or examine the ambivalence about or resistance to the imperative to breastfeed that women have shown over many years. The exceptions are those writers who draw upon data from women's own accounts of their breastfeeding decisions and experiences (see, for example, Carter 1995, Hoddinott 1996, Hoddinott and Pill 1999, Maclean 1990, Murphy 1999). These writers often challenge the accepted wisdom that 'breast is best' for both mother and infant. They argue that breastfeeding decisions and experiences are complex, related to such factors as a woman's physical heath, the health of her baby, the needs of her other children and family members, the family's living conditions and other demands on the woman's time and energy. They demonstrate that rather than being an individual act, breastfeeding (or the decision to bottle feed) is structured through prevailing sociocultural meanings and economic conditions.

Carter (1995), for example, highlights the resistance that women have shown over many years to the medical imperative to breastfeed. She analyses women's experiences of breastfeeding across a number of generations. Carter notes that for many women in the period from the 1920s onwards, 'breastfeeding was associated with exhaustion, poverty, discomfort, embarrassment and restriction as well as authoritarian hospital practices' (1995: 90). Indeed, for the majority of women interviewed by Carter, breastfeeding represented hard work. For some women, bottle feeding actually offered some respite from the demands of childcare, as it could be carried out by fathers or others.

Both Hoddinott (1996) and McIntosh (1985) conducted studies of women from lower socio-economic groups. They concluded that the personal and social context within which breastfeeding takes place is more important than knowledge and attitudes about breastfeeding in determining whether or not a woman decides to breastfeed. Further, while there is evidence that the return to paid employment has an impact upon breastfeeding decisions, in reality this tends to reflect socio-economic conditions. In Australia and other Western societies, many women who have completed a high-school or tertiary-level education or hold higher-status occupations possess a degree of control and autonomy over their employment options. These women are more likely to receive paid maternity leave, have the option to work fewer hours and have more flexible working conditions, all of which facilitate breastfeeding (Hills-Bonczyk et al. 1993, Galtry 1997, Lindberg 1996)[2].

It has been argued by other commentators that breastfeeding decisions and practices are embedded within, and thereby draw meaning from, a specific social and cultural milieu (Baumslag and Michels 1995, Maher 1992, Morse and Harrison 1987). In Western cultures, powerful discourses and expectations continue to

---

2   In Australia all public sector employees have access to a period of paid maternity leave (that varies from nine to 12 weeks in duration) and additional unpaid leave up to a total of 12 months full time or 24 months part time. In private sector employment, however, women are not always provided with paid maternity leave. Some employers in this sector offer to keep a position open for women but situations still exist where women have to resign from their job when they leave to have their baby. It is becoming very commonplace for women not to commence paid maternity leave until they are 37 to 39 weeks pregnant, allowing them to have a longer period of paid leave after the birth. Men are also entitled to paid paternity leave that can be shared with their female partner. Again, while this is an option available to those in public sector employment, it is rare that men in private sector employment have this opportunity. None of the couples in our research took the opportunity to share maternity/paternity leave. While the majority of women in Australia initiate breastfeeding there are no specific provisions made for breastfeeding women in the workplace. The Australian Council of Trade Unions (ACTU) has produced a document entitled 'Achieving Mother Friendly Workplaces' which provides guidelines maintaining and supporting breastfeeding in the workplace. The Australian government has recently funded the development of a work-based strategy to increase awareness of the needs of breastfeeding women.

prescribe the appropriate length of time women should breastfeed and where and in front of whom they should expose their breasts to do so (Morse and Harrison 1987, Murphy 1999).

One of the most commonly voiced sociocultural accounts relates experiences of breastfeeding to the cultural meanings attached to the breast. Some commentators argue that the preoccupation in Western societies with the breasts as objects of sexual gratification is particularly influential in women's decision whether or not to breastfeed (Baumslag and Michels 1995, Palmer 1988, Rodriguez-Garcia and Frazier 1995, Van Esterik 1989). In Western societies the breasts are fetishized as powerful symbols of feminine sexuality, which has important implications for how women feel about exposing their breasts to feed in private or public domains (Young 1990).

It is not surprising, therefore, that a number of empirical studies identify the discomfort that women face when trying to breastfeed in overcrowded living conditions because of the need to expose the breasts to others' gaze (Carter 1995, McIntosh 1993). The thought of embarrassment and discomfort at breastfeeding in public is used by some women as a justification for their decision to bottle feed and as something that must be overcome or 'managed' to preserve modesty by those who decide to persevere with breastfeeding (Hoddinott and Pill 1999, Murphy 1999, Stearns 1999). Other studies have also identified the dissatisfaction or distress women may experience in relating to the physical sensations of breastfeeding. McNatt and Freston (1992) found that women who had not felt successful or satisfied in their feeding experience described discomfort and a lack of pleasure in breastfeeding as reasons they were not 'successful'.

Further, the continual demands made of a mother from her breastfeeding infant can be experienced as physically and emotionally exhausting. Balsamo et al. (1992) found that, for many of their interviewees, breastfeeding on demand was often conceptualized as 'chaotic and dangerous' for women and the baby was portrayed as 'encroaching' on a sense of self. Maclean (1990) also describes the dramatic changes breastfeeding brings to women's lives and their dislike for their lactating breasts. Britton (1997) and Morse and Bottorff (1989) note the feelings of distress or revulsion that some women describe in response to the sensations of the 'let down' reflex and the leaking of breast milk.

Breastfeeding, Embodiment and Subjectivity: Our Research

To further explore that ways in which women experience breastfeeding, particularly in relation to notions of selfhood and embodiment, we draw upon empirical data and analysis from a recent qualitative and longitudinal study of first-time parenthood. 25 women living in Sydney and their partners participated in a study of first-time parenthood. A series of semi-structured interviews from late pregnancy until three years following the birth of their first child were conducted with each participant[3]. Interviews were carried out just before the birth of the child, between two and 10 days after the birth and then at the intervals of four to six weeks, 10 to 14 weeks, five to six months, one year, 18 months, two years and three years after the birth. Our discussion here focuses on data from the earlier interviews (up to five to six months following the birth).

The questions asked of the female participants focused on their expectations and experiences of first-time motherhood. Breastfeeding was but one of the many aspects of these expectations and experiences that were explored in the interviews. Nonetheless, our analysis of the interview data revealed that breastfeeding was central to these women's experience of motherhood, especially in the first few weeks and months following the birth.

In contrast to the varying degree of commitment to breastfeeding found among women in the work of Hoddinott (1996) and Murphy (1999), all these Australian women portrayed breastfeeding as a crucial part of maternal identity. Prior to the birth, all of them said that they intended to breastfeed, and the majority was strongly committed to breastfeeding. This commitment made by the women we interviewed may, in part, be attributed to their socio-economic status (predominantly middle-class)[4]. However, it also is reflected in comparative breastfeeding figures for Australian women overall, who are more likely to initiate and continue to breastfeed than either British or American women (Murphy et al. 1999).

All the women in our study believed that breastfeeding was 'natural', and therefore desirable, crucial to their relationship with their baby and best for their baby's health. Furthermore, breastfeeding represented 'good' mothering. Most women were prepared to 'persevere' with breastfeeding to achieve their identity as a breastfeeding mother. This is particularly clear in Jane's account: 'I think [breastfeeding] is a major motherhood thing, that you have to try and persevere

---

3   This study was funded by two Australian Research Council Large Grants awarded to Lesley Barclay and Deborah Lupton, with Virginia Schmied as an associate investigator. Recruitment into the study took place progressively between late 1994 and early 1997. Both women and men in a couple expecting their first child were interviewed (although only the data from the interviews with the women are drawn on here). Most of the couples who took part (17 of the 25) were volunteers attending antenatal classes at a metropolitan Sydney hospital. Limited snowball sampling and the use of other contacts were also used as recruitment strategies, and eight couples were recruited this way. The age of the female participants at the first interview ranged from 23 to 35 years, with a mean age of 28.2 years (very close to average age for Australian first-time mothers giving birth).

4   The majority of female participants (15) were employed in white-collar occupations such as clerical, administrative, personal service and health care work. While some of these women held post-school qualifications, none had completed a university degree. The other 10 held one or more university degrees: of these, one was a doctoral student, two were speech therapists, one a dietitian, one a research scientist, two were management consultants, two were teachers and one was a research assistant.

and accomplish'. Breastfeeding was something that the women wanted to master, to get under control.

As a result of their strong commitment to breastfeeding, all the women participating in this study began by breastfeeding their babies. One woman stopped feeding at five days because she was experiencing difficulties, and four other women weaned between six and 12 weeks. Three months after the birth, 20 women continued to exclusively breastfeed. At six months, 18 women were still feeding, and 12 women continued to feed their babies to between one to two years of age.

None of the women in this study initially planned to combine breast and formula feeding. Only four women returned to paid work within the first six months. Two weaned their babies before returning to work, while the other two intended to express breast milk once back at work. Both of these latter women found, however, that in practice expressing breast milk was difficult and their infants were weaned quite soon after their return to work.

Following the birth, the women talked in great detail about breastfeeding. They reiterated their commitment to breastfeeding and the discourses of bonding and the child-centred account of 'breast is best'. In their accounts, the embodied experience of breastfeeding emerged, as not only shaped by the dominant discourses of childcare and motherhood, but importantly also as representative of an extra-discursive, sensual and highly emotional experience that was difficult to describe in words. Phrases such as 'nobody told me breastfeeding would be like this', 'it's hard to explain it' and 'I can't describe it' were common. None of these women had been able to imagine or prepare for the intensely embodied nature of breastfeeding. As Sally put it:

> Because you don't have that much sort of physical, not contact physical association with things that you do in life so much – [breastfeeding] is one thing that is so … that's all there is to it, it's so physical that – well I don't think that I have ever done anything that makes you feel so much a part of what you are doing. It's very strange.

It was evident from our data that most of the women in the study responded to breastfeeding in one of two contrasting ways. For some women, the breastfeeding experience was pleasurable and intimate, a vital means of emotional connection to their infants, but for others it was difficult, unpleasant and disruptive. In the remainder of the discussion we examine these very different ways of experiencing breastfeeding.

'Still Part of Me': Breastfeeding as a Source of Intimate Connection

Bottorff (1990) argues that the image of breastfeeding as 'gift giving' is seen as a motivation for many women to 'persist' with breastfeeding. Within this embodied closeness or intimacy, a woman and her baby 'become one'. This feeling of companionship and closeness makes breastfeeding easier to practise and to continue: 'it becomes almost effortless' (1990: 206).

This sense of pleasurable connection was indeed evident in the accounts of some women in our study. At differing times following the birth, about a third of the interviewees spoke of a sense of connectedness, continuity or oneness between themselves and their baby. This was a powerful experience, described as 'wonderful' by these women. They spoke of feelings of interdependence, harmony and intimacy shared with their infant. Lyn, for example, described breastfeeding in the following way: '[it's] a special kind of moment, when you breastfeed, and you look down and they're looking at you and you think, "Oh, this is when they need you the most". You know, they really need you. It's a wonderful thing to breastfeed'.

In their descriptions of their breastfeeding and relationship with their babies, other women used the imagery and metaphors of harmony, intimacy, giving of self and exclusivity. Kerry described herself and her baby as a 'package', Julie saw her baby as 'still part of me' and Sally explained she would feel 'alien' if she did not breastfeed. They were comfortable with, indeed actively enjoyed, 'sharing' their body with their baby. To maintain this intense embodied and emotional relationship, these women participated in subtle but powerful practices that excluded others. Most commonly this consisted of establishing 'special times' with the baby where the two were alone. As Lyn described it: 'I like the morning feeds: he lies up in bed with me and I feed him in bed and then take all his clothes off and he'll have a kick and we talk. That's my favourite time, when it's just me and him'. Similarly, Kerry said that she particularly enjoyed sleeping in the spare bed with her baby when he wouldn't settle in the middle of the night.

In breastfeeding their infants, these women said that they were gaining personal rewards greater than they had thought possible. Megan described the pleasure she gained from gazing at her baby while he breastfed: 'there's just some really beautiful moments, just looking at [him]. It's the closeness, that intimacy'. A desire for 'skin to skin' closeness prompted Christine to bathe with her baby. She elaborated on the sensual nature of her breastfeeding experience: 'I fed him in the bath. But it was such a nice feeling! I was lying in the bath and I thought, well, "Oh, this is lovely!" Their bodies are just so perfect'. Cecily also savoured some of the pleasurable moments of breastfeeding: 'I love the closeness, the warmth and I love looking at his little face if he comes down to the breast and he's got it in his view and even his mouth gets ready. He latches on, gets his mouth in the position and he starts to breathe [faster] and get excited'.

These profoundly pleasurable experiences, continuing for some women for many months beyond birth, challenge the assumption of psychodynamic separation of the body/self of the mother and baby at birth or within the first month following birth that is described in early psychoanalytic work (for example, Deutsch 1944, Bibring et al. 1961, Rubin 1984). These women articulated few or no difficulties with the notion that their bodies/selves and that of the babies were inextricably interlinked, the boundaries between self and Other blurred. They saw neither their selves nor that of their babies as autonomous from each other or in conflict with each other.

In her analysis of women's literary writings of childbirth, Cosslett (1994) also describes an embodied connection and intimacy between a mother and her breastfed baby. She draws upon examples of breastfeeding and mothering that celebrate the unity between a woman and her infant. Breastfeeding may be experienced and articulated as a sense of continuity and intimacy between mother and baby. The separation that has occurred at birth may be restored by the interdependence fostered in a breastfeeding relationship. The uncertainty of the boundary between mother and child, the fluidity of self and Other is reintroduced via this harmonious embodied experience.

The Infant as 'Other': Breastfeeding as a Disrupted and Disconnected Experience

Not all the women in our study shared the connected, harmonious and sensual embodiment of breastfeeding. Indeed the women who enjoyed this experience, particularly in the early weeks, were in the minority. Other women articulated an embodied experience of breastfeeding that highlighted the ambiguities and tensions existing between the positive breastfeeding rhetoric and the experiences of women. Many of these women struggled with the contradictions between their experiences of breastfeeding, pro-breastfeeding discourses and the prominent notions of rational autonomy that are privileged in Western societies. They spoke vividly of the demands they felt breastfeeding placed upon them. For example, Helen spoke of 'the never-ending supply and demand – at the moment, he cries, I'm there, if he wants a feed, I'm there. And sometimes it gets demanding and very draining. But I'm on call and I think that I'm more on call because there is not much [my partner] can do'.

The nature of the breastfeeding relationship necessitated the women's constant proximity to their baby. The baby was always with them, occupying their thoughts as well as making physical demands. As the person responsible for the care, particularly feeding of the baby, these women undertook a huge amount of 'worry' or 'thinking work' (Walzer 1996). They breastfed their infants often feeling that despite the rhetoric there was little reward or recognition for their efforts. They felt they were restricted from participating in activities they had previously enjoyed, and resented this.

Many women described a sense of loss of self and agency occurring as a result of breastfeeding and other demands made by their infants. As Maggie explained, 'I feel like I'm sort of just hanging around waiting for [my baby] to wake up and be fed. To a certain extent my life's gone on hold at the moment'. Maggie's baby was six weeks old when she described these feelings of disruption to self, and she stressed that she had not realized the extent to which it would happen. This was a common sentiment amongst many of these women at this stage of their baby's life. Donna described herself as 'not my own person, I am his person'. These women started to realize how much their lives had changed, talking of being 'confined' to domesticity and the private world. They recognized that mothering and breastfeeding centred on the private world and they yearned to have time away from their baby, to be part of public life again. The demands of their breastfeeding infant and their commitment to 'intensive' mothering (Hayes 1996), disrupted their personal bodily routines and patterns. They always had to be there. These women talked about wanting their 'body back' or their 'old life back'. Petra, for example, talked of 'having to be on tap all the time', but she was prepared to put up with this because she was adamant that breastfeeding was crucial for her baby's health. Alternatively, Jenny and Prue were not prepared to put up with the constant demands of breastfeeding, and weaned their babies from the breast at eight and 12 weeks respectively.

For some women, the experience of breastfeeding was sometimes described as a 'distorting' one. They commented that breastfeeding had changed their breasts in undesirable ways. Not only had the size and shape of their breasts changed, but the sensations of their breasts and nipples were different. Their breasts were described as 'strange', 'heavy' and sometimes painful, even excruciating. The known boundaries or borders of the breast changed as the heavier, larger breast looked and felt different both clothed and unclothed. So distressing were these changes to their 'known breasted experience' (Young 1990), that it was common for women to objectify their lactating breasts and breast milk, noting that 'the stuff just pours out', the breast 'deflated', the breast milk had 'curdled'. The feeling of alienation between self and body was more common when women experienced breastfeeding difficulties such as blocked ducts, cracked nipples or mastitis, or the baby appeared 'unsatisfied' after feeding.

The searing pain in nipples and breasts experienced by several women in our study was often attributed by them to the 'uncivilized' behaviour of the infant. A number of the women provided vivid descriptions of the way their infant, constructed as 'the Other', would bite or chew on their nipple or fight and scratch at the breast. For one woman, 'it was a battleground'. Some women found themselves crying because of the pain they felt each time they attempted to breastfeed. Thus, not only did their breasts 'distort', but, there was (an)Other constantly attached to the breast, causing discomfort and pain. Even the sensations associated with the 'let-down' reflex, commonly described in popular and professional texts as 'pleasant tingling sensations' were not comfortable for some women. Sally, for example, particularly disliked the sensation associated with her let-down reflex:

> I never realized it would hurt so much. It's not an act that has no sensation to it at all. I had no concept that it would actually pinch and the let down would even be painful. That tingling, it's not even a nice tingling, it's like an electrical sort of tingling, it's like, ohh, yuk. Yeah I can understand why some women just don't

want to experience it. It still hurts as [my baby] gets on [the breast] when I'm not using the [breast] shield, and I have to grit my teeth.

The involuntary or uncontrolled flow of breast milk from a woman's body is a powerful symbol of the 'distortion' to known body boundaries or borders. Leaking breast milk highlights the ambiguity of inside and outside, self and Other. Some of the women in this study were surprised by the amount of milk that 'leaked' from their breasts, particularly at times unrelated to feeding the baby. They described feeling sticky, messy, dirty, embarrassed and uncomfortable and resented having to 'pad up' (use nursing pads) and wear particular clothing that would camouflage the leaking milk. Many of the women had not realized breast milk could leak so frequently and profusely and they felt compelled to control it in some way, not to let it show.

In some women's breastfeeding experiences, the boundaries of self and Other were also constantly challenged through the incessant demands of the baby to feed from the mother. Jenny described how her baby was always 'at' her. Prue could not find the words to describe what it was about breastfeeding she did not like, but noted that she 'just did not like the baby being at my breast'. The disrupting and distorting experience of breastfeeding gave some women a feeling their relationship with their baby lacked harmony, that they were somehow working in opposition to each other.

Some of these women desperately wanted to develop a sense of connectedness and harmony with their infant through breastfeeding, and persevered despite their discomfort and pain for this reason. Jane, for example, spoke vividly of the difficulties that she experienced with breastfeeding. Yet she also believed so firmly that breastfeeding brings a mother 'closer' to her child, and therefore persevered with it: 'So I suppose it was just that I felt like I was missing out on something, that closeness or something and maybe you know, it might affect [my baby] later, which is probably a load of garbage'. Jane decided to wean at six weeks. Other women, however, persevered for many weeks, even months in order to achieve a connected and harmonious breastfeeding relationship. Women such as Katrina, Sally and Marianne talked of achieving this relationship and experience and were 'glad' they had persevered. Others persevered with breastfeeding well beyond six months for pragmatic reasons, but never talked of experiencing an embodied connection and harmony.

The women who vehemently disliked breastfeeding described a need to 'disconnect' from the infant, striving for separation and individuation from their baby. In describing their baby they used metaphors of intrusion and devourment, talking of being, suck[ed] dry' and the baby as 'the rotten sucking little leech', the 'child from hell'. They felt as thought they existed only for the use of this antagonistic, parasitic creature. The demands of the 'uncivilized' infant for constant attention and proximity encroached on these women's sense of self, their autonomy and independence. This lack of tolerance for the ambiguity between the identity of mother and child and a desire for separation from the infant is also found in Cosslett's (1994) analysis of literary writings on childbirth. She notes that the imagery of the baby growing at the mother's expense, 'using up' the mother, violent and devouring, is prominent in women's literary accounts of breastfeeding.

Discussion: Contradictions and Tensions in Breastfeeding

The empirical data, upon which we have drawn, positions breastfeeding as an embodied relationship that has implications for feminine subjectivity. Like pregnancy, breastfeeding blurs or challenges the boundaries between mother and child, between self and Other. As we noted in the Introduction, some feminist theorists have argued that this blurring may offer the potential for women to explore a new, positive form of femininity and sexuality. This approach to breastfeeding is, however, problematic on two counts.

First, representation of breastfeeding as fostering connectedness and intimacy between mother and child can contribute to an overly romanticized discourse of maternal identity. Some accounts support the notion of an 'authentic' or 'true' feminine self that is partly discovered and experienced via breastfeeding (see Dignam 1995, Hatrick 1997, Van Esterik 1989). Dignam, for example, believes women who are breastfeeding may use the intimacy engendered via the practice as an 'identity tool' through which the self can be more fully defined (1995: 480). This need to discover the authentic self is given precedence over the ability to negotiate or tolerate ambiguity and uncertainty of selfhood.

Second, advocating breastfeeding as a connectedness between mother and child is challenging for feminist debates of equality and fails to acknowledge or accommodate the diversity in women's embodied experience of breastfeeding. It did indeed appear to be the case that for some of the women in our study, breastfeeding their babies afforded them a highly pleasurable sensual and emotionally charged experience. Through their bodies' communion with that of their babies these women achieved a delight in closeness and the blurring of notions of selfhood and Otherness. Breastfeeding, for many of these women, continued the harmonious interconnection that they had felt when carrying their babies during pregnancy. Their experiences reflect the ideals proffered by feminists keen to celebrate the unique capacities of the female body to provide sustenance for another body.

But these women were in the minority among our interviewees. It would seem that, despite the arguments of Chodorow (1978) and others, women do not automatically develop a sense of self that is able to desire and tolerate connectedness and interdependency. Almost two-thirds of the women in our study found breastfeeding to be a disrupting, distorting and disconnected experience, and for some, it was experienced as excruciating, violent and mutilating. Far from breastfeeding contributing to mutual sensual pleasure between themselves and their infant and to a strong bond, it undermined their pleasure and confidence in mothering and led to feelings of alienation from their infant. Indeed, one of the most interesting and unpredictable findings of our study was the extent to which women tended either to 'love' or 'hate' breastfeeding from early on in their mothering experiences and did not tend to change their attitudes to any great extent over time.

Why did many of the women we interviewed respond so negatively to breastfeeding after so earnestly expressing the desire to breastfeed before their baby was born? Breast discomfort or the pain endured from damaged nipples or mastitis was certainly a factor, but did not account for all the negative feelings expressed. Some women did not find breastfeeding painful, but still vehemently disliked it. Nor was the embarrassment about exposing their breasts to others that was identified in other research concerning women's reluctance to breastfeed (reviewed in the Introduction) a dominant factor. Very few women in our study mentioned this issue in their accounts of the positive and negative aspects of breastfeeding.

Rather, for many of the women in our study who were ambivalent, disliked or hated breastfeeding, it would appear that the negative meanings they attributed to the demands of the feeding infant and the accompanying feelings of encroachment of body/self were central. In their accounts of devourment, intrusion and alienation, the demands of their bodies made by their babies and the uncertain or blurred boundaries between a mother and her breastfeeding baby were experienced as intolerable. These women sought to regain control over their lives, over their bodies, to regain their sense of autonomous self. For many women, there was comfort in a return to a dualist understanding of mind and body, self and Other. These women demonstrated the need to restore certainty to their body boundaries and to 'civilize' or train the baby as an independent being who would make fewer demands of them.

That this was the case is not surprising, given there is little tolerance for ambiguity between self and Other in Western societies. Feminist critiques have consistently exposed the marginality of women's bodies compared with the ideal of the masculine, contained, autonomous and civilized body (for example, Douglas 1966, Ehrenreich and English 1979, Jacobus et al. 1990, Martin 1987). The male body in late-modern Western culture is culturally represented as controlled, contained with rigid boundaries between self and Other. In contrast, the female body is constantly portrayed as uncontrolled, unclean and lacking defined boundaries, and therefore as inferior.

The work of Douglas (1966), Kristeva (1982) and Grosz (1994) alerts us to the 'horror' or intense discomfort felt in response to the leaking, permeable and absorptive feminine body, in which boundaries between inside and outside and self and Other are constantly blurred, constituting 'a formlessness that engulfs all form, a disorder that threatens all order' (Grosz 1994: 203). For centuries, female bodily secretions or flows such as menstrual blood, breast milk and amniotic fluid have been portrayed as uncontrollable and uncontained. Feminist critiques have described the various ways in which women are incited to manage, 'civilize' and 'sanitize' their bodies (Bordo 1988, Doane 1990, Martin 1987, Poovey 1990,

Treichler 1990). These indeterminate, unbounded states and uncontrolled flows are invested with cultural meaning as dangers, as pollutants, dirt or contaminants.

That which is marginal or different is always located as a source of danger and vulnerability to the self (Douglas 1966). For Kristeva, this dirt or disruption to order is the 'abject'. The abject transgresses borders, it is 'in between' and ambiguous: 'It is not a lack of cleanliness or health that causes abjection but what disturbs identity, system, order' (Kristeva 1982: 4). Kristeva contends that the feminine – and particularly the maternal-body is the epitome of the abject body. Female subjectivity and embodiment are represented as a threat to the clean and the proper. The maternal body, in particular, is a figure that incites both idealization and fascination and anxieties and fear because of its ambivalent status as 'two bodies in one'. As Kristeva remarks, 'A mother is a continuous separation, a division of the very flesh' (1986: 178). In this ambiguity, the maternal body is subject to many cultural taboos and is typically marginalized as Other to the ideal of the contained, autonomous body.

In theories of mothering, whenever issues of bonding, separation, autonomy, merging, individuation or symbiosis emerge, the heterosexual male functions as a guarantor of order, a gatekeeper between public and private spheres. Adams notes 'Women, and especially mothers, represent the disorderly matter that must be sorted out, assembled and disassembled, bonded and broken down' (1995: 426). Women who find breastfeeding a pleasurable and sensuous experience threaten the strict borders between motherhood and sexuality. Images of women in Western society persist with the dichotomy of Madonna and Whore. As Young states, Woman is either 'sensual mother or sexualized beauty' (1990: 197). Motherhood is associated with one type of love and sexuality with the other. For a woman to enjoy or take sensual pleasure in her infant's body is crossing the border of motherhood and sexuality, raising stirrings of the incest taboo (Young 1990).

Breastfeeding, therefore, remains a vexed feminist issue. Advocating breastfeeding not only for the health benefits for baby and mother, but also for the immense pleasure and intimacy that can be gained and for its contribution to 'authentic' femininity, can be hazardous in its link to biology, essentialism and conservative arguments about women's reproductive and nurturing roles. As our findings demonstrate, even if on a 'rational' level women strongly believe in breastfeeding, they respond with extremely strong reactions to the actual embodied experience that have little to do with 'rationality' but more to do with deeply-felt emotions and sensations. These reactions, if negative, are surprising and distressing for the women involved. They feel a sense of failure and a loss of control for not conforming to the ideal of the contented and fulfilled mother suckling her baby.

The attempt to privilege the positive sensual and relational aspects of breastfeeding is enormously challenging, as in doing so it is difficult not to 'exclude or dishonour those who do not or cannot and without contributing to a new moralism that is just as coercive as the old' (Blum 1993: 306). Feminist frameworks that promote breastfeeding as a source of female empowerment and alternate subjectivity limit our understanding of difference and diversity among women (Carter 1995). Incited by the desire to experience a different form of sexuality, an 'authentic' feminine identity and a more rewarding experience of mothering, women may embark upon breastfeeding as an avenue for self-definition. If they are unable to achieve this ideal, women are susceptible to disappointment and feelings of failure and a sense that somehow they are 'bad mothers'.

References

Adams, A. 1995. Maternal bonds: recent literature on mothering. *Signs*, 20, 414–28.

Australian Bureau of Statistics. 1996. National Health Survey 1989–1990.

Balsamo, F., De Mari, G., Maher, V. and Serini, R. 1992. Production and pleasure: breastfeeding in Turin, in *The Anthropology of Breastfeeding: Natural Law or Social Construct*, edited by V. Maher. Oxford: Berg, 59–90.

Baumslag, N. and Michels, D.L. 1995. *Milk, Money and Madness: The Culture and Politics of Breastfeeding.* Westport: Bergin and Garvey.

Bibring, G., Dwyer, T., Huntington, D. and Valenstein, A. 1961. A study of the psychological process in pregnancy and of the earliest mother-child relationship. *Psychoanalytic Study of the Child*, 16, 9–24.

Blum, L. 1993. Mothers, babies and breastfeeding in late capitalist America: the shifting contexts of feminist theory. *Feminist Studies*, 19, 291–311.

Bordo, S. 1988. Anorexia nervosa: psychopathology as the crystallization of culture, in *Feminism and Foucault: Reflections on Resistance*, edited by I. Diamond and L. Quinby. Boston: Northeastern University Press.

Bottorff, J. 1990. Persistence in breastfeeding: a phenomenological investigation. *Journal of Advanced Nursing*, 15, 201–209.

Britton, C. 1997. Letting it go, letting it flow: women's experiential accounts of the letdown reflex. *Social Science in Health*, 3, 176–186.

Carter, P. 1995. *Feminism, Breasts and Breast-feeding*. Houndmills: Macmillan.

Chodorow, N. 1978. *The Reproduction of Mothering: Psychoanalysis and the Sociology of Gender*. Berkeley: University of California Press.

Commonwealth Government of Australia. 1993. Goals and Targets for Australia's Health in the Year 2000 and Beyond. Report prepared for the Commonwealth Department of Health, Housing and Community Services.

Cosslett, T. 1994. *Women Writing Childbirth: Modern Discourses of Motherhood*. Manchester: Manchester University Press.

Dettwyler, K.A. 1995. Beauty and the breast: the cultural context of breastfeeding in the United States, in *Breastfeeding: Biocultural Perspectives*, edited by P. Stuart-Macadam and K.A. Dettwyler. New York: Aldine De Gruyer, 167–208.

Deutsch, H. 1944. *The Psychology of Women: a Psychoanalytic Interpretation (Volumes 1 and 2)*. New York: Grune and Stratton.

Dignam, D. 1995. Understanding intimacy as experienced by breastfeeding women. *Health Care for Women International*, 16, 477–485.

Doane, M.A. 1990. Technophilia: technology, representation and the feminine, in *Body Politics: Women and the Discourses of Science*, edited by M. Jacobus, E. Fox Keller, and S. Shuttleworth. New York: Routledge, 163–176.

Douglas, M. 1966. *Purity and Danger: An Analysis of the Concepts of Pollution and Taboo*. London: Routledge and Kegan Paul.

Ehrenreich, B. and English, D. 1979. *For Her Own Good: 150 Years of Experts' Advice to Women.* New York: Anchor Press, Doubleday.

Galtry, J. 1997. Suckling and silence in the US. The costs and benefits of breastfeeding. F*eminist Economics*, 3, 1–24.

Grosz, E. 1994. *Volatile Bodies: Towards a Corporeal Feminism*. Sydney: Allen and Unwin.

Hatrick, G. 1997. Women who are mothers: the experience of defining self, *Health Care for Women International*, 18, 263–277.

Hays, S. 1996. *The Cultural Contradictions of Motherhood*. New Haven: Yale University Press.

Henschel, D. and Inch, S. 1996. *Breastfeeding: A Guide for Midwives*. Hale: Books for Midwives Press.

Hills-Bonczyk, S.G., Avery, M.D., Savik, K. et al. 1993. Women's experience with combining breastfeeding and employment. *Journal of Nurse-Midwifery*, 38, 257–266.

Hoddinott, P. 1996. *Why Don't Some Women Want to Breastfeed and How Might we Change their Attitudes?* MPhil Thesis, Cardiff University of Wales, College of Medicine.

Hoddinott, P. and Pill, R. 1999. Qualitative study of decisions about infant feeding among women in the East End of London. *British Medical Journal*, 318, 30–34.

Jacobus, M., Fox Keller, E. and Shuttleworth, S. 1990. *Body Politics: Women and the Discourses of Science*. New York: Routledge.

Kristeva, J. 1982. *Powers of Horror: An Essay on Abjection*. New York: Columbia University Press.

Kristeva, J. 1986. Stabat mater, in *The Kristeva Reader*, edited by T. Moi. Oxford: Basil Blackwell, 160–186.

Lindberg, L. 1996. Trends in the relationship between breastfeeding and postpartum employment in the United States. *Social Biology*, 43, 191–202.

Maclean, H. 1990. *Women's Experience of Breastfeeding*. Toronto: Toronto University Press.

Maher, V. 1992. Breastfeeding in cross-cultural perspectives: paradoxes and proposals, in *The Anthropology of Breastfeeding: Natural Law or Social Construct*, edited by V. Maher. Oxford: Berg, 1–33.

Martin, E. 1987. *The Woman in the Body: A Cultural Analysis of Reproduction*. Boston: Beacon Books.

McIntosh, J. 1985. Barriers to breast feeding: choice of feeding method in a sample of working class primiparae. *Midwifery*, 1, 213–224.

McNatt, M.H. and Freston, M.S. 1992. Social support and lactation outcomes in postpartum women. *Journal of Human Lactation*, 8, 73–77.

Meershoek, S. 1993. The economic value of breastfeeding. *Breastfeeding Review II*, 8, 354–357.

Morse, J.M. and Harrison, M.J. 1987. Social coercion for weaning. *Journal of Nurse-Midwifery*, 32, 205–210.

Morse, J.M. and Bottorff, J.L. 1989. Leaking: a problem of lactation. *Journal of Nurse-Midwifery*, 34, 15–20.

Murphy, E. 1999. 'Breast is best': infant feeding decisions and maternal deviance. *Sociology of Health and Illness*, 21, 187–208.

Murphy, E., Parker, S. and Phipps, C. 1999. Motherhood, morality, and infant feeding, in *A Sociology of Food and Nutrition: the Social Appetite*, edited by J. Germov and L. Williams. Melbourne: Oxford University Press, 405–419.

Palmer, G. 1988. *The Politics of Breastfeeding*. London: Pandora.

Poovey, M. 1990. Speaking of the body: Mid-Victorian constructions of female desires, in *Body Politics: Women and the Discourses of Science*, edited by M. Jacobus, E. Fox Keller, and S. Shuttleworth. New York: Routledge.

Riordan, J.M. 1997. The cost of not breastfeeding: a commentary. *Journal of Human Lactation*, 13, 93–97.

Rodriguez-Garcia, R. and Frazier, L. 1995. Cultural paradoxes relating to sexuality and breastfeeding. *Journal of Human Lactation*, 11, 111–115.

Royal College of Midwives. 1996. *Successful Breastfeeding*. London: Churchill Livingstone.

Rubin, R. 1984. *Maternal Identity and the Maternal Experience*. New York: Springer.

Sichtermann, B. 1983. *Femininity: The Politics of the Personal*. Cambridge: Polity Press.

Smith, J. and Ingham, L.H. 1997. The economic value of breastfeeding, in Australia. Paper presented at *'Breastfeeding: The Natural Advantage' Nursing Mothers' Association of Australia International Breastfeeding Conference*, Sydney, 23–25 October, 200–222.

Stearns, C. 1999. Breastfeeding and the good maternal body. *Gender and Society*, 13, 308–325.

Stuart-Macadam, P. and Dettwyler, K. 1995. *Breastfeeding: Biocultural Perspectives*. New York: Aldine De Gruyter.

Treichler, P. 1990. Feminism, medicine and the meaning of childbirth, in *Body Politics: Women and the Discourses of Science*, M. Jacobus, E. Fox Keller and S. Shuttleworth. New York: Routledge.

Van Esterik, P. 1989. *Beyond the Breast-Bottle Controversy*. New Brunswick: Rutgers University Press.

Virden, S.F. 1988. The relationship between infant feeding method and maternal role adjustment. *Journal of Nurse-Midwifery*, 33, 31–35.

Walker, M. 1993. A fresh look at the risks of artificial infant feeding. *Journal of Human Lactation*, 9, 97–107.

Walzer, S. 1996. Thinking about the baby: gender and the division of infant care. *Social Problems*, 43, 219–234.

Young, I.M. 1990. *Throwing like a Girl and Other Essays in Feminist Philosophy and Social Theory*. Bloomington: Indiana University Press.

Chapter 2
Menstruation and Dene Physical Practices[1]

Audrey Giles

It is also a piece of policy with the women, upon any difference with their husbands, to make that [menstruation] an excuse for a temporary separation ... This custom is so generally prevalent among the women, that I have frequently known some of the sulky dames leave their husbands and tent for four or five days at a time, and repeat the farce twice or thrice a month, while the poor men have never suspected the deceit, or if they have, delicacy on their part has not permitted them to enquire into the matter (18th-century arctic explorer Samuel Hearne cited in Abel 1993: 22).

Introduction

In this chapter, I use data collected from 13 months of ethnographic research conducted between 2002–2004 in the *Dehcho* (Mackenzie) region of the Northwest Territories (NWT), Canada to explore Kristeva's (1982) assertions concerning menstruation and abjection. Drawing on Foucault's understanding of constraints, I assert that Dene menstrual practices are not solely driven by ideologies of pollution that inhibit women's activities, but that menstrual blood can also symbolize and be indicative of the medicine power that Dene women possess. Through the use of examples of swimming in a lake in a Dene community and Dene hand games, I further Kristeva's writings on menstruation and abjection, and particularly maternal power, by showing that Dene women's and community members' responses to menstrual blood are constructed in and by very particular social and cultural contexts. As noted by other authors about women in other social and cultural milieus, men's power is often only possible when women agree that their power should support male power and keep things symbolically and imaginarily clean so that men's powers are not weakened. In this chapter, I extend this argument to small communities in Canada's sub-arctic.

---

1 This chapter is an adaptation of two previously published papers:
Giles, A. 2004. Kevlar®, Crisco®, and menstruation: 'tradition' and Dene games. *Sociology of Sport Journal,* 21(1), 18–35. Giles, A. 2005. A Foucauldian approach to menstrual practices in the Dehcho, Northwest Territories, Canada. *Arctic Anthropology,* 24(2), 9–21.

Placing the Communities and their Residents

Aboriginal peoples, particularly those who reside in remote northern communities, are often displaced from non-Indigenous people's imaginations. As a result, it is not surprising that very few people can locate the three locations at which I conducted my research on a map: Trout Lake-Sambaa K'e[2], JMR-Tthedzehk'edeli, and Fort Simpson-Liidlii Kue. The fact that the communities of Trout Lake-Sambaa K'e and JMR-Tthedzehk'edeli are so tiny that they do not appear on many maps likely does not help the situation.

Trout Lake-Sambaa K'e can be found nestled in the southwest corner of the NWT, just above the upper reaches of British Columbia's border. In the summer months, this community of 65 residents is accessible only by air, while a winter road helps to break-up the isolation during the colder months. Trout Lake-Sambaa K'e bills itself as being one of the most traditional communities in the NWT. For example, in the *Deh Cho Visitors Guide*, Chief Dennis Deneron is quoted as saying, 'We're strongly active with our traditional activities' (Northern News Service 2002: 24); traditions involving menstruation are no exception.

To the northeast of Trout Lake-Sambaa K'e, on the bank of the Mackenzie River, lays the community of JMR-Tthedzehk'edeli. With 52 residents, JMR-Tthedzehk'edeli is one of the smallest communities in the NWT. Though tiny in size, JMR-Tthedzehk'edeli looms large within anthropological literature, but under the pseudonym June Helm (2000) used in her research over fifty years ago: Lynx Point. The 'Lynx Point people' and Helm's study of them, including their menstrual practices, feature prominently in many texts about Dene peoples (e.g., Abel 1993, 1998, Coates and Powell 1989, Goulet 1998; Morrison 1998).

Fort Simpson-Liidlii Kue, a community of 1,200 people that is located at the confluence of the Mackenzie and Liard Rivers, is an historic gathering and trading place for Aboriginal peoples in the Dehcho region, and later gained prominence for Eurocanadian traders when it became a post for the North West Company and later the Hudson's Bay Company. The North West Company built Fort of the Forks soon after 1800 (Morrison 1998). 'The Forks' was renamed Fort Simpson when the North West Company was absorbed by the Hudson's Bay Company in 1821 (Abel 1993). Currently, the community serves as the regional centre for the Dehcho and houses, among other things, a high school that has boarders from neighbouring communities in which high school is not offered, a sizable health centre, and offices for various branches of local and regional Aboriginal governments, as well as the Federal and Territorial governments.

Indigenous residents of Trout Lake-Sambaa K'e, JMR-Tthedzehk'edeli, and Fort Simpson-Liidlii Kue are Dene – specifically, Slavey – and Métis (mixed Aboriginal and European ancestry) peoples. According to Abel, the Slavey are

---

2   I use both the English and South Slavey names for each community in order to acknowledge the rich history and culture residents had prior to and have had after the arrival of Europeans.

'found along the Mackenzie between Great Slave Lake and Fort Norman (now known as Tulita), along the Liard River to Fort Nelson, and through northern British Columbia and Alberta to Hay River' (1993: xvii). Familial and political ties between all three communities are strong; many community members are related, and the Bands in all of these communities are members of the Dehcho First Nations. As these communities have close ties, it is not surprising that their cultural practices, including those related to menstruation, are also similar.

Menstrual Practices

Discourses concerning menstruation as 'dirty, vile, impure, and pollution' (O'Keefe 2006) have had significant impacts on women of European descent. Indeed, from the third century onwards Christian religious leaders have maintained that menstrual blood is impure, unclean, and even 'God's curse' (Phipps 1980: 300). Such beliefs played a prominent role within Eurocanadian-derived discourses about women and appropriate activities for women. For example, in the early 1900s, menstruation and women's reproductive organs were viewed as incapacities. Indeed, according to Lenskyj (1986: 25), menstruation 'reinforced the existing power relations between men and women: women experienced this monthly "incapacity", men did not'. Women's 'god-given responsibilities for child-bearing and mothering' (Kidd, 1996: 120) were privileged over engagement in sport and recreation, with some gynaecologists threatening that 'violent exercise, especially during menstruation, caused [uterine] displacement' and could 'exacerbate existing uterine problems' (Lenskyj 1986: 27). Though by the middle of the twentieth century doctors were prescribing physical activity as a way of relieving symptoms of menstruation (Lenskyj 1986), and though attitudes towards female reproductive capabilities and the impact of exercise have changed, Eurocanadian women still tend to view menstruation as an embarrassing and often 'dirty' problem that needs to be dealt with, often in a secretive manner.

Though the discourses outlined above have shaped women of European descent's reaction to menstrual blood and their involvement in physical activity, it is fallacious to assume that all women have been subjected to discourses such as these and, hence, that they would have identical reactions to menstruation. Indeed, here I hope to demonstrate that understandings of menstruation vary between European and Aboriginal cultures and, as such, responses to menstrual blood and its consequent impact on activities also differ.

Several authors (Abel 1993, Giles 2004, 2005, Goulet 1998, Helm 2000) have documented historical menstrual practices among Slavey peoples, some of which continue to be practised today. Suza Tetso, a Dene woman from the Fort Simpson-Liidlii Kue area who is a recognized authority on Dene culture, explained the rites of passage associated with the first onset of menses for young women that were practised in the past:

As soon as they get their cycle … [t]hey're instructed, they're taught from a very young age and they're aware of it, they get a stick and they hit the tree and they make noise so that as soon as the grandmother or auntie or mother knows that noise, they go to where she's at, build a little hut, a shelter around her and they leave her there and she doesn't leave that spot, and that's where she'll stay for up to a year … by herself, hunting, gathering food … So what happens is that she stays there and the teachers come. The mother comes and teaches her a sewing technique of some kind and stays with her for maybe a few days or how long it takes her to master that skill. When she masters that skill, the grandmother comes and visits her, but they don't stay, they visit her every day. They talk to her and they teach her stories. They do that sometimes for a month, that same person comes. When she masters another skill, that person leaves and another person comes. Then that person comes and teaches a different sewing technique, so she learns from the women in the whole community. One by one they come, and this woman is created, her skills are created from all the Elders and the people who have these skills and they leave. When she's ready to come into the community, it's a whole celebration where she comes and there's gathering, they're a prayer offering and a prayer song and she's brought back into the community where she does a dance once around the circle and that's where she's starting her life (Personal communication, 12 February 2004).

Menstrual practices continued into adulthood, during which time Dene women would sequester themselves in either a hut or tent outside of the main settlement or in a room in a house for the duration of their menstrual cycle:

The women are taught that when they have their cycle, they're not allowed in public. [You would] [n]ever see women out when you know women are on their cycle, the mothers, grandmothers, aunts, daughters; they're supposed to stay in their own corner. They have their own washroom. They're not supposed to walk on the same path as men. They have their own washroom, their own exit, their own cup, their own dishes, they had a little bowl … to drink water out of because they're not allowed to drink like that, with their hand or cup, they had a little bowl that they used. They could be in their homes, when they're in their tent, she stays in a corner and she doesn't leave that corner for up to a week or maybe two weeks, until her cycle is finished, totally finished, then she can leave. [S]he'll make other people sick when she [is in contact with men] because the man's power and his connection to the animals and his spiritual gifts are what he uses to provide for the family. Before the men go out [hunting], they have visions and dreams of the animals and where they need to go. If a woman walks over the man's path, even his trail where he walks, she will interfere with that connection of the hunter and the animal.

During my own fieldwork, I found that menstrual practices are followed to different extents in the communities with which I conducted research. For instance, while most, if not all, women in Trout Lake-Sambaa K'e used to remain sequestered while menstruating, today, instead of remaining segregated, most female residents of Sambaa K'e now avoid going anywhere that they do not have to go; refrain from eating fish, birds, and berries; and do not go boating while 'on their time'. Residents of Trout Lake-Sambaa K'e believe that this behaviour is an important way for women to show respect towards fellow community members as well as to maintain health-related practices.

Helm's fieldwork in JMR-Tthedzehk'edeli from 1951–52 led her to the conclusion that 'certain beliefs and practices (in JMR-Tthedzehk'edeli) have a common underlying theme, the danger of blood and the concomitant need to handle it carefully' (2000: 276). Helm found that during menstrual taboos required women to sit in one corner of their house and abstain from all activities, including household chores. If these practices were not followed it would 'bring tuberculosis to her husband and the children and (apparently the more common explanation) would bring bad luck to her husband in his trapping, snaring, and hunting' (2000: 276–277). During my own fieldwork in JMR-Tthedzehk'edeli and Fort Simpson-Liidlii Kue, several community members shared with me that, though menstrual practices are not continued to any great extent in the communities in contemporary times, they did take place in the past.

Based on the above, it would be relatively easy to understand menstruation as being inherently filthy; certainly, many anthropologists have taken such an approach. Discourses of pollution are prevalent in many ethnographic accounts of menstruation. Buckley and Gottlieb (1988) found that most ethnographic reports of menstrual practices and beliefs view menstrual blood as 'symbolically dangerous and otherwise defiling' (1988: 4). Buckley and Gottlieb further noted that these 'analyses have great predictability, for again and again they centre on the concepts of taboo (supernaturally sanctioned law) and pollution (symbolic contamination)' (1988: 4). While notions of pollution and taboo have been used as the primary explanations for menstrual practices, other authors explain menstrual practices in terms of power. For instance, Anderson (2000) asserts that Aboriginal women's segregation during menstruation is based not on impurity, but instead on the enhanced power that women have during this time. Along similar lines, Irwin notes that many North American Indigenous societies have viewed menstrual blood as having a detrimental impact on men's hunting ability, as 'menstrual blood is not thought of as polluting but as clashing with a man's power(s)' (1984: 177). Though many of the interviewees in my research made reference to menstruation as being taboo and/or polluting, many of them also made comments that follow Anderson's emphasis on women's enhanced power during menstruation. In both cases, however, it is important to note that women's power is used to support men's power to enable apparent group benefits. In order to recognize the ways in which Dene menstrual practices can be understood as producing not only discourses of pollution but also those of power, I turn to Foucault's work on constraints.

Foucauldian Constraints

According to Foucault, 'power establishes a network through which it freely circulates, this is true only up to a certain point... But I do not believe that one should conclude from that that power is the best distributed thing in the world' (1980: 99). One of the effects of the legacy of colonialism towards Aboriginal peoples in Canada's North is the weight that colonial discourses carry; Cairns (1988) argues that Eurocanadian discourses are often privileged over those stemming from Aboriginal people and practices. I extend this argument to Dene menstrual practices; it is often assumed that what is contingently true for the dominant group (e.g., Eurocanadian women's reactions to menstrual blood) must be true for colonized groups (e.g., Dene women). One of the ways through which research can disrupt colonial, mainstream discourses is through the surfacing of subjugated knowledges, which Foucault describes as 'a whole set of knowledges that have been disqualified as inadequate to their task or insufficiently elaborated: naïve knowledges, located low down on the hierarchy, beneath the required level of cognition or scientificity' (1980: 82). In the following passage, Foucault elucidates the enormous potential for this sort of knowledge:

> It is through the re-emergence of these low-ranking knowledges, these unqualified, even directly disqualified knowledges ... , which involve what I would call a popular knowledge (*le savoir des gens*) though it is far from being a general commonsense knowledge, but is on the contrary a particular, *local*, *regional knowledge*, a differential knowledge incapable of unanimity and which owes its force only to the harshness with which it is opposed by everything surrounding it ... it is through the re-appearance of this knowledge, of these local popular knowledges, these disqualified knowledges, that criticism performs its work.

By surfacing subjugated knowledge about Dene women's menstrual practices we are able to challenge metanarratives that dismiss Indigenous knowledge about and reactions to menstruation.

Dene menstrual practices can be considered disciplinary practices. While many of Foucault's musings about discipline are strongly tied to aspects of French, and more generally European, history, the application of his understanding of discipline to Dene women and menstrual traditions is revealing. According to Foucault, 'discipline produces subjected and practiced bodies, "docile" bodies' (1977: 138). It is important to note that Foucault's use of the term docility does not imply passivity. Rather, docile bodies are skilled, disciplined bodies produced by particular configurations of time, space and movement, and thus able to exercise power within particular discourses. Indeed, such an approach allows us to view femininity as active.

Foucault (1980) understands power as constraints on action that are both enabling and inhibiting (Fraser 1989, Shogan 1999). Such a view allows for constraints to be seen as productive, rather than just oppressive. By way of example, Shogan (1999: 4) has examined the ways in which game rules serve to constrain athletes' actions:

> Game rules enable certain actions and limit other actions by placing constraints on what athletes are allowed to do. Some of these constraints prohibit certain actions while others prescribe actions. Together these constraints on athletes' actions produce what counts as the skills in a sport.

The 'no holding rule' in hockey, for example, can be used to illustrate her point: while such a constraint might enable the defender to defend the goal, it inhibits the offensive player's ability to score a goal. As a result, constraints prohibit certain forms of action while simultaneously making others possible.

In taking a Foucauldian approach to menstruation, rather than viewing past and current menstrual disciplinary practices as resulting in exclusively inhibitory effects, we must also question the ways in which these practices, and the power relations implicated in such practices, are productive of enabling discourses about and for Dene women. Below, I explore the ways in which menstrual traditions apply to swimming in Trout Lake and Dene hand games, both of which are illustrative of the ways in which constraints can be simultaneously inhibiting and enabling.

Swimming in Trout Lake

If you examine a map carefully, you will notice that Trout Lake, the lake on which the community by the same name is found, is shaped like a person lying on his or her side in the foetal position. This impression in the ground is said to have been made by the giant most often referred to as 'Yamoria'. For many people, the association with the giant is what makes the lake sacred. Indeed, community members have a deep respect for the lake. According to Dennis Deneron,

> The legend about the lake here, you have to pay respect to the lake and then it will respect you. Give a piece of clothing or tobacco or that, it'll be good to you … I remember my grandma told me a story about the lake, she said that there are water people who live in the lake. A long time ago, before outboard motors came along, you see just globs of fish fat that float right up on shore, and then when it's a nice calm day you can hear drum dances underneath the lake, (water) dogs are howling.

Another important tradition concerning Trout Lake involves women refraining from swimming in it. Sarah Ann Jumbo recalls,

[When I was young] me and my sisters, we really wanted to go swimming, but whenever we wanted to go swimming, go to the water, my mom used to chase me down from the beach and scare us back to the camp with spruce boughs because girls weren't allowed to go in the water because it was a place where the giant slept, and we weren't allowed. My brothers were allowed to go swimming, and we girls really wanted to go swimming, but mom always told us not to.

Similarly, Elder Julie Punch remembers,

The only time we went out in the water was when it was wavy to get some water for drinking, just go down from the knee, that's the only time we could go in the water ... When we were growing up [women] weren't allowed to go in the water. When we went in the water, we'd always get in trouble with some Elders telling us not to go in the water because ... there's fish in the water and water's for drinking and there's fish...and the fish is old. It's an old lake.

Various reasons for women refraining from swimming came to light during the semi and unstructured interviews I conducted with 21 participants of Trout Lake-Sambaa K'e's 65 community members. These reasons included: hurting fishes' spirits; a negative influence on the female swimmer's reproductive abilities, particularly the birthing process; that if boys and girls or men and women swam together, it would have a negative impact on the man's hunting ability; and that, according to one member of the younger generation, 'they said that a long time ago older girls shouldn't go swimming in the water because there's something in the water or something (often reported as being a big beaver or monster). And girls were swimming in the water and that's why there's something in the water that came back' (Anonymous, 16 July 2002).

I asked several Elders how they felt about girls swimming in the lake in present times, a practice that was becoming increasingly common, especially when a travelling waterfront supervisor from the region would visit in the summer months. Elder Julie Punch said,

I really don't have much to say about that, because in the past the Elders were very strict. Now, the younger people are growing up, they're turning away from the story that was being kept. They're more into the white man's world today and they can just go into the water whenever they want.

Conversely, her husband, Joe Punch, said 'Swimming, that's against the Dene law (for girls), you know'.

Some members of the younger generation expressed frustration with traditions concerning women and swimming. One young woman, who asked not to be identified, reported the following recollection from her youth:

Men, like, they'd go swimming every day if they wanted to. But women, they're not supposed to go swimming too often ... I think it's because women get their monthly cycle every month and stuff like that, eh. You need time to get it all settled or whatever before you can go back in the water and stuff like that because everybody drinks the water and they get fish from the water too. I thought that that was pretty unfair because sometimes it would get really, really hot. And that time too we didn't have showers and bathtubs like we do now, we used to live in log houses ... we had no bathtubs, no running water, nothing. So in the hot weather, it gets really hot and no trees around, no shade, nothing, we had to stick it out in the hot weather and (boys) can go live in the lake.

According to Sarah Ann Jumbo, women's use of the lake has changed in recent years: 'Now the girls they just go in the water whenever they want, when it gets hot, and when the lake is calm they just go in the water whenever they want'. This statement, however, appears to only be true to a point. All of the women I spoke with said that they would not swim while menstruating; they reported that they continued to follow the practice of not swimming (or even boating) while menstruating.

By examining the above selections from the interviews that I conducted, we can see how menstrual traditions can be viewed as constraints in a Foucauldian sense. Certainly, menstrual practices create and reinforce discourses that inhibit many of Trout Lake-Sambaa K'e's female residents from participating in aquatic-based activities; however, these practices also produce what can be considered to be enabling discourses and discursive practices. By exercising non-participation in swimming, the community's women have kept the legend of the lake alive, and they have produced discourses of tradition and power pertaining to the lake, as well as of women and their responsibility for community health. While Joe Punch's comment that girls swimming in the lake is against the 'Dene law' might seem to feed into strictly inhibitory discourses, it, like his wife's comment, speaks to women's power and the important role that women have and exercise by following menstrual practices and refraining from swimming in the lake. These discourses however, also a paradoxical effect. In addition to producing Dene women as traditional and powerful, however, menstrual practices also enable and support men's power through the circumscription of women's activities.

Hand Games

Hand games, also known as stick gambling, have a rich history in Denendeh[3], and oral histories of past hand games participation continue to exist. Hand games involve a moosehide drum, which many Dene people view as sacred. Most residents of the three communities that I interviewed reported that, in the past, women did

---

3   Denendeh is term the Dene use for the region in which they live.

not play the drum or hand games, and that women's participation in either activity could potentially harm men's hunting abilities. Fort Simpson-Liidlii Kue Elder William Antoine reported that '[o]nce in a while Elderly ladies would go in to the hand games, but the younger ladies don't … The Elders told the younger girls, ladies, not to join in. The grandparents and the parents would get mad at them and the Elders won't let them'. Another resident of Fort Simpson-Liidlii Kue explained that '[i]t's just the younger ladies' mothers are still teaching them stuff and they don't want to distract their attention to something else. It has something to do with the monthlies, too, because in the old days women tended to keep to themselves'. A female resident of Trout Lake-Sambaa K'e reported, 'before, like, a long time ago women weren't allowed to play it, to play handgames or to play the drum or stuff like that'. Similarly, Yvonne Jumbo shared with me, 'my grandma told me that, that the drum is sacred. But back then they relied on their medicine people, so they used the drum for some sort of praying, for healing, so she said women are not supposed to play the drum'. By way of a final example, another young woman in Trout Lake-Sambaa K'e reported that she played hand games when she was a child, but 'as I got older I started reading the rule books of the Dene games, and most of them, there's only men playing, no women are supposed to play. It's because of women's time of the month and stuff'. Indeed, most residents reported that menstruation indicated a time of special power (either enhanced power or more potentially dangerous power) and, as a result, precautions about activities during this time need to be taken.

Though almost all of the individuals I interviewed reported that women did not participate in hand games in 'the old days', which is a finding that supports other research (e.g., Heine 1999), interestingly, the most detailed oral traditions about hand games that were relayed to me pertained to instances in which women did in fact play. Dolphus Jumbo of Trout Lake told me the following story involving two groups of Dene people who met on a trail many years ago:

> [By winning hand games] one tribe took everything from another tribe – blankets, guns, everything. So the men lost. The men said "you can't take everything. That's our livelihood, we live on it". Blankets and everything. So one of the women stood up and said "let us give it a try". So they did. They won the whole thing back on top of what the others have – guns, axe, knives, everything. And then one of them, when they're losing everything, one of the Elders said, "let's stop here, we need that stuff". But the women said, "you took everything from our men, so we have to take everything". Eventually that's what they did.

Suza Tetso related another oral tradition of women's involvement in hand games:

> This one gathering, women were getting food and watching the kids and the men were gone … they'd be playing hand games, it went on for days and things needed to be done that didn't get done. Everyone had a role and were needed, so

the women were starting to get really upset. "This has gone on too long", they said. The women said okay ... stopped what they were doing, got together, went to where the men were playing hand games. They went over there and stopped in there and said, "stop this game! You're needed over here. You need to go hunting, check the nets, do all these things. Dogs need to be fed. You have a lot of responsibility, you men have to take responsibility. Stop the game now, let's get back to life". And they didn't want to stop. So the women were really upset, so they said "we'll challenge you. We'll take you on. If we win, you stop and everyone goes back to what they need to do and don't play this game again, not for a long time, because you have responsibilities". So the men just laughed at the women. "Ha-ha, you can't beat us"! And the women were really angry and said, "no, we'll challenge you right now". [The men said] "no, we don't want to play, we're playing this game here, we don't want to play with the women". So what happened was that the women challenged them and they said no, and the women said "because you are afraid to lose to the women because we're good at what we do and you know it, that's why you're afraid to challenge us". And the men just laughed and they had no choice ... So the women challenged them and the women said, move, we're going to take over this game. They got in there. You can imagine what these women are like, they're traditionally dressed and some of them had handkerchiefs and stuff like that and they were playing. And my grandfather's telling my mother this story, saying all these women they started playing hand games ... leaning over like this ... and you're singing. And my grandfather's telling my mother this saying they ... were right into the game and their breasts were just bouncing up and down and they didn't care, they were just getting into it! They were playing and playing and they beat the men at their own game. The game stopped right there and then they all went back to their work. And the only reason they didn't want the women to play is that there's nobody else to do the jobs at the camp. They didn't have anybody else to do it. If the women and the men did it, nobody's going to raise the children or feed the dogs, so they left all the work to the women and the women said no. Because it's an equal system that keeps the balance of the family where everyone does their part, even the little kids.

While neither of these oral traditions explicitly state the reasons why women were not involved in hand games in the past, the fact that the stories of women's involvement in hand games are remembered as exceptions to typical instances of hand games speaks to the fact that, in the past, women played such games infrequently.

In the above interview segments, much like those relating to swimming in Trout Lake, we see that women's activities are curtailed not due to the psychic horror of menstruation, but due to inhibitory discourses surrounding activities and the ways in which women, and particularly women following disciplinary practices concerning menstruation, should participate. Thus, it would be relatively easy to overlook the ways in which some residents of the Dehcho view menstrual practices as being productive of enabling discourses that acknowledge women's power and its importance to community health and balance, and instead focus on what some might view as sexism or discriminatory behaviour, or the inherently 'filthy' and 'polluting' aspects of menstruation. In doing so, however, much of the understanding of the richness of women's power and place in society becomes marginalized.

Re-thinking Responses to Menstruation

I will confess that as an atheist feminist, my initial reaction to hearing local stories and histories concerning monsters in Trout Lake and of menstruating women causing irreparable harm to men should they participate in hand games was to use post-positivistic, Western liberal feminism to transform such information into a secular story, one that did not rely upon 'invisible powers'. In writing histories of physical practices in the communities with which I conduct research, I initially felt that I had to explain away the 'supernatural' in order to be taken seriously within academic discourses. Chakrabarty points out that '[a] secular subject like history faces certain problems in handling practices in which gods, spirits, or the supernatural have agency in the world' (2000: 72). I was quite happy to rationalize away the impact of power derived from menstruation; my Eurocanadian, secular upbringing and education had taught me to ignore such forms of power or to view them as something only used by the ignorant, those who did not have access to the answers science can provide. Indeed, the academic world in which I inhabit is largely disenchanted and calendrical (Chakrabarty 2000), viewing history as something that happens along a timeline that is shared throughout the world. As Chakrabarty (2000) notes, the timeless qualities of spirits and mysterious powers are forced out of the post-positivistic world of academia in order to generate sameness throughout the world. By forcing spirits and powers into a universal language and explaining them away, one is able to view these local manifestations as individual examples of a universal phenomenon (i.e., ignorance of science). As a result, sameness is created, which gives us access to a universal language, one that, through translation, erases difference and perpetuates the idea of a single, universal world history – and, by extension, uniform responses to phenomena like menstruation. By transforming information from the spiritual world through secular, scientific language (e.g., Western liberal discourse), the goal is to develop one consistent story, the one that is the 'Truth'.

In terms of my own research, the transformation of interview material through post-positivistic, Western liberal feminism might look something like this: local residents claim that there is a monster in the water that appears when women, especially menstruating women, enter the water. Also, local residents say that women should not play hand games and should stay home when they are menstruating to avoid harming the community members' health, which is clearly linked to patriarchy and also the abjection associated with menstruation. Through this transformation of the stories that I was told, the participants in the research study would have become the confessors (Foucault 1978), I would have become the interpreter, and the tale that I wove would have become represented as 'what really happened' or 'the truth'. This story, in all likelihood, would have supported existing research on the subordination of women in physical practices as well as what Kristeva (1982) identifies as the defilement associated with menstruation. Local knowledge would have been subjugated, and colonial power relations that victimize Indigenous communities would have been re-inscribed.

Notably, a Foucauldian approach does not engage in such post-positivistic transformations. By choosing not to force stories of Dene power through Eurocanadian-based, secular, scientific discourse, and by instead embracing a Foucauldian approach, constraints concerning menstruation become visible as being both enabling and inhibiting, and criticism that is rooted in local knowledge is able to do its work. The circulation of power, and its exercise and employment through a net-like organization (Foucault 1980), is recognized, as are the ways in which individuals are always 'simultaneously undergoing and exercising this power. They are not only its inert or consenting target; they are also the elements of its articulation' (Foucault 1980: 98).

Without asking Dene women why they do not figure prominently in the cultural landscape of some forms of physical practices, it is easy to come to the conclusion that they are absent because they are oppressed as a result of the management of inherently abject and polluting menstrual blood. While some Dene women argue that that is indeed the case, others point to the fact that it is their power, which is enhanced during menstruation, and not their disempowerment due to pollution that results in their abstinence in participating in certain activities. In fact, rather than displaying their oppression, by deciding not to participate in hand games and aquatic activities, Dene women might actually be displaying their agency and autonomy and proliferating enabling, rather than or in addition to inhibiting, discourses concerning Dene women, their bodies, and power. If the typical Western liberal feminist goal of 'equality' and 'empowerment' were to be expressed in attempts to have women participate in aquatic activities in Trout Lake and hand games, it is paradoxical that such empowerment might come about only by failing to acknowledge the power that some Dene people associate with menstruation.

Conclusion

While a Foucauldian approach does not provide a panacea to the politics of research in post/neocolonial settings, it does offer some exciting opportunities for problematizing the metanarratives that have been produced about menstruation. In particular, this approach allows the re-emergence of subjugated knowledges, which most certainly contribute to Indigenous knowledge projects that have as their focus the disruption of mainstream discourses that largely ignore or attempt to (re)colonize Indigenous peoples and their practices. Further, this approach has the added benefit of acknowledging women and mothers' important role in rejecting menstruation as abject.

In the 88 interviews that I conducted between 2002 and 2004, not one participant spoke of menstrual blood as being 'unclean'. While quite a few participants identified menstrual blood as being potentially harmful to a man's medicine power, as illustrated above, that harm need not come from exposure to filth, but can instead be considered as being a result of Dene women's enhanced power during menstruation. The impact of colonisation, too, cannot be ignored in examining menstruation in Dene communities, as some suggest that discourses concerning the polluting aspect of menstruation appeared only when missionaries who did not understand the nuances of Dene culture arrived in the North. Certainly, my findings coalesce with Kristeva's (1982) understanding that menstruation can be constructed as abject in patriarchal contexts, but that there are also social and cultural contexts that can enable women to play an important role in understanding what counts as proper and improper as well as clean and unclean.

References

Abel, K. 1993. *Drum Songs: Glimpses of Dene History*. Montreal and Kingston: McGill – Queen's University Press.

Abel, K. 1998. Prophets, priests, and preachers: Glimpses of Dene History, in *Out of the Background: Readings on Canadian Native History* (2nd ed.), edited by K. Coates and R. Fisher. Toronto: Irwin Publishing, 118–149.

Anderson, K. 2000. *A Recognition of Being*. Toronto: Second Story.

Buckley, T. and Gottlieb, A. 1988. Introduction: a critical appraisal of theories of menstrual symbolism, in *Blood Magic: The Anthropology of Menstruation*, edited by T. Buckley and A. Gottlib. Berkeley, CA: University of California Press, 4–50.

Cairns, A.C. 1988. *Citizens Plus: Aboriginal Peoples and the Canadian State*. Vancouver: UBC Press.

Chakrabarty, D. 2000. *Provincializing Europe: Postcolonial Thought and Historical Difference*. Princeton: Princeton University Press.

Coates, K. and Powell, J. 1989. *The Modern North: People, Politics and the Rejection of Colonialism*. Toronto: James Lorimer & Company.

Foucault, M. 1977. *Discipline and Punish*. New York: Vintage Books.

Foucault, M. 1978. *The History of Sexuality Volume I: An Introduction*. New York: Vintage Books.

Foucault, M. 1980. Two lectures, in *Power/Knowledge: Selected Interviews and Other Writings, 1972–1977*, edited by C. Gordon. New York: Pantheon Books, 78–108.

Fraser, N. 1989. *Unruly Practices: Power, Discourse, and Gender in Contemporary Social Theory*. Minneapolis: University of Minnesota Press.

Giles, A.R. 2004. Kevlar®, Crisco®, and menstruation: 'tradition' and Dene games. *Sociology of Sport Journal*, 21(1), 18–35.

Giles, A.R. 2005. A Foucauldian approach to menstrual practices in the Dehcho, Northwest Territories, Canada. *Arctic Anthropology*, 24(2), 9–21.

Goulet, J.A. 1998. *Ways of Knowing: Experience, Knowledge, and Power among the Dene Tha*. Vancouver: UBC Press.

Heine, M. 1999. *Dene Games: A Culture and Resource Manual*. Yellowknife, NWT, Canada: The Sport North Federation & MACA (GNWT).

Helm, J. 2000. *The People of Denendeh: Ethnohistory of the Indians of Canada's Northwest Territories*. Iowa City: University of Iowa Press.

Irwin, L. 1994. *The Dream Seekers: Native American Visionary Traditions of the Great Plains*. Norman: University of Oklahoma Press.

Kidd, B. 1996. *The Struggle for Canadian Sport*. Toronto: University of Toronto Press.

Kristeva, J. 1982. *Powers of Horror*. New York: Columbia University Press.

Lenskyj, H. 1986. *Out of Bounds: Women, Sport, and Sexuality*. Toronto: Women's Press.

Morrison, W.R. 1998. *True North: The Yukon and Northwest Territories*. Toronto: Oxford University Press.

Northern News Service. 2002. Trout Lake. *Deh Cho Visitors Guide*. Yellowknife: Northern News Service.

O'Keefe, T. 2006. Menstrual blood as a weapon of resistance. *International Feminist Journal of Feminist Politics*, 8(4), 535–556.

Phipps, W.E. 1980. The menstrual taboo in the Judeo-Christian tradition. *Journal of Religion and Health*, 19(4), 298–303.

Shogan, D. 1999. *The Making of High Performance Athletes*. Toronto: University of Toronto Press.

Chapter 3

'What it Means to See': Reading Gender in Medical Examinations of Suicide

Katrina Jaworski

Introduction

Examining the practices required for investigating suicide, Holmes and Holmes ask: 'How does one determine whether a death is a suicide? … For example, does the death appear to be self-inflicted?' (2005: 113). For Holmes and Holmes (2005), the post-mortem examination is crucial to verifying whether what appears as lethal is an actual cause of death. Typically carried out by a pathologist, this is how suicide is determined on medical grounds. My concern with seeing what appears as self-inflicted is not about disputing whether post-mortem practices should be part of verifying suicide. Nor is it about challenging specific science-based practices integral to the medical examination of deceased bodies. Instead, my concern is to do with an enduring understanding that the body exists as a neutral, autonomous, stable and visually mappable tableau for displaying suicidal intent.

Drawing on Michel Foucault's (1973) work on the medical gaze, supplemented with resources from visual culture, I will argue that the assumption made about the body as neutral, autonomous and stable is incited by the workings of the medical gaze through which suicide is rendered as masculine and masculinist. I will also argue that there is a gendering of suicide via the autopsy, which means that it fails to sustain self-destruction as ontologically secure. As an effect of power, what it means to see suicide bodies is discursively entangled with gender, and cannot be easily separated from it. I will begin by summarizing a contemporary understanding of suicide and situating the issue of what it means to 'see' on the basis of medical knowledge. I will then analyse selected photographic images portraying the examination of deceased bodies and depicting particular methods of suicide. Furthermore, I will interrogate the interpretation of lethality as a neutral measure of suicidal intent by deploying elements of Kristeva's notion of the abject. My aim is to call into question the visual intelligibility of completed suicide to show how what is rendered neutral cannot exist outside social and cultural norms that condition how knowledge about suicide is constructed.

A few terms need addressing before I proceed. I take gender to refer to the interpretation of cultural and social codes such as masculinities and femininities: a discursive means through which fleshy depths of bodies are etched with meanings (Grosz 1990, 1994, 1995). The analysis of what it means to see gender is informed by gendering, or the *process of materializing* the act of suicide (Butler 1993). I am arguing that how suicide is rendered produces it as masculine and masculinist, the latter referring to an exclusively gendered subject position in Western philosophy, articulated as male, rational, abstract, objective, neutral, white, heterosexual, and universal, transcending time and the material body (Hekman 1990, Lloyd 1984, 1996). In other words, these are the prime conditions under which a valid subjective position is recognized and established.

Suicide as a Deliberate and Lethal Material Act

Suicidology – or the study of suicide – broadly defines suicide as the act of deliberately taking one's own life in a way that is voluntary, intended and self-inflicted (Brown 2001). Understanding suicide as deliberate and intended is influenced by gender. Statistical data, as one example, shows that more men than women complete suicide, whereas more women than men attempt suicide (Australian Bureau of Statistics 2004). In this way, men are viewed as completers and women as attempters. Based on outcome, determined by mortality rates, suicide is understood as a male and masculine phenomenon (Canetto and Lester 1998; Dahlen and Canetto 2002; Range and Leach 1998).

The interpretation of suicide methods plays an important role in understanding suicide. Traditionally, men prefer to use methods considered more lethal, such as firearms, whereas women prefer to use less lethal methods such as drug overdoses. Methods such as firearms are considered not only more visually and physically violent, but also male, masculine and *active*. Methods such as drug overdoses, however, are viewed as female modes of engaging with suicide that are less visually and physically violent and lethal as well as more feminine, reactive and *passive*. Where the former is viewed as serious and 'real', the latter is viewed as reactive, manipulative and attention-seeking, configured by a fear of bodily disfigurement (Brockington 2001, Canetto and Lester 1995, Canetto and Sakinofsky 1998). Rich, Kirkpatrick-Smith, Bonner and Jans (1992), and Stack and Wasserman (2009), contend that women in particular are concerned about the damage to visible parts of their bodies, such as the face. To a degree this is shaped by the process of socialization, where traditionally women more than men are taught to be aware of the appearance of their bodies. Social norms concerning gender are therefore part of particular concerns about direct impacts on female bodies.

An important element that frames the interpretation of suicide methods is lethality. Kral (1998: 223) situates the connection between lethality and suicide methods by noting that lethality has been taken to mean 'the likelihood that the method used would cause death in a particular individual. The term has been used rather loosely in the literature to mean a specific method, a set of behaviours, or a description of the person'. Despite the reference to it as socially and culturally interpreted, as shown in Rosen and Heard's (1995) analysis of self-inflicted injuries, lethality is also viewed as medically neutral. Lethality relates to different physical levels of injury inflicted on the biological body through wounds on the neck, arms, wrists and abdomen. What is important about different physical wounds for researchers such as Rosen and Heard (1995) is whether they have the potential to be lethal. This is certainly echoed by Peterson, Peterson, O'Shanick and Swann (1985) who argue for instance that gunshot wounds are the most serious and lethal signs of suicide. Here too the location of wounds on the body plays a significant role. It becomes clear that the more dangerous a wound is, the more likely it is that its selection will be interpreted as lethal. It is also clear that lethality as a marker of suicide and the body as a physical tableau are viewed as neutral.

Seeing and Knowing: Foucault's Reading of the Medical Gaze

The threshold between the end of the 18th century and the beginning of the 19th century witnessed an increase in efforts to observe, measure and record the natural and social environments. Such efforts were of particular interest to Foucault (1973) who sought to document the shift towards hospital-based medical teaching and research in France at the end of the 18th century. This shift occurred as a result of the replacement of traditional methods of diagnosis with empirically motivated anatomical dissection of the corpse. From being a largely public spectacle, dissecting deceased bodies became a hospital-based private practice (Armstrong 1997, Barker 1984, Young 1997).

Foucault (1973) was interested in the idea of how medical truth became visible. Disease and suffering, he argued, was 'not conjured away by means of a body of neutralized knowledge; they have been redistributed in the space in which bodies and eyes meet' (Foucault 1973: xi). Isolating and reducing the body to 'the plane of visible manifestations', the gaze of the doctor could now penetrate the body via the 'technique of the corpse' to reveal signs and symptoms of disease (Foucault 1973: 19, 141). It was not so much that disease suddenly changed. Rather, new forms of visibility reorganized disease into new patterns which now could be mapped onto different bodily surfaces and organs. For Foucault, the new forms of visibility were 'the result of a recasting at the level of epistemic knowledge *(savoir)* itself, and not at the level of accumulated, refined, deepened, adjusted knowledge *(connaissances)*' (1973: 137). The gaze not only dealt with diseases afflicting individuals; it became the means through which individual truths could be established. Bringing individual truths into existence was an effect of power and knowledge.

The clinic was the means through which medical truths became visible. The clinic did not emerge out of nowhere. Instead, repetitive and rigorous practices of examining, observing and measuring disease gave rise to this space (Foucault 1973). The clinic, therefore, was a significant site of practice because direct physical examination of bodies allowed the physician to qualify the nature of disease on and in the body (Osborne 1994). The individual patient, whose body was rendered as the source and object of illness, could be treated as a single case available for scrutiny and capable of comparison with other cases (Armstrong 1983, Foucault 1973, Young 1997).

What is Visually Mapped as Self-Inflicted

To pursue the gendering of suicide, in post-mortem practices, I want to examine black and white photographic images of deceased bodies taken from a medical text entitled, *Post-Mortem Procedures,* published in 1979 by Geoffrey Gresham and Franklin Turner. As a text, *Post-Mortem Procedures* is distinctly visual, relying heavily on visual depictions of deceased bodies and bodily organs. Nevertheless, the text also contains detailed explanations of images. Most of the discussion is focused on describing relevant details necessary to verify whether the deceased has suicided (Gresham and Turner 1979: 110). Such details include determining the extent of injury and damage, the significance of various wounds, bruises and marks, and the techniques required to examine various forms of self-infliction on the body. What is represented in various images exemplifies what is known of different methods and, importantly, arrays the signs the pathologist should look for when examining deceased bodies. Photography then is a significant mechanism through which the evidence of suicide is captured and represented. In this sense, photography is part of rendering suicide visually and medically intelligible.

Rendering suicide, however, is not a matter of mechanically capturing the evidence. This is because, as Evans and Hall (1999), Mirzoneff (1999) and Tagg (1999) argue in various ways, the production of photographs heavily relies on institutional practices that define and mobilize their use. Furthermore, what is displayed in and by images is configured through institutional relations of power where images 'exert power and act as instruments of power' (Sturken and Cartwright 2001: 93). Taking photographs is enabled by the power to access and capture something on camera (Tagg 1999). Thus, depicting and representing something can never be thought of as neutral. What is seen in a photograph is not simply the result of what literally appears, captured by the camera's lens at some point in time. Rather, what appears is conditioned by the means through which an image is made available, how it becomes circulated in different sites of practice, and by the values attributed to qualify what is represented (Jenks 1995, Mirzoneff 1998, Van Dijck 2005). Thus, reading any visual depictions of suicide is likely to be already discursively conditioned the moment the deceased body is framed by the camera's lens.

The configuration of autopsy space in which the body is examined also plays an important role. Gresham and Turner (1979: 27) describe various aspects of what they refer to as 'the dissecting room'. This room must be arranged in such a way as to enable efficient visual description and measurement of the corpse. It must contain various features such as tables and instruments; be of the right colour; and have ample light to illuminate the details on deceased bodies (Gresham and Turner 1979: 25). It seems that the medical gaze must have specific conditions under which the pathologist can make the facts of death transparent (Wagner 2004). Yet, rendering something transparent is not only dependent on what evidence the body yields. It is also closely connected to the attentive manner in which the medical gaze functions under particular spatial conditions. In some sense then, the autopsy space becomes an interrogation room, where deceased bodies are *framed* as yielding their secrets to determine whether what appears is indeed self-inflicted.

While the selected images speak of different methods of suicide, all visually portray death as essentially final. The first image below locates the chest as a bodily site on which a wound inflicted by a bullet from a shotgun is displayed. While the second image is a close up of the first, both images focus on measuring the wound, drawing attention not only to the external width of the wound but also to the extensiveness of bruising.

Even though the surface of the skin is no longer intact in both images, the second image in particular focuses on the presence of fluid around the inscription bearing the mark of the gun's barrel. The caption underneath the images explains the presence and significance of relevant inscriptions. Gresham and Turner (1979: 110) state that '[p]roof of suicide by shooting rests, in part, by demonstrating that the individual could have done it himself'. Photographic images of the same hand serve the purpose of illustrating that the deceased was directly responsible for the wound caused by the discharge of the shotgun.

The two images draw attention to the marks or abrasions on the thumb due to the recoil of the shotgun's trigger. The external measurement of abrasions appears important. In contrast to the caption explaining the wound on the chest, the caption explaining the abrasions on the thumb identifies the body of the deceased as male. It is difficult to tell why this is so. Is it a matter of wording which identifies particular details? Is it a matter of ensuring that the relationship between the chest and thumb is clear? Or is it because, unlike the chest, the hand is presumably a less distinctive sign qualifying the deceased body as male?

For Gresham and Turner (1979: 110), '[i]n all cases of hanging a ligature mark on the neck and the appearance of the mark are of considerable help in deciding whether the strangulation was suicidal or not'. The ligature mark is the focus of the image below depicting suicide by hanging.

The image frames the neck as the site bearing the ligature mark. Although impossible to tell, since the image is black and white, the colour of the mark is described as brown. While the focus predominantly rests on the mark itself, further emphasized by measuring its length, the knot of the rope is included. The knot is important because '[t]he way in which the knot has been tied often helps to identify the person who tied it' (Gresham and Turner 1979: 110). Further, the image captures facial hair, indicating that the deceased body is possibly male. This, however, does not seem relevant. The caption underneath situates the position and colour of the ligature mark on the neck and stresses the importance of not disturbing the knot.

The final image selected here is quite distinct from the previous images. This image captures a dissected area of the body, identified as the pelvic brim.

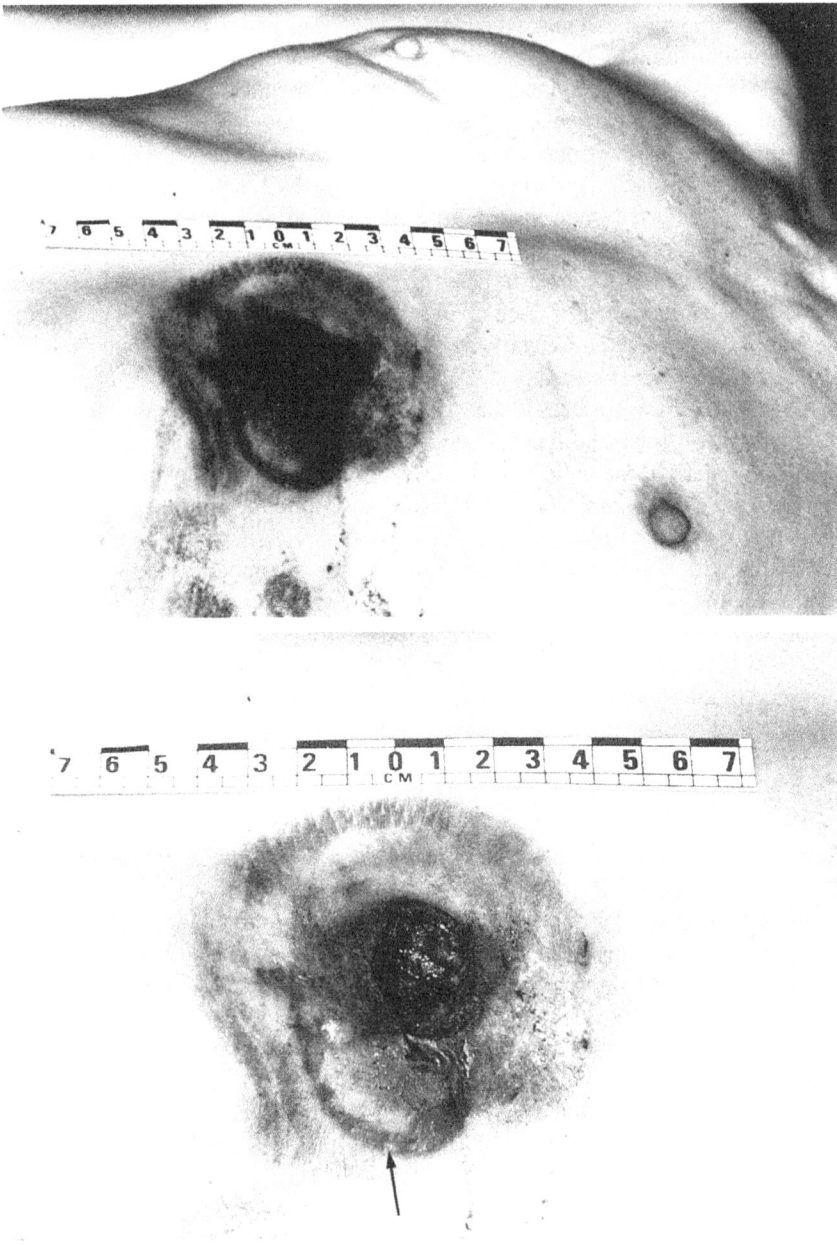

Figure 3.1/3.2 Wound caused by the discharge of a 12-bore shotgun. A
fine spray of powder marks surrounds the hole. The mark
of the undischarged barrel can be seen in the second figure
(arrowed).

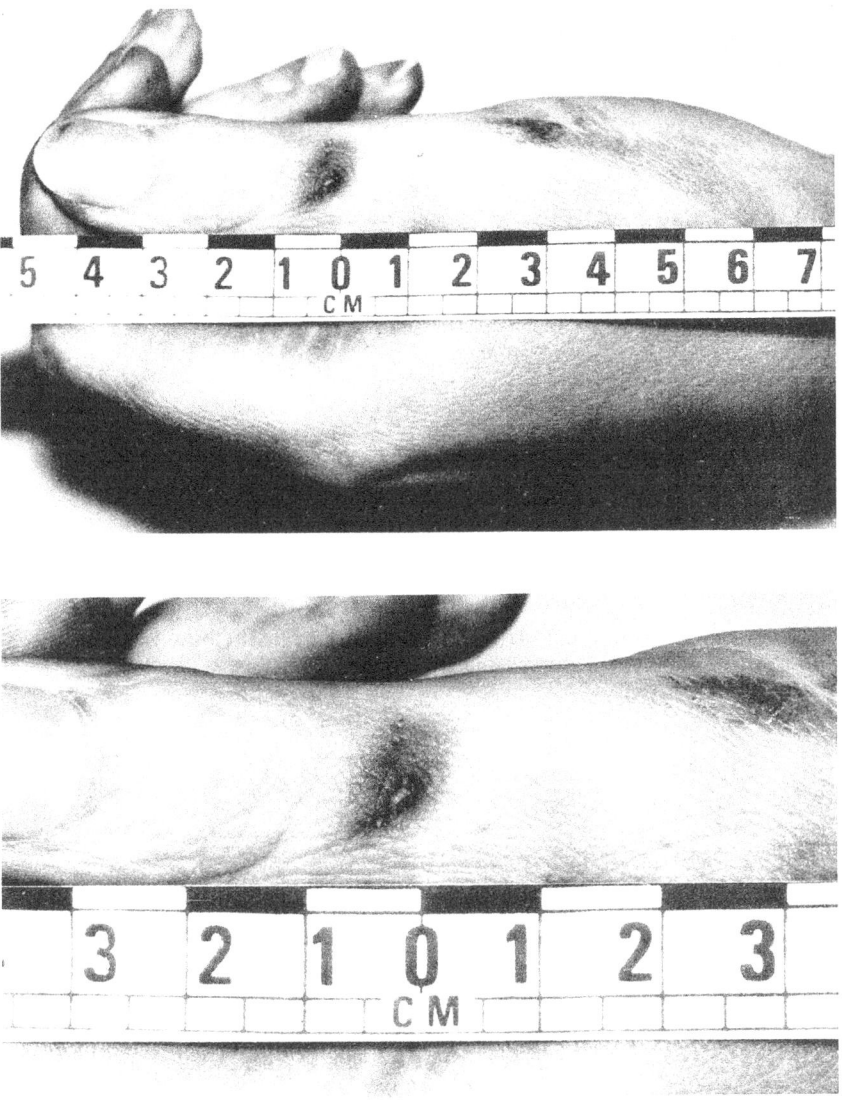

Figure 3.3/3.4 Abrasion of the thumb due to recoil of the trigger of a 12-bore gun used to kill himself. This indicates the victim pulled the trigger.

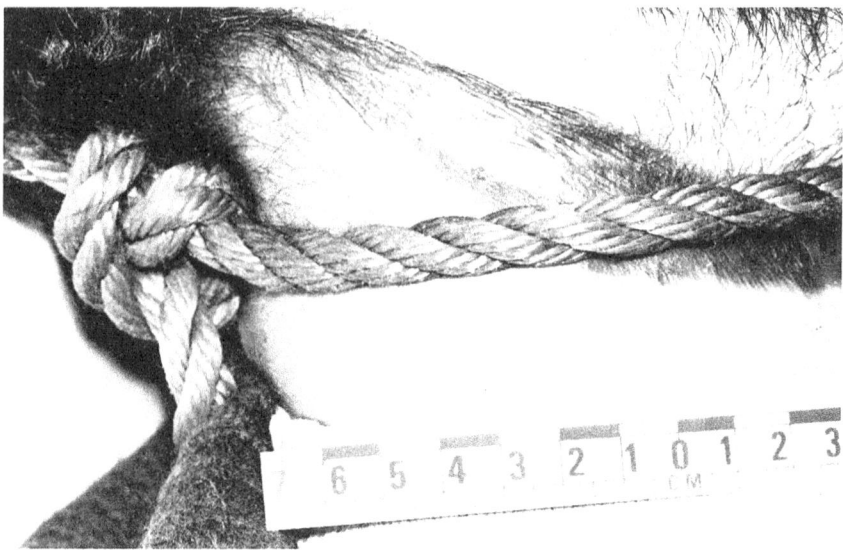

Figure 3.5   Showing the noose which has dropped away from the brown
ligature mark. It is important not to disturb the knot.

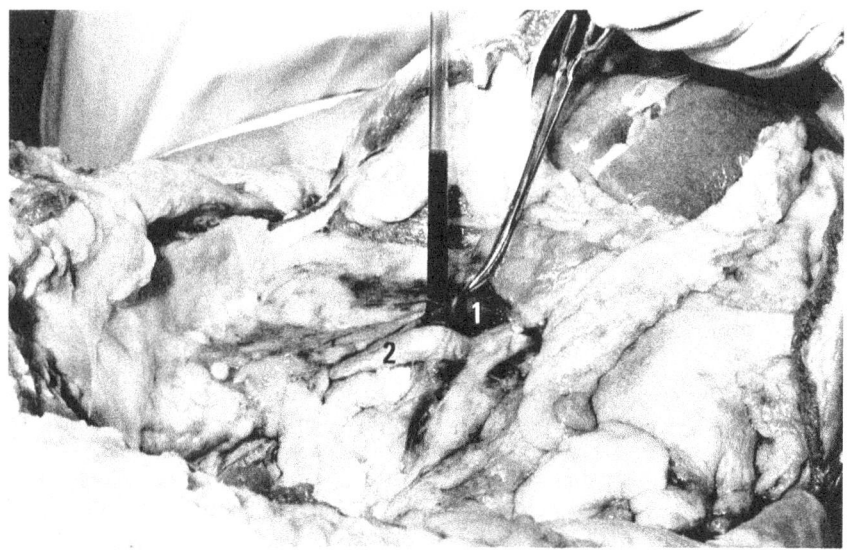

Figure 3.6   Blood is removed from the right iliac vein with a wide-bore
pipette (1 – iliac vein; 2 – right common iliac artery).

Unlike the previous examples, the method of suicide is more difficult to recognize since the image does not bear particular external inscriptions through which self-infliction might be interpreted. Instead, the image represents a body cut open, revealing various internal organs and tissues. The focus rests primarily on the manner in which particular instruments remove fluids. The discussion in the text indicates that this is an example of self-poisoning, a method acknowledged as relatively common at that time (Gresham and Turner 1979: 110). The discussion also suggests that self-poisoning requires a number of samples for toxicological analysis which should be collected by using specific instruments. While '[b]lood and urine are always taken for analysis; whole organs such as brain, liver, kidneys, stomach … are not always required' (Gresham and Turner 1979: 110). Although other methods of suicide may require internal examinations as well, it seems that the gaze of the pathologist invades the body at a deeper level in order to qualify death by self-poisoning, and requires technological extension and intensification of the diagnostic 'gaze'.

What has been described canvasses the visuality of suicide on the basis of particular methods, made available to the reader by the medical gaze and framed by the camera's lens. The gaze travels across and draws attention to bodily surfaces, decoding lethality and intent by observing, examining, measuring and documenting various inscriptions. It is as if to verify it, suicide must be 'named by being tagged or branded' on bodily surfaces (Grosz 1990: 65). In suicide recognized in this manner, the deceased body is 'inspected, palpated, poked into, cut open … transformed into an object of scrutiny' (Young 1997: 1). Suicide materializes by being mapped onto and through the surfaces of the corporeal body as the object and source of scrutiny. The signs, be it 'external' or 'internal', I am arguing, are privileged since what is recognized as visible is interpreted as essential, and in turn, as evident truth. The problem with such privileging is that it presupposes the body is an ontologically secure point of reference for suicide – an inert prediscursive given through which lethality and, in turn, suicidal intent, are rendered transparent and self-evident. Presupposing the body as a prediscursive given, I want to suggest, implicitly ignores that the body has to be turned into a particular kind of body in order to verify suicide. What is additionally overlooked is the possibility that autonomy itself may be generated by norms which privilege bodies as more or less autonomous, so that what is visually inscribed can represent violence. Such norms belong to the masculinist ways of knowing which, despite privileging the mind over the body, require a certain kind of body to render the activities of the mind coherent.

In a way, the corporeal body could well be the point of origin for interpreting suicide throughout post-mortem practices. The body certainly appears as neutral, its surfaces stripped of any cultural meaning. What the images depict is framed as the raw basis on which particular methods and their signs of lethality are visually displayed. This could be feasible, provided that the manner in which the body has been rendered visible did not depend on the workings of the medical gaze, was not influenced by the camera's lens, or by space to which the body is brought for interpretation. By saying this, I do not mean that the body is unreadable, but rather that the way particular meanings materialize is dependent on something other than the body – that something being the medical gaze. This means that rather than simply responding to deceased bodies bearing the mark of suicide, the medical gaze is part of constituting and regulating that which it sees, as an effect of its own power to see. Lethality as a transparent measure of suicidal intent cannot for instance be thought outside the power of the medical gaze and its capacity to constitute the visibility of particular corporeal inscriptions.

One point crucial to this argument is the recognition that any rendering of the corporeal body as the source for interpreting the transparency of lethality cannot be thought of outside gender norms operating in photography. 'When we are thinking about photography', Evans writes, 'we should keep in mind the way it is often discursively put to use in order to make appearances equate with reality' (2001: 107). Evans (2001) insists that the manner in which photography is used to situate something as real cannot be divorced from positivism, which seeks to establish essential and universal truths, ignoring the contexts in which such truths are produced and the purposes they serve. For Evans (2001: 109), '[t]he realism of photography seems to justify the essentialist assumptions of masculine forms of institutionalized knowledge'. This is because, as Evans further explains, 'the whole apparatus of sexual difference … appears to be uniquely based on the centrality of 'vision', of what can be *seen*. These differences are made to seem 'real' and therefore 'true' – and unchangeable – because the difference we can 'see' … appears to ground their 'truth' beyond history' (2001: 109 [original emphasis]). My argument then is that if the display of lethality by the photographic images appears transparent, then this too has something to do with the operation of masculinist norms, encoded into the visual display of bodily surfaces. What may appear unmediated and in turn, 'true', may already be conditioned by gender, even if it appears simultaneously as resting outside gender. In this sense, the gendering of suicide can be shown to be epistemologically entangled with gender norms, since what it means to 'see' via photography cannot be disentangled from gender with absolute certainty.

Is the framing of the corporeal body as a neutral and transparent object of medical examination shaped by medical models of the body? Shildrick (1997: 15) claims that the medical model presumes that 'the body is some kind of stable and unchanging given, differentiated simply by its variable manifestation of signs and symptoms of health or disease'. This certainly appears to be the case here, for deceased bodies are treated by the gaze as autonomous, stable givens, differentiated only by different types of lethal inscriptions. For scholars such as Lupton (1994), Shildrick (1997), Cartwright (1998) and Shildrick and Price (1998), the medical interpretation of the body as neutral and autonomous is a gendered effect of medicine's power, reducing it to the status of a malfunctioning machine. This particular gendered effect is sustained by the mind/body dualism and its emphasis on the body as neutral and autonomous – and unlike the cultured mind (Shildrick 1997). It is also shaped by a largely unchallenged bias towards acceptance of the male body as the normative standard upon which gender differences can be established in medical knowledge (Cartwright 1998, Eckman 1998). Hence if lethality is configured as neutral to verify suicidal intent, this process cannot be divorced from the masculinist privileging of the male body in medical knowledge. This is especially so because suicide depends on how the body is rendered intelligible in post-mortem examinations. Thus, the very visibility of suicide may actually be dependent on the invisibility of these gendered norms through which suicide is bound to masculinist ways of knowing. This is likely to produce from the same discursive strategy two effects: an over-determined view of suicide as inherently a male act, and an ongoing uncertainty as to whether female acts of self-harm are 'true' suicides. As such, it is possible to see the visible appearance of self-infliction of lethal harm as inciting the production and reproduction of suicide as masculine and masculinist.

Seeing Suicide Through the Abject

To further pursue the gendering of suicide in post-mortem practices, I now want to consider whether what appears as self-inflicted can also be read as abject. In *Powers of Horror*, Julia Kristeva (1982) examines three forms of abjection, one of which involves the corpse. 'The corpse', writes Kristeva, 'is something rejected from which one does not part'. 'It is thus not lack of cleanliness or health that causes abjection but what disturbs identity, system, order. What does not respect borders, positions, rules. The in-between, the ambiguous, the composite' (1982: 4).

The images analysed here frame what is inscribed on and through bodies as unsettling, confronting and horrifying. The images can be described in such terms not only because what appears signals a tragic end to life, but also because the border between life and death has been disrupted. The deceased bodies can be read as representing this disruption because they no longer visually display signs of vitality and life. The bodies – dead yet not out of sight – disturb order, even if the inscribed wounds and marks have been made sense of in order to verify suicide. Perhaps the bodies also disturb order precisely because they have been made sense of – have been rendered intelligible. The bodies in the photographic images are abject because, as Kristeva (1982) points out, what is abject draws attention to and heightens fragility and vulnerability. The display of fragility and vulnerability revealed is not 'real', yet the effects, incited by the powers of the medical gaze and those of its affiliates, are so compelling that what they represent seems 'real' enough.

More specifically, fluidity and seepage at the entrance to the wound caused by the shotgun death depict disruption through a lack of bodily order. The presence of blood here does not signify life, or the possibility of living, as it can elsewhere, but rather is an element representing the loss of life. The presence of blood is abject because it materializes bodily surfaces as fragile and vulnerable. The body is no longer whole and intact – the border between the exterior and interior surfaces has been disrupted – an interiority which opens the carapace of the male body surface to both destabilizing fluidity and feminizing penetrability (Grosz 1994, Williams 1998). Something similar can be said of the image that displays the dissection of the pelvic rim in relation to self-poisoning. The body is cut open to gain access to the inner cavities to obtain a blood sample for toxicological analysis. The image displays exposed interior organs and tissues. The body is no longer proper; it represents a threat to stability and order as it is no longer contained. The exterior surface cannot hold back the internal organs. Instead, the body is leaky. It threatens decay.

What the remaining images represent can also be interpreted as abject. The abrasions on the thumb and fingers from pulling the shotgun's trigger may not necessarily be as confronting as the wound on the chest. Yet the abrasions and marks are not signs of health and vitality. This is the hand that extinguished life; it introduced disorder, fragility and death. The image depicting the ligature mark displays the impact of strangulation. It focuses on skin discolouration at close range, inscribed by the noose still attached to the neck. The noose and the ligature mark draw attention to being strangled – to the body suspended and lifeless.

Depending on the method of suicide, the photographic images represent different forms of fragility and vulnerability, yet each in the context of rendering the signs on the body as medically intelligible. In a way, the reason the images are horrifying and transgressive is not only because of particular inscriptions, but also because suicide is generally understood as a private act, a very deliberate turn away from the social, and not witnessed by another party. Hence, at one level, the images are a breach of the intense privacy of the act, compelling us to imagine more vividly that a human being actively carried out the act of violence upon themselves. Nevertheless, even though someone actively chose suicide, the abject introduces an element of passivity. This, I think, is already strengthened by the power of the medical gaze which, as Foucault (1973: 130) describes, responds to disease as 'the passive, confused object' that must be made readable. In a sense, to become readable, what is inscribed on the fleshy surfaces of the body must also be framed as passive rather than active. 'Passivity' and 'activity', as two significant terms which are part of understanding suicide, may not be entirely distinct on a conceptual level. The medical site of practice that seeks to eradicate ambiguity and confusion in suicide appears paradoxically to introduce an element of ambiguity.

Reading the selected photographic images as abject thus challenges the medical interpretation of the body in suicide. Grosz (1994), Shildrick (1997) and Williams (1998) contend that the medical conceptualization of the body is understood not only as neutral and stable, but also as a bound and solid container. This masculinist container, Williams (1998: 69) argues, resists 'external forces, while holding back internal ones from expansion and intrusion'. It resists the threat of being aligned with corporeality, inscribed as female, feminine, dependent, passive and leaky (Grosz 1994, Shildrick and Price 1999). This, I think, is significant, particularly in relation to the visual example of the wound caused by the use of the shotgun.

In this instance, the body is identified as male, confirmed by the corresponding images. What can be said then of a sexed-gendered body that is not meant to seep or leak – a body which even in suicide is actively responding to difficult circumstances, rather than passively reacting to them? In being read as abject, is the male body vulnerable, fragile and passive – terms frequently invested in the interpretation of female bodies in suicide?

More specifically, what can then be said of active methods of suicide such as firearms which are more commonly associated with being male and masculine? On the one hand, it can be argued that interpreting the wound caused by a shotgun as abject actually strengthens the connection between male bodies, masculinity, lethality and violence. That is, what visibly appears as violent can still be taken as lethal and thereby, as serious, active, male and masculine. On the other hand, reading the wound through the lens of the abject indicates that the use of active methods binds suicide to the corporeal body, a body which in the context of passive methods is read as feminine, dependent and passive. By saying this, I want to assert several points. First, the boundary between what is active and passive in suicide may not be entirely clear-cut and obvious. As such, passive and active become terms which in gendering suicide are visually implicated in one another. Secondly, it seems that gendered meanings surrounding the interpretation of 'passive' suicides enter the interpretation of 'active' suicides. Thirdly, if active acts appear to transcend the material conditions of the corporeal body aligned with female bodies and femininity, then it seems that such transcendence is not entirely successful. This is because the appearance of the male body in the representation of death by a firearm appears to be bound to the material conditions of the corporeal body. Thus, something about gender is already present at the scene of bodily infliction. This does not mean that the facticity of suicide cannot be understood as lethal. Rather, lethality as a neutral measure of suicidal intentions is dependent on gender.

If the abject contributes significantly to interrogating the framing of active methods, can it also contribute to interrogating passive methods, such as overdoses? To some degree it can be said that the dissected body discussed earlier, identified as the site for self-poisoning, is rendered even more passive. Although there is no way of knowing whether the body is male or female, would self-poisoning be so closely aligned with the material conditions of the body if it were identified as female? Would the method of suicide be read as passive and feminine, rather than active and masculine? Would the same assumptions be made, regardless of the fact that the deceased did commit suicide? Would the intent to suicide be considered active and serious? Posing these questions indicates that perhaps what is important in the gendering of suicide is not only whether bodies are male or female, but whether they can be identified and culturally interpreted as male or female.

Paradoxically, if unlike most men, most women choose active and violent methods of suicide less often because they fear bodily disfigurement, then in the event of self-poisoning leading to death, disfigurement and violent spasms of bodily disruption seem unavoidable. What this might suggest, then, is that the constitution of disfigurement is bound to particular contexts through which a range of meanings are attributed. That is, the rendering of disfigurement is bound not only to those who engage with the act of suicide, but also to those who, as in the case of post-mortem examinations, either further disfigure or introduce disfigurement for the purpose of verifying suicide. Why extrusion of blood, rather than the purging of vomit, urine or faeces, should be considered 'more' abject must surely rest on cultural contexts in which the piercing of the body's surface (gunshot wound) is somehow worse than exteriorizing the (abject) interior. If in an *essentializing* discursive frame the female body 'is' abject, then enhancing its abjection, through poisons or through medical sectioning, is acceptable. If the male body 'resists' abjection, then representations of penetrative suicidal acts, such as gunshot wounds, risk both destabilizing fluidity and abjection, and must be mitigated – through consideration of a 'strong modality' act.

The analysis of the abject in relation to gender in suicide raises questions. Despite the violence it bears, why is it that the gendered male body remains hidden from view in the interpretation of suicide as 'active'? If blood, fluidity and seepage are present in methods such as firearms, why is so little said about their relevance? Why focus only on blood and disfigurement as disincentives for female suicide, when both seem to be absent in even more abject methods such as overdoses? Finally, why not speak of disfigurement in active methods in ways that move beyond acknowledging violence as of no real concern to most men?

Conclusion

By scrutinizing the effects produced via the workings of the medical gaze in post-mortem practices, the analysis has shown that what is configured as visible and lethal is important to how knowledge of suicide is constructed. I have argued that the medical gaze constitutes the corporeal body as a mappable, autonomous territory through which lethality, and thereby suicidal intent, can be verified. I have also argued that lethality as a transparent measure of intent is dependent on discursive conditions, invoking suicide as masculine and masculinist. Wounds, cuts and abrasions carry meanings. These meanings cannot be made separate from gender as gender conditions their configuration. Thus, the gendering of suicide undermines suicide as an ontological given. Visibility reveals the already gendered invisibilities operating in determining the visibility of the act of suicide.

Deploying the notion of the abject, I have problematized terms such as active and passive which are often positioned as binary opposites in understanding suicide. It now becomes apparent that the male body risks being interpreted as fragile and vulnerable, elements more closely aligned with what is female, feminine and passive. Perhaps then the production of particular understandings and terms protects the male body from being recognized as vulnerable, in order to continue to legitimize and privilege the normativity of the male body, and so the performance of male gender in the production of knowledge of suicide. Instead of protecting the male body from being recognized as vulnerable, perhaps those researching suicide in health related fields ought to respond to it in ways that are gender-aware, in ways that aim not only to prevent suicide, but also to prevent the normative gendered interpretations of suicide. Rather than *silencing* the corpse, perhaps those researching suicide ought to recognize more readily the body's fragility, be it male, female, masculine, feminine, active, passive. Perhaps then, via the abject, we can see hope for thinking otherwise.

References

Armstrong, D. 1983. *Political Anatomy of the Body: Medical Knowledge in Britain in Twentieth Century*. Cambridge: Cambridge University Press.

Armstrong, D. 1997. Foucault and the sociology of health and illness: a prismatic reading, in *Foucault, Health and Medicine,* edited by A. Petersen and R. Bunton. London: Routledge, 15–30.

Australian Bureau of Statistics. 2004. *Suicides: Recent Trends, Australia* 1993–2003, Cat. No. 3309.0.55.001. Canberra: Australian Government Publishing Service.

Barker, F. 1984. *The Tremulous Private Body: Essays on Subjection.* Michigan: The University of Michigan Press.

Brockington, I. 2001. Suicide in women. *International Clinical Psycho-pharmacology*, 16(2), S7–S19.

Brown, R.M. 2001. Suicide, in *Encyclopedia of Death and Dying*, edited by G. Howarth and O. Leaman. London: Routledge, 438–442.

Butler, J. 1993. *Bodies that Matter: On the Discursive Limits of 'Sex'.* London: Routledge.

Canetto, S.S. and Lester, D. 1995. The epidemiology of women's suicidal behavior, in *Women and Suicidal Behavior*, edited by S.S. Canetto and D. Lester. New York: Springer Publishing Company, 35–57.

Canetto, S.S. and Lester, D. 1998. Gender, culture, and suicidal behavior. *Transcultural Psychiatry*, 35(2), 163–190.

Canetto, S.S. and Sakinofsky, I. 1998. The gender paradox in suicide. *Suicide and Life-Threatening Behavior*, 28(1), 1–23.

Cartwright, L. 1998. A cultural anatomy of the visible human project, in *The Visible Woman: Imaging Technologies, Gender, and Science*, edited by P.A. Treichler, L. Cartwright and C. Penley. New York: New York University Press, 21–43.

Dahlen, E.R. and Canetto, S.S. 2002. The role of gender and suicide precipitant in attitudes towards nonfatal suicidal behavior. *Death Studies*, 26, 99–116.

Eckman, A.K. 1998. Beyond 'The Yentl Syndrome', in *The Visible Woman: Imaging Technologies, Gender, and Science*, edited by P.A. Treichler, L. Cartwright, and C. Penley. New York: New York University Press, 130–168.

Evans, J. 2001. Photography, in *Feminist Visual Culture*, edited by F. Carson and C. Pajaczkowska. New York: Routledge, 105–120.

Evans, J. and Hall, S. 1999. What is visual culture?, in *Visual Culture: The Reader*, edited by J. Evans and S. Hall. London: Sage Publications, 1–7.

Foucault, M. 1973. *The Birth of the Clinic: An Archaeology of Medical Perception*. Trans. A.M. Sheridan Smith. New York: Vintage Books.

Gresham, G.A. and Turner, A.F. 1979. *Post-mortem Procedures (An Illustrated Textbook)*. London: Wolfe Medical.

Grosz, E. 1990. Inscriptions and body-maps: representations and the corporeal, in *Feminine/Masculine/Representation*, edited by T. Threadgold and A. Cranny-Francis. North Sydney: Allen & Unwin, 62–74.

Grosz, E. 1994. *Volatile Bodies: Toward a Corporeal Feminism*. North Sydney: Allen & Unwin.

Grosz, E. 1995. *Space, Time and Perversion: The Politics of Bodies*. North Sydney: Allen & Unwin.

Hekman, S.J. 1990. *Gender and Knowledge: Elements of a Postmodern Feminism*. Boston: Northeastern University Press.

Holmes, R.M. and Holmes, S.T. 2005. *Suicide: Theory, Practice, and Investigation*. Thousand Oaks: Sage Publications.

Jenks, C. 1995. The centrality of the eye in Western culture: an introduction, in *Visual Culture*, edited by C. Jenks. London: Routledge, 1–25.

Kral, M.J. 1998. Suicide and the internalization of culture: three questions. *Transcultural Psychiatry*, 35(2), 221–233.

Kristeva, J. 1982. *Powers of Horror: An Essay on Abjection*. Trans. L.S. Roudiez. New York: Columbia University Press.

Lloyd, G. 1984. *The Man of Reason: 'Male' and 'Female' in Western Philosophy*. London: Methuen.

Lloyd, G. 1996. The Man of Reason, in *Women, Knowledge and Reality: Explorations in Feminist Philosophy,* edited by A. Garry and M. Pearsall. New York: Routledge, 149–165.

Lupton, D. 1994. *Medicine as Culture: Illness, Disease and the Body in Western Societies*. London: Sage Publications.

Mirzoneff, N. 1998. What is visual culture, in *The Visual Culture Reader*, edited by N. Mirzoneff. London: Routledge, 3–13.

Mirzoneff, N. 1999. *An Introduction to Visual Culture*. London: Routledge.

Osborne, O. 1994. On anti-medicine and clinical reason, in *Reassessing Foucault: Power, Medicine and the Body*, edited by C. Jones and R. Porter. London: Routledge, 28–47.

Peterson, L.G., Peterson, M., O'Shanick, G.J. and Swann, A. 1985. Self-inflicted gunshot wounds: lethality of method versus intent. *American Journal of Psychiatry*, 142(2), 228–231.

Range, L.M. and Leach, M.M. 1998. Gender, culture, and suicidal behavior: a feminist critique of theories and research. *Suicide and Life-Threatening Behavior*, 28(1), 24–36.

Rich, A.R., Kirkpatrick-Smith, J., Bonner, R.L. and Jans, F. 1992. Gender differences in the psychosocial correlates of suicidal ideation among adolescents. *Suicide and Life Threatening Behavior*, 22(3), 364–373.

Rose, N. 1994. Medicine, history and the present, in *Reassessing Foucault: Power, Medicine and the Body*, edited by C. Jones and R. Porter. London: Routledge, 48–72.

Rosen, P.M. and Heard, K.V. 1995. A method for reporting self-harm according to level of injury and location on the body. *Suicide and Life Threatening Behavior*, 25(3), 381–385.

Shildrick, M. 1997. *Leaky Bodies and Boundaries: Feminism, Postmodernism and (Bio)Ethics*. London: Routledge.

Shildrick, M. and Price, J. 1998. Introduction, in *Vital Signs: Feminist Reconfigurations of the Bio/logical Body*, edited by M. Shildrick and J. Price. Edinburgh: Edinburgh University Press, 1–17.

Shildrick, M. and Price, J. 1999. Breaking the boundaries of the broken body, in *Feminist Theory and the Body*, edited by J. Price and M. Shildrick. Edinburgh: Edinburgh University Press, 431–444.

Stack, S. and Wasserman, I. 2009. Gender and suicide risk: the role of wound site. *Suicide and Life-Threatening Behavior*, 39(1), 13–20.

Sturken, M. and Cartwright, L. 2001. *Practices of Looking: An Introduction to Visual Culture*. Oxford: Oxford University Press.

Tagg, J. 1999. Evidence, truth and order: a means of surveillance, in *Visual Culture: The Reader*, edited by J. Evans and S. Hall. London: Sage Publications, 244–273.

Van Dijck, J. 2005. *The Transparent Body: A Cultural Analysis of Medical Imaging*. Seattle: University of Washington Press.

Wagner, S.A. 2004. *Color Atlas of the Autopsy*. London: CRC Press.

Williams, S.J. 1998. The transgression of corporeal boundaries. *Body & Society*, 4(2), 59–82.

Young, K. 1997. *Presence in the Flesh: The Body in Medicine*. Cambridge: Harvard University Press.

Chapter 4

Fearing Sex: Toxic Bodies, Paranoia and the Rise of Technophilia

Dave Holmes and Cary Federman

Introduction

For more than two decades, the fight against AIDS has used powerful prevention messages throughout the media for the promotion of safe sex practices. Western nations, including Canada and the US, are today confronted by a fresh outbreak of HIV and other sexually transmitted infections, despite the efforts of health care professionals and organisations engaged in campaigns of prevention. Although these campaigns constitute critical elements in the struggle against HIV/STIs, we believe that these campaigns are also capable of engendering *iatrogenic* effects.

In effect, while the HIV prevention strategy promotes safe sex practices, the very same strategy is capable of inducing a generalized fear of others. All the while created by a system of thought within which everybody is potentially toxic and dangerous. The creation of (potentially) toxic bodies has had the effect of marginalising certain groups within society. Some groups are targeted more than others, which gives rise, among other things, to a homophobic outbreak, where gay and bisexual men are labelled as carriers of a new and deadly disease. From a fear of contagion at the anatomo-political (individual) level, the whole society is suddenly 'at risk' of contamination, thus extending this fear at a bio-political (population) level. According to French sociologist, Jean Baudrillard (1996), the whole strategy of the prevention of AIDS shifts the problem from the biological to the social body.

> The promotional infectiousness of information is just as obscene and dangerous as that of the virus. If AIDS destroys biological immunities, then the collective *theatricalisation* and brainwashing, the blackmailing into responsibility and obligation, are playing their part in propagating the epidemic of information and, as a side-effect, in reinforcing the social body's immunodeficiency (140).

Not unlike the medical literature regarding degeneration that was popular at the end of the 19th century, where the fear of the insane individual or degenerate body was extended to the social realm, and became a more generalized fear of the crowd (the 'social body'), made up of sexual adventurers, immigrants and political dissenters, the individual homosexual today comes to stand for an entire pathological outbreak, and represents both a biological and political threat to the larger community. As William Eskridge (2000) has written, though the language of the anti-homosexual community has shifted away from the language of contagion, the new discourse of no promotion of homosexuality, or no promo homo, still employs a discourse of fear of the act itself.

In the domain of HIV and STI prevention, we would argue that public health prevention messages might have contrary effects, notably on the expression of social interactions, in particular, sexual ones. These perverse effects could give rise to a new form of pathology even more 'socially' dangerous than the various sexually transmitted infections (STIs) health professionals wish to prevent. Along with Baudrillard, Paul Virilio (1997) argues that public (health) policies might have created new forms of disease, such as *cyberpathology* or *technophilia*, where cybersexuality replaces all forms of intimate (sexual) encounters. We are now, more than ever, hooked on technology (Stone 2001). In fact, 'skin-to-skin' sex is slowly being replaced by extensive new possibilities from sexual on-line chatting to 'face to face' on-line masturbation. With cybersexuality, individuals no longer truly connect; they disintegrate (Virilio 1998). The choreography of sexual intercourses has been changed but the effects poorly explored. The rise of the mechanical in order to satisfy sexual urges constitutes one of these effects. After the psychiatric parade of 'unnatural' perversions (zoophilia, etc.), new forms of desire emerge: mechanical ones.

> Defeat of the fact of making love, here and now, to the benefit of a mechanical medium in which 'distance' once more becomes *distantio*, distension and dissension between partners (Virilio 1997: 113).

The objective of this paper is to discuss the possible (perverse) effects of HIV/STIs prevention through the work of major European theorists such as Baudrillard, Foucault, Kristeva and Virilio, and exemplify to what extent sexual encounters are flavoured by a paranoid aura. We will also discuss the contribution of the health care *apparatus*, namely that of its agents, in the whole circuitry of *technophilia*.

The Construction of Toxic Homosexual Bodies

We all know that society establishes various procedures in order to categorize individuals deciding, along this very subjective process (often under the guise of scientific 'truths'), who is 'normal' and who is not. Canguilhem (1966), Foucault (1972, 1975, 1978) and Goffman (1975), among others, extensively discussed and criticized these scientific assumptions and their implications for stigmatized persons. Health care professionals, as bearers of scientific and expert knowledge, constitute one of the main cogs of these scientific 'truth' claims. For example, health care providers know what constitutes a 'normal' dying process. Any deviation from accepted norms regarding death implies specific intervention. In doing so, health care professionals perpetuate the normalisation of death and feed the discourse that supports it.

Being identified as disabled or different carries a significant stigma in our society where imperfections of any sort, be they physical, psychological or social, force the stigmatized persons to deal with stereotypes that are imposed upon them (Kleinman 1988, Gilman 1985). Stereotypes mark deviant bodies. They constitute further inscriptions on an already territorialized entity. As such, they represent another psychic and social burden for stigmatized persons as they reinforce unrealistic representations of so-called deviant selves.

According to social psychology and psycho-sociology, stereotypes constitute forms of ideological manifestations of collective and socialized thought (Mannoni 1998). Stereotypes are thus the building blocks of collective thought, and contribute to a system of social representations. These collective representations reassure, and act as certainties to which one can adhere (Mannoni 1998). Stereotypes therefore seem like 'truths' that are sanctioned by a particular group, and which are then imposed onto each member of the group, in an intuitive and spontaneous manner. Hannah Arendt (1995) reminds us that the values that feed stereotypes can be detected in official institutional discourse, and may serve as propaganda in ideological contexts.

The tragic appearance of AIDS in the early 1980s has produced (and to some extent continues to produce) irrational and visceral responses in all segments of society (Patton 1986, 2002). The male homosexual community was particularly hard hit by the disease itself and by the outbreak of homophobic discourse where male homosexuals were said to be carriers of a new plague.

For decades, the social construction of homosexuality as a deviant sexual practice has been linked to a discourse of contagion, contamination and pollution (Stychin 1995). Homosexuals are said to be polluted because they have 'developed some wrong condition or simply crossed some line which should not have been crossed and this displacement unleashes danger' (Douglas 1988: 113). 'Danger-beliefs' centred on notions of danger, pollution and toxicity constitutes means of *governmentality* (Douglas 1988, Foucault 1991). In effect, the language of disease, and furthermore the language of contagion and toxicity associated with the construction of epidemics such as AIDS, constitute a means of social control (Douglas 1996).

The coupling of the homosexual body with contagion and toxicity has now been exacerbated by the linkage of AIDS with male homosexuality. The construction of homosexual bodies as toxic is clearly demonstrated in many forms of media. Indeed, homosexuals are portrayed as vessels of AIDS and therefore as extensions of that disease (Gilman 1993). Moreover, AIDS is seen as the tangible proof of the toxic and dangerous nature of homosexuality. The potential toxicity of homosexual bodies demands the creation of a *dispositif* (apparatus) for the protection against the destructive 'Other'. The homosexual body as a carrier of a virus (or bacteria) has become a potential threat to others. In the age of AIDS, gonorrhoea and syphilis, the governance of personal sexual conduct is mandatory. Public health organisations deploy their energies toward the practice of safe sex, rendering imperative the use of condoms. Yet the condom comes to represent 'a very thin and precarious partition' between 'culture and anarchy' (Pick 1989: 223). It is of a piece with the nineteenth century's medicalization and *pathologization* of the subject, a generalized move by educators and doctors into a regime of self-surveillance, discipline and punishment. The intrusion of public health in private matters is not, therefore, a new phenomenon. History has shown that 'the epidemic provides an occasion and a rationale for multiplying points of intervention into the lives of bodies and populations' (Singer 1993: 117).

Contemporary public health discourse makes us regard any potential sexual partner as possibly infected by HIV or an STI. The principles of *universal health precautions* constitute, in our view, a supplemental ingredient which only intensifies the paranoia already latent in all sexual relationships. Afflicted more than any other group by the stigmatisation of HIV/STIs, the homosexual community continues to cause fear among the general public because the homosexual body itself is always already considered potentially toxic. It therefore threatens to infect the body politic as well. According to commodity culture, the gay male body remains tied to the transmission of HIV/STIs. Indelibly marked by stigma, the homosexual, as potentially toxic matter, shares with among others such as the mentally ill, the prison inmate, and the disabled a marginal kingdom where exclusion provoked by the fear of Otherness reigns.

Deviance is put to further effect when it takes a physical form because of our highly visual and superficial culture. Physical appearance is used as a signifier of the 'Other', and it plays an important role in the patterns of social interaction (Curra 2000). But non-physical deviance also plays an important role in shaping social interactions between the stigmatized person and the *collectivity*. Not only is deviance of any sort the object of surveillance, inquiry and intervention, because it breaks the social order, but it is also often an object of disgust, repulsion and fear. Far from a general lack of knowledge, we assert that differences induce fear and abjection which in turn can create several constructions, such as the toxic homosexual body. The clean and proper body (*corps propre*), as described by Julia Kristeva, is challenged by transgressive ones, such as homosexuals. So-called 'normal' individuals try to shore up a defensive position, a defence perimeter that would protect their bodies from the potentially filthy toxic ones. This defensive position is taken on as a matter of integrity and security, as an attempt to strengthen their subjectivity (Kristeva 1982).

So the anxiety grounded in the permeable line between us (inside) and the 'other' (outside) is constant and infinite. The subject is struggling, and as such is always in the process of defining him- or herself, while protecting his or her boundaries. In order to do so we push away from the proximity of our 'normal' body the 'toxic' ones. 'Rituals directed at maintaining boundaries between the self and the "other", the subject and the object, are thus attempts to ward off abjection by establishing separation, maintaining one's own body as "clean and proper"' (Lupton 1999: 139).

According to Lupton, the notion of contempt explains the virulent and often irrational feelings to which marginalized groups are exposed (Lupton 1999). Like many marginalized groups in society, homosexuals constitute a potentially biological hazard. The stigma that some groups of people must bear constitutes an important and influential element that transforms the nature of the relationship between them and other members of society. The pervasive culture of fear promoted at the individual, collective and institutional levels, which resonates in cinema, for example (*Shivers, Rabid, Outbreak, Cabin Fever, 28 Days Later*), is responsible for what some authors (Melley 2000, Lyon 1994, O'Donnell 2000) refer to as 'postmodern paranoia'. The classic symptoms of these various contagious agents include red blotches or rash, fever, psychotic dementia, grand mal seizure and haemorrhages from bodily orifices (Preston 1994). But death could also come under the guise of sex: 'erogenous sores, sexual frenzies and death spasms, resulting in an epileptic spattering of semen more often than blood' (Langeteig 1997: 139).

This being said, Virilio (1997) argues that sex is slowly but surely disintegrating. Fearing sex is an emerging social problem, created in part by the promotional infectiousness of information and prevention slogans (Baudrillard 1996). Herein, it requires us to have the courage and the humility to rethink the entire public health prevention paradigm.

Fear and Postmodern Paranoia

In the context of a society that still pushes homosexual sex to the outer regions of acceptable behaviour because of fear of contamination, into the bedroom but not part of the bedroom, that is, to where the TV and computer screen are, into the realm of cybersex, is there any distinction to be made between the state's exercise of power over subjects and the care of the self, between the requirements of self-surveillance and paranoia? Baudrillard categorized America in 1986, still the beginning of the AIDS crisis, as: 'Protect everything, detect everything, contain everything – obsessional society' (Baudrillard 1986: 40). Normal Americans, Justice Antonin Scalia argued in *Lawrence* v. *Texas* (2003), do not want persons who openly engage in homosexual conduct as partners in their business, as scoutmasters for their children, as teachers in their children's schools, or as boarders in their homes. They view this as protecting themselves and their families from a lifestyle that they believe to be immoral and destructive.

Scalia fears what Elias Canetti calls, 'the touch of the unknown' (Canetti 1984: 15). Such a person, Canetti (1984: 15) writes, 'wants to *see* what is reaching toward him, and to be able to recognize or at least classify it'. The Court in *Lawrence,* Scalia wrote, has accepted 'the legal profession's anti-anti-homosexual culture', thereby demonstrating that the Court 'is seemingly unaware that the attitudes of that culture are not obviously "mainstream"' (602).

Underlying Scalia's opinion that to be anti-homosexual is to be 'mainstream', is the idea that homosexuality is a classifiable condition, something toxic, that it spreads like a disease upon contact, and that homosexuals are dangerous because they (and not us) engage in sodomy, which, in the context of a homosexual accused of sodomy, conjures up notions of anal rape, molestation and disease. The mainstream, which Scalia has taken upon himself to protect, and which he feels is under direct attack by both homosexuality as an idea, and by homosexuals as persons, is the place where thought is easily understood, where toxicity is contained, where the structures of our thought and the edifice of constitutional law have not been 'dismantle[d]' by degeneration (Lawrence 2003: 604). The pure edifice of the anti-homosexual culture is the unmediated space where degeneration has not yet occurred. Fear is at the door of the law, but it is the only thing we've got to protect us from the 'other'. This 'other' was theorized by Kroker and Kroker (1988: 22) as a 'panic body' that is 'an inscribed surface onto which are projected all the grisly symptoms of culture burnout'. This body is 'incited less by the languages of accumulation than fascinating, because catastrophic, sign of self-[extermination], self-liquidation and self-cancellation'.

When the Court's majority in *Lawrence* limited its decision to the case at hand, and declared that protecting homosexual activity under the fourteenth amendment's liberty clause would not involve the government giving 'formal recognition to any relationship that homosexual persons seek to enter', in other words, the Court's majority denied that one could understand its decision as opening the door to state-sanctioned homosexual marriage, Scalia tartly replied: 'Do not believe it' (Lawrence 2003: 604).

'Do not believe it' means: the homosexuals are lying. It means: trust us, because we have the moral high ground – the law, the family and cleanliness are on our side. It means: 'the "properly" unified, coherent, "normal" self of our civilisation is by definition heterosexual – one whose object-choice is not its own mirror image, the homo –, but rather its binary other, the hetero' (Byers 1995: 12–13). Paranoia and homophobia are thus related, because they are

> Matters of maintaining the body's sealed-off coherence and solidity against all sorts of threats of invasion and dissolution: threats of Deleuzian schizophrenia and Kristevan abjection, of feminism and feminisation, gender trouble and homosexuality, of fluidity, dissemination and termination (Byers 1995: 15).

Paranoia of the non-clinical variety exists because the gap between structure and agency – between causal explanations that clearly delineate ways of thinking about heredity and environmentalism, nature and nurture – can no longer be closed by reference to one system that can explain behaviour. Postmodern paranoia recognizes the death (and not just the incredulity) of grand narratives and the monumental. Postmodern paranoia is thus not a mere pathological response to one's understanding of modernity (Lyon 1994, Oldham and Bone 1994); rather, it is 'an integral part of what constitutes postmodern history' (O'Donnell 2000: 149).

Paranoia inhabits the space torn asunder by structural and individual explanations of phenomena.

If we follow the lines drawn by Stephen Kern in his book, *The Culture of Time and Space, 1880–1918* (1983), as well as the arguments of Jameson (1995) and Harvey (1990), it is modernity itself that has fragmented lived experience to the point that achieving a unity of experience can only be had either by force or by sheer accident. Lyotard (1984), for example, wonders what kind of unity Habermas has in mind when he argues in favour of bridging the gap between 'cognitive, ethical and political discourses' (72). In Italy, as the English historian Daniel Pick demonstrates, the gap between 'heredity and milieu' (Pick 1989: 140) that dominated scientific discourse from the end of the nineteenth century through the first quarter of the twentieth century was closed by fascism. Postmodern paranoia, then, derives from a breakdown in the representation of meaning given to things within a critical moment in modernism, without giving in to the 'fascism that causes us to love power, to desire the very thing that dominates and exploits us' (Deleuze and Guattari 1983: xiii). It begins with a recognition that the 'principle of ordering ceases to be resemblance and becomes relations of identity and difference' (Gutting 1989: 146). With modernity, signs lose their privileged place in the order of things. Meanings shift from the world to the individual mind. Postmodern paranoia is therefore a symbolic fabrication; it is a recognition (by the self) that the self has no foundation in reality.

In the context of the health profession's concern with homosexual toxicity, we have achieved what Jameson (1995: 38) calls 'high-tech paranoia', which reduces critical inquiry into the problem of knowledge and power to narratives of technology's capillary capabilities. The computer provides the comfortable space created by the received view that all bodies are potentially toxic. Each communication from the public health industry is a message that needs to be decoded. The deterroritorialized homosexual body reterritorializes itself within the safety of on-line sexual images and computer codes. Safety reigns in this terminal zone of eyes, hands, mouths and anuses without bodies. Secrecy supplants openness. Fear becomes the dominant agent of knowledge. Power is omnipresent and omniscient because surveillance is everywhere (Yar 2003). Conspiracy theories arise, according to Fenster (1999: xiii–xiv), 'when the political is interpreted within a specific, conspiratorial narrative frame by those for whom politics is inaccessible and its meaning is impenetrable or secret' for O'Donnell (2000: 14):

> Paranoia as manifested in contemporary narrative can be further considered as the multifarious contradiction of a postmodern condition in which the libidinal investment in mutability, in being utterly other, contests with an equally intense investment in the commodification of discrete identities.

To be 'utterly other' is to engage in a practice of the self, mediated through technology. But the libidinal investment in mutability has been shortchanged. The push to cleanse the homosexual body of its illnesses by opening up on-line sex is the paranoid fantasy of the late twentieth century's desire for a regime of order, cleanliness, discipline and punishment.

Collateral Damage: The Rise of *Technophilia*

Communication technologies provide a cyborg habitat where new behaviours emerge. For example, cyberspace constitutes a social system that can be sexually charged without skin-to-skin sex (Holmes 1997). A book titled, *The War of Desire and Technology and the Close of the Mechanical Age* (Stone 2001), addresses this issue of having sex without meeting a real person. While advocating for mechanical-sex, because it offers new possibilities, Stone (2001: 38) is nevertheless interested in 'how people without bodies' have sex.

Technology is considered to be one of the key components of postmodern culture (Lane 2000, Terry 1997). According to Baudrillard (1983), whose interest lies in the subject's experience of technology as part of everyday life, technology is now able to produce three levels of distinct simulation. The first level is an obvious copy of the real. The second level of simulation blurs the boundaries between the real and the representation (copy). Finally, the third level is one of complete simulation where the fake precedes the original (Lane 2000). By entering in the third level of simulation, humankind creates the 'hyper-real'. For example, technological 'advances' permits the creation of wars (Baudrillard 1995) by TV networks and thus mask what is going on for 'real' on the battlefield. The perfect crime has been achieved: the real is dead (Baudrillard 1996). Technology constitutes a new way to be 'in the world' which has been amputated from symbolic dimensions. Baudrillard argues that the relationship between the person and the symbolic, ritualized behaviours are actually disappearing (Lane 2000). The complexity of the world now resides in technological objects at the expense of persons, where technology destroys social interactions. To make this point clearer, Virilio (1997) links cybersex to the technological replacement of the emotions. Moreover, technological 'progress' is a euphemism from a Baudrillardian perspective, because technology has rapidly become non-functional, non-utilitarian, and designed according to fantasy and desire (Lane 2000).

Sometimes used interchangeably with virtual reality (VR), cyberspace 'specifically denotes the real and imagined space in which individuals meet in electronically mediated and simulated space…it requires the construction of computer-mediated worlds in which communication can occur' (Holmes 1997: 234). Cyberspace no longer refers to a futuristic concept or dream; it has now penetrated our lives. Since the mid-1990s, a renewed world order expands 'on the shimmering surface of our computer screens' (Nunes 1997: 163). Cyberspace disposes of the 'real' for the 'hyper-real' (the third and last level of simulation, according to Baudrillard). Contemporary analysis of cyberspace comprehends it as a site of excess connection and a site of (bodily) fragmentation (Stone 2001, Vasseleu 1997).

We have come to a point where electric and biological currents are entangled, where intimacy in cyberspace can replace sexual intercourse with 'real' bodies (Virilio 1997). Stone (2001) offers a more benign view of the prospects of disentangling computers from humans. She implies that individuals in cyberspace are playfully interacting, and developing a 'mutual discourse' regarding different ways of interacting. She sees cyberspace as an opportunity for further explorations of human behaviour and contact. As a consequence, computers are not only hardware tools but arenas 'for social experience' (Stone 2001: 15).

On the other hand, if in cyberspace the risks of getting HIV and STIs are annihilated, so is the risk of the degrading of social interactions (Baudrillard 1996, Vasseleu 1997, Virilio 1997). For these critics, technology's penetration of human bodies leads almost inevitably to the extinction of human relations. Cyberspace gives human beings the very possibility to alter themselves in numerous ways, and allows people to experience their most pleasurable fantasies, and at the same time, their worst nightmares (Springer 1996). To be sure, popular culture frequently represents cybersex only as a pleasurable experience (Springer 1996). Yet internet sexual encounters are both social and anti-social simultaneously. On the one hand, they allow for a connection to a global community. But on the other, they are anti-social because they imply that face-to-face communication becomes an 'attenuated level of human association' that is 'no longer valued in cultural representation' (Holmes 1997: 39). In the era of cyberspace, sexual encounters are something you can plug in or turn off as you wish. Cybersex is a form of *telepresence* which protects the subject, not only from sexually transmitted infections, but also from the vulnerability of being there in the flesh with others. The ultimate achievement of cybersex is 'un-reality without risk'. Cybersex allows partners 'to overcome their reciprocal proximity without risk of contamination, the electromagnetic prophylactic outdoing by a long shot the fragile protection of the condom' (Virilio 1997: 104). In cyberspace the subject is freed from material constraints, including social ones, and has been offered new sexual possibilities characterized by freedom. But what type of engagement does cybersex promote? Cyberspace opens up untapped sexual territories for those who fear (for various reasons) skin-to-skin sexual intercourse. But these renewed possibilities are as dangerous as the diseases health care providers want to protect us from.

Fear of toxic 'Others' has led some to find refuge before a computer screen which permits the exploration of new ways to practise sexual urges. The interface between human bodies and computers is the privileged site where electronic culture transmits its virus – words and images – in the human host, 'enforcing its toxic message … on the very cells' (Burroughs cited in Langeteig 1997: 142). In the domain of cultural studies, the postmodern subject is defined as being fractured, *liminal* and extreme; a terminal of 'high-tech system where the human being is endangered: an end-of-the world scenario aptly summed up in the phrase *crash culture*' (Langeteig 1997: 137).

In effect, virtual reality (VR) is not so much protective as it is an addictive sex-charged space. The virtual subject, as a no risk sexual subject, encounters neither resistance nor fear of contamination in cyberspace. His body is not engaged in the world but serves as a plain surface for sexual exchanges. The VR subject is a victim of what Virilio (1991: 72) calls 'constitutive dispersal' where bodily boundaries have collapsed into an 'open system in which nobody can find any perceptible, objective limits'. The virtual subject has become prosthetic (Cooper 1997), as he or she collapses into 'the complex circuitry of a high-tech system to become a *machinic* subjectivity' (Guattari 1992: 29).

If the use of cyberspace as an area of plenitude, desire, and joy only occurs with the removal of the desiring subject from the problems of real sex (and real diseases), how will it be possible, then, to mediate between the fake and the real world when dealing with sex (Cooper 1997)? The manner in which virtual reality technology operates must be thoroughly delineated. Cybersex removes the desiring subject from the complexity of sexual practices that have constituted a meaningful experience in the 'real' world. The generalized social fear as it pertains to HIV/AIDS and other STIs, induced to some degree by radical prevention messages, might be responsible for what Virilio (1997) calls *cyberpathology* or *technophilia*. As such, sex in cyberspace could constitute an escape route in response to a generalized fear of contamination. 'Only a new way of getting pleasure can save us' declares one of cyberculture's advertising slogans (Virilio 1997: 111). Once vital, copulation is slowly replaced by an option: remote-control (media) masturbation. The very act of interacting with a computer matrix is a solitary one, but it is still considered a sexual act, 'a masturbatory fantasy expressed in terms of entering something but lacking the presence of another *potentially polluted* human body' (Springer 1996: 68 [italics added]).

Germphobia has created mutual repulsion between partners, wiping out sexual attraction for new pathological expressions. The rise of *technophilia*, a nascent long-distance-sex-disease, is 'a game of pathological inertia' that provides a sense of comfort without the risks of getting HIV and other STIs (Virilio 1997). Fear of 'others', particularly marginalized 'Others', is slowly winning the battle over skin-to-skin sexual encounters.

At issue in the debate of sexual disintegration is the annihilation of social interactions. Springer (1996) suggests that we have been engaged in self-destruction since the arrival of AIDS and nuclear energy and that, sexual encounters in cybersex constitutes a response to these fears. 'Human bodies are already vulnerable to unprecedented threats of AIDS ... nuclear annihilation, overpopulation and environmental disasters ... to stimulate human consciousness electronically indicates a desire to redefine the self' (Springer 1996: 71). From fear of toxic bodies to sexual diversion through cybersex, is it possible that we have entered into an irreversible phase of sexual disintegration under the reign of prevention campaigns? According to Springer (1996) it should not come as a surprise at a time when paranoia over human contact in response to the 'hills vibes' is common, human interaction should occur through computer screens, with participants unable to touch each other.

Final Remarks

The representation of the rendered toxic subject by technology has been widely accounted for in the discourse of the human sciences. Research on that topic in the health sciences is almost non-existent, despite the physiological or psychological effects of addiction to computers. Cyber (sex)-addiction not only generates physiological and psychological trauma but social ones. It is responsible for what Baudrillard calls *electronic encephalisation* and *lobotomy*.

To paraphrase Virilio, we thought we were safe because we were not moving. The virtual parasitism of cybersex gives us an *avant-goût* of the horrors of our postmodern human condition. Some fearful persons now prefer the risks of toxic communication to the risks of gonorrhoea. Some persons trade the potential virulent/bacterial contamination of HIV/STIs for the one provided by cybersex(ual) intercourse. Cyberspace is now the new way of life and cybersex the new path toward orgasms, even if the virtual subject, as Baudrillard writes, disappears into the network of its empty (sexual) communications.

The rise of *technophilia* confirms that a crash is happening in cyberspace and that the death of the vital subject has occurred simultaneously with the birth of the cyber one. The terminal addict described by William Burroughs in *Naked Lunch* is close to the terminal subject: 'with a spine like a frozen hydraulic jack … his metabolism approaching Absolute Zero … the addict regards his body impersonally as an instrument to absorb the medium in which he lives' (Burroughs 1992: 67). Postmodern humans are political surfaces; they experience interactions without distance as if life was reduced to immediacy and the flat surface of the computer or television screen (Baudrillard 2001, Springer 1996).

Here we are at the close of the mechanical age (and at the birth of the virtual one), a time where technology merges with neurology and genitals, all hovering on the edge of a stunning socio-sexual annihilation. It is true that cyberspace is a location for transformation, a cyborg factory, in which bodies are becoming mechanical. Stone (2001) writes that cyber means steer, a space between 'promise and danger' and of 'desire and technology' (183).

The continued use of fear (of contamination, of pollution, etc.) by public health professionals with regard to HIV/STIs prevention constitutes a powerful pedagogical activity against the 'concretisation' of risks. But it is also a means by which other risks can arise. It is important to problematize the public health discourse which constitutes an *apparatus* that is able to induce fear of 'others' by its very strategies. As such, public health discourses can be constructed as being both sources of positive and negative outcomes when it comes to health matters. Health providers working as agent of governmentality (Federman and Holmes 2000, Holmes and Federman 2003, Holmes and Gastaldo 2002) and working at the intersection of individuals, populations and public health authorities must remain aware of the potential 'perverse' effects of their (healthy) discourse, which also has the power to draw distinctions between natural and unnatural, clean and filthy, civilized and non-civilized, as well as to induce a degree of fear of 'other' such that it can create new, 'pathological' possibilities.

References

Arendt, H. 1995. *Les origines du totalitarisme: le système totalitaire.* Paris: Seuil.

Baudrillard, J. 1983. *Simulations.* New York: Semiotext(e).

Baudrillard, J. 1986. *America.* London: Verso.

Baudrillard, J. 1995. *The Gulf War Did Not Take Place.* Sydney: Power Publications.

Baudrillard, J. 2001. L'élevage de la poussière. *Libération.* Février.

Burroughs, W. 1988. *The Western Lands.* New York: Picador.

Burroughs, W. 1992. *Naked Lunch.* Concord: Grove Press.

Byers, T. 1995. Terminating the postmodern: masculinity and homophobia. *Modern Fiction Studies*, 41(1), 5–33.

Canetti, E. 1984. *Crowds and Power.* New York: The Noonday Press.

Canguilhem, G. 1966. *Le normal et le pathologique.* Paris: Presses Universitaires de France.

Cooper, S. 1997. Plenitude and alienation: the subject of virtual reality, in *Virtual Politic*, edited by D. Holmes. Thousand Oaks: Sage, 93–106.

Curra, D. 2000. *The Relativity of Deviance.* Thousand Oaks: Sage.

Deleuze, G. and Guattari, F. 1983. *Anti-Oedipus.* Minneapolis: University of Minnesota Press.

Douglas, M. 1988. *Purity and Danger: An Analysis of Concepts of Pollution and Taboo.* New York: Routledge.

Douglas, M. 1996. *Risk and Blame: Essays in Cultural Theory.* New York: Routledge.

Eskridge, W. 2000. No promo homo: the sedimentation of antigay discourse and the channeling effect of judicial review. *New York University Law Review*, 75, 1327–1411.

Fenster, M. 1999. *Conspiracy Theories: Secrecy and Power in American Culture.* Minneapolis: University of Minnesota Press.

Federman, C. and Holmes, D. 2000. Caring to death: health care professionals and capital punishment. *Punishment and Society*, 2(4), 439–449.

Foucault, M. 1972. *Histoire de la folie à l'âge classique.* Paris: Gallimard.

Foucault, M.1975. *Surveiller et punir.* Paris: Gallimard.

Foucault, M. 1978. *Histoire de la sexualité: la volonté de savoir.* Paris: Gallimard.

Gilman, S. 1985. *Difference and Pathology: Stereotypes of Sexuality, Race, and Madness*. Ithaca: Cornell University Press.

Goffman, E. 1975. *Stigmates: les usages sociaux des handicaps*. Paris: Les Éditions de Minuit.

Grosz, E. 1992. Lived spatiality: Insect space/virtual sex. *Agenda*, 26(7), 5–7.

Gutting, G. 1989. *Michel Foucault's Archeology of Scientific Reason*. Cambridge: Cambridge University Press.

Harvey, D. 1990. *The Condition of Modernity: An Enquiry into the Origins of Cultural Change*. London: Blackwell Publishers.

Holmes, D. 1997. *Virtual Politics*. Thousand Oaks: Sage.

Holmes, D. and Federman, C. 2003. Killing for the state: the darkest side of American nursing. *Nursing Inquiry*, 10(1), 2–10.

Holmes, D. and Gastaldo, D. 2002. Nursing as means of governmentality. *Journal of Advanced Nursing*, 38(6), 557–565.

Jameson, F. 1995. *Postmodernism, or the Cultural Logic of Late Capitalism*. Durham: Duke University Press.

Kern, S. 1983. *The Culture of Time and Space, 1880–1918*. Cambridge, MA: Harvard University Press.

Kleinman, A. 1988. *The Illness Narratives: Suffering, Healing and the Human Condition*. New York: Basic Books.

Kristeva, J. 1982. *Powers of Horror*. New York: Columbia University Press.

Kroker, A. and Kroker, M. 1988. *Body Invaders: Panic Sex in America*. New York: St. Martin's Press.

Lane, R.J. 2000. *Jean Baudrillard*. London: Routledge.

Langeteig, K. 1997. Horror *autotoxicus* in the red night trilogy: ironic fruits of Burrough's terminal vision. *Configuration*, 5, 135–169.

Lawrence v. Texas. 2003. 539 US. 558.

Lupton, D. 1999. *Risk*. London: Routledge.

Lyon, D. 1994. *The Electronic Eye: The Rise of Surveillance Society*. Minneapolis: University of Minnesota Press.

Lyotard, J.F. 1984. *The Postmodern Condition*. Manchester: Manchester University Press.

Mannoni, P. 1998. *Les représentations sociales*. Paris: Presses Universitaires de France.

Melley, T. 2000. *Empire of Conspiracy: The Culture of Paranoia in Postwar America*. New York: Cornell University Press.

Nunes, M. 1997. What Space is Cyberspace?, in *Virtual Politics*, edited by D. Holmes. Thousand Oaks: Sage, 163–178.

O'Donnell, P. 2000. *Latent Destinies: Cultural Paranoia and Contemporary U.S. Narrative*. Durham: Duke University Press.

Oldham, J. and Bone, S. 1994. Paranoia: historical considerations, in *Paranoia: New Psychoanalytic Perspectives*, edited by J. Oldham and S. Bone. Madison: International Universities Press, 3–15.

Patton, C. 1986. *Sex & Germs: The Politics of AIDS*. Montreal: Black Rose Books.

Patton, C. 2002. *Globalizing AIDS*. Minneapolis: University of Minnesota Press.

Pick, D. 1989. *Faces of Degeneration: A European Disorder, c. 1848–1918*. Cambridge: Cambridge University Press.

Preston, R. 1994. *The Hot Zone*. New York: Bantam Books.

Rheingold, H. 1991. *Virtual Reality*. London: Secker and Warburg.

Singer, L. 1993. *Erotic Welfare: Sexual Theory and Politics in the Age of Epidemic*. New York: Routledge.

Springer, C. 1996. *Electronic Eros: Bodies and Desire in the Post-Industrial Age*. Austin: University of Texas Press.

Stone, A.R. 2001. *The War of Desire and Technology at the Close of Mechanical Age*. Cambridge, MA: Massachusetts Institute of Technology.

Stychin, C.F. 1995. Unmanly diversions: The construction of the homosexual body (politic) in English Law. *Osgoode Hall Law Journal*, 32(3), 527–536.

Terry, J. 1997. *Processed Lives: Gender and Technology in Everyday Life*. London: Routledge.

Vasseleu, C. 1997. Virtual bodies/Virtual worlds, in *Virtual Politics*, edited by D. Holmes. Thousand Oaks: Sage, 46–58.

Virilio, P. 1991. *The Lost Dimension*. New York: Semiotext(e).

Virilio, P. 1997. *Open Sky*. New York: Verso.

Yar, M. 2003. Panoptic power and the pathologisation of vision: critical reflections on the Foucauldian thesis. *Surveillance & Society*, 1(3), 254–271.

Chapter 5

Eroticizing the Abject: Understanding the Role of *Skeeting* in Sexual Practices

Patrick O'Byrne

Introduction

In contrast to conventional definitions of health care, which position it as the provision of caring and curative services for already-present health concerns on an individual (case-by-case) basis, there is also a public health component of health care which aims to improve the health status of entire populations through the enaction of preventative interventions (Last 2001, Lupton 1995, Shah 2003). As part of the development of the latter style of health care, public health departments began to appear in the middle of the 1900s, and often with the mandate of infectious disease control (Lupton 1995). Unsurprisingly, the most successful of these public health infectious disease strategies were those that required the least amount of effort from the general population; take for example, water purification, waste removal, or mass vaccination (Lupton 1995). Nevertheless, despite knowledge about the proven effectiveness of such *passive* public health interventions, Western countries have recently begun to more readily invest in the development of health interventions that aim to directly modify the behaviour of individuals who are identified as being *at-risk* for future ill health (MacIntyre and Ellaway 2001). However, Emmons (2001) and Glass (2001) identify that such individually based initiatives rarely improve health at the population level, and they believe that this may be the case because most of the behaviour modification strategies that have been tested to date have not been based on clear understandings of the cultural significance/meaning of the behaviours and outcomes that have been targeted for modification. According to Bennett and Hodgson (1995), such cultural understandings help mitigate potentially unanticipated reactions.

In the realm of sexually transmitted infection (STI) and HIV public health work, one such unintended outcome which may have arisen as a result of health workers ignoring the cultural significance of the behaviours they are trying to change/eradicate is *skeeting*[1] – which is a sexual practice that may have increased

---

1   In this context, the term skeeting refers to the sexual practice of dispersing ejaculate onto or around, but not into, a sexual partner. It is a withdrawal technique that is driven by desires for the external dispersion of ejaculate, not wishes to prevent the potential consequences associated with unprotected internal ejaculation. This informal term arose

in popularity, in part, as a result of public health interventions which treat semen exclusively as a dangerous bodily fluid, one that is implicated in both STI/HIV transmission and pregnancy. Stated differently, public health workers' blatant disregard of the meaning and significance of semen, in particular for men who have sex with men, disregards its erotic significance during sexual contact (Holmes and Warner 2005), and thus, may have resulted in an increased occurrence of *skeeting*. This further supports Glass' (2001) suggestion that public health interventions, which are not based on cultural understandings, may produce unexpected outcomes. Of particular interest in the case of *skeeting*, however, is that the erotic appeal of semen previously noted by Holmes and Warner (2005) is maintained, just in a novel way that incorporates public health messaging about bodily fluid exchange, membrane permeability, and STI/HIV transmission. Although research has been undertaken to understand many other sexual practices, such as, intentional unprotected anal sex and internal ejaculation (*barebacking*) (Bolous et al. 2006, Elford 2006, Holmes et al. 2007, Holmes and Warner 2005, PHAC 2005), very little research has addressed the topic of why some individuals chose to ejaculate on (rather than in) their sexual partners.

Therefore, as a preliminary and exploratory evaluation of this topic, the findings of a research study undertaken at two Canadian gay circuit parties (GCP) are analysed below. To situate the practice of *skeeting*, the concept of abjection will be utilized to ground an understanding about the processes which occur when individuals encounter substances/objects that are no longer part of them or someone else (for example, blood, vomit, faeces, semen), and the resulting repulsion/attraction that is caused by encountering such separated substances/objects (Kristeva 1982). The ultimate outcome will be that the concept of abjection will be used to situate the act of *skeeting* as a harm reduction method that balances the erotic (driven toward) nature of semen, and the simultaneous repulsion that it causes by its potential to serve as a vector of illness and infection.

Theoretical Framework – Abjection

As not to re-hash everything that was stated by Rudge and Holmes (in this collection) regarding Kristeva's (1982) concept of abjection, only a summary will be presented here. Specifically, only that which is most salient about abjection in relation to *skeeting* will be presented. This is: (1) individuals construct their self-identity by dichotomizing and sorting their external and internal environments into that which is either similar (clean) or dissimilar (unclean); (2) this sorting process produces a simultaneous attraction and repulsion that arises when individuals encounter those substances/objects that they have been classified as

---

as slang because its original definition denotes a competitive shooting game in which clay targets (skeets) are launched into the air and marksmen are required to unholster their guns and fire rapidly at them.

dissimilar; (3) this process of classification first appears when a baby differentiates its mother from itself (that is, my mother is dissimilar/separate from me), and the developing individual continues this sorting process in relation to additional objects; (4) the process of abjection is a mechanism of identity creation and maintenance throughout the lifespan; and (5) this identity maintenance is achieved by labelling objects as either clean or dirty (that is, similar or dissimilar) (Kristeva 1982, McAfee 2004). This fifth point is a return to step one above.

One further point about abjection that is important in this discussion is that the abject serves as a mechanism to sever an individual's associations with dissimilar objects in an effort to maintain cleanliness and propriety (McAfee 2004). Such a rejection of the abject ensures that the unclean and the self remain discrete in order to maintain the individual's self-identity through spatial and/or social segregation. This produces spaces of abjection (e.g., quarantine or ostracism), and also precisely delineates the areas within which abject objects are permitted to exist. These spaces show that it is not an absolute lack of cleanliness or a potential to produce unhealthy outcomes that causes the anxiety and discomfort associated with objects of abjection, but rather, that these emotions occur when objects that are seen as potentially problematic do not respect their designated borders, and remain in-between, ambiguous, or composite (Kristeva 1982). This indeterminateness produces the wavering emotions of concurrent temptations and condemnations: summons and repulsions.

Within this context, semen is a readily available example of this phenomenon because it has acquired a special social status that often persists without any analysis of the socially mediated explanation that is given to describe people's feelings toward it (Kristeva 1982). Indeed, within the sexual health domain, the explanation of these feelings toward semen seems to be an uncritical transference of the underlying evolutionary perspective[2] frequently used to explain common human aversions to faeces and vomit. However, different cultures experience abjection in relation to different objects, thus bringing the evolutionary explanation into question. For example, in Western societies, in relation to STI/HIV transmission, it can be suggested that there is a greater stigma attached to bisexual, than to homosexual, men notwithstanding that both groups have sex with men. The purposed explanation for this difference is the societal belief that bisexual men act as vectors of infection between the homosexual and heterosexual populations (Ekstrand et al. 1994). They are the bridge for HIV between the marginalized to the mainstream. That is, bisexual men are an abject sexual group because

---

2   The evolutionary perspective delineates that feelings of repulsion toward faeces and vomit must have made 'our ancestors' more fit to survive, thus explaining why the ever-present feelings of disgust toward these objects increase when they are not appropriately contained within their spaces of abjection. For example, a disgust of faeces increases if/when it is not located within its designated spot – the toilet. From this perspective, because of its potential to transmit diseases, these feelings exist as the result of a biological adaptation to keep away from human excrement.

they transgress imposed sexual boundaries. This further supports Kristeva's (1982) suggestion that location is, in fact, a highly important factor in relation to abjection.

In addition to the importance of spatial separation, the factors which produce abjection also apply to the body, with its physically established boundaries and varying loci of permeability (Kristeva 1982). Moreover, since the relatively recent invention of the microscope, scientists have had to redefine the causes of many human illnesses based on discoveries about the integrity of human epithelial membranes and about infectious disease transmission/acquisition. Ill health is no longer a form of cosmic retribution; it is now understood to be the outcome of behaviours that expose an individual to infectious agents (Lupton 1999, 2004). Further complicating this issue is that the absence of signs and symptoms for most STIs/HIV prevents members of the general population from being able to easily identify infected bodies (abject bodies, that is) by sight (Lupton 2004). Thus, the microscopic discovery of many infectious agents has produced not readily identifiable stigmatized groups (those with infectious diseases) (Evans 2001), while mainstream public health campaigns related to STIs/HIV have promulgated the message that each and every person is a potential and hidden threat to everyone's health – including their own. This invisibility of infectious agents means that a specific STI/HIV is not regarded as an abject object; this position is assigned to the infected individual and his or her bodily secretions (for example, saliva, mucous, urine, faeces, and anal, vaginal and penile discharges, including semen). Semen, however, is unique as an abject substance. Unlike blood and excrement, which often signals death, injury, disease, or elimination, semen has traditionally been associated with life and procreation. In antiquity, for example, the Greeks believed that losing one's sperm was associated with a loss of vitality (Abbott 2000), and that the health complications associated with an untreated gonococcal infection in men was caused by a loss of semen. Indeed, a direct translation of the word gonorrhea from Greek into English reveals that this term means 'flowing seed/semen' (*gonos* 'semen' + *rhoia* 'flux') (New Oxford American Dictionary, Digital Version).

However, after the advent/discovery of HIV, and other STIs, semen now plays the dual role of creating life, while also functioning as a vector of illness and infection, or at least, as a visible manifestation of this potential transmission. In this way, a conflicting situation arises in which a potential or actual sexual partner may be an object of abjection – that is, a sexually desired, but dangerous, entity. Thus, the movement of semen from one individual to another could constitute a practice that breaches the rules of propriety. That which was supposed to remain separate has transgressed boundaries that are supposed to be maintained as inviolable. Within the context of safer sex, the bodily fluids of each individual are required to remain distinct: bounded by a condom or, at least, kept external to the body (see PHAC 2006). Such externality, however, includes an elimination of potential contact between bodily fluids and vulnerable sites, such as the permeable membranes of the mouth, eyes, nose, urethra, vagina, anus, or open wounds/sores. Hence, within the modern context, semen must not breach the protective epithelial layer of others.

This has resulted, at least within the context of this chapter, in the suggestion that the erotic allure, but public health induced fear, of semen may produced an increase in the popularity of the erotic art of *skeeting* as a harm reduction method.

Methodological Considerations

At this point, the methodological processes of the research project, including the recruitment strategies, the study design, the data collection methods, and finally, the data analysis techniques will be presented.

Recruitment

Participants were recruited for self-administered questionnaires and semi-structured interviews at two gay circuit parties (GCPs) which ran on consecutive nights. In addition, direct recruitment and poster distribution for the interviews also occurred in bathhouses, gay bars, clubs, gyms, and sexual health clinics in three Canadian urban centres that are home to the largest Canadian Anglophone and Francophone communities.

Study Design

This project was undertaken within the paradigm of critical theory, from a poststructuralist perspective. The precise design was ethnography, and as such, the outcome was the collection of information about the environmental aspects of history, culture, gender and sexuality. Attention was also given to the environment, social interactions and the culmination of all the physical/non-physical connections that produced the overall ambience of the GCP. Such an approach allowed for an interactive and qualitatively driven research project, which located the researcher far from the taken-for-granted assumptions propagated by current public health discourses, such as, what Lupton (1995) calls the 'imperative of health'. This critical ethnographic design (Hammersley and Atkinson 2005) provided information about the motivation of individuals who engage in sexual practices that are incomprehensible within the paradigm of contemporary mainstream public health mandates.

Data Collection Methods

Self-Administered Questionnaire

Non-probability sampling created a convenience sample. While such an approach can be considered a methodological limitation, in this situation, this technique was unproblematic because the main purpose of the questionnaire within this research project was for the recruitment of interview participants – not to make generalized statements about GCP-goers. Therefore, representative sampling was unimportant within this context. The sample was thus created from individuals who self-selected to complete a self-administered and anonymous questionnaire. Moreover, this survey had been previously piloted in a research undertaken in Canadian gay bathhouses (Holmes, Gastaldo and O'Byrne 2007, Holmes, O'Byrne and Gastaldo 2005, Holmes et al. 2008). Specifically, it was findings from this previous research project that identified the need to add questions to the self-administered questionnaire (see Holmes and Warner 2005). This was done in an effort to, first, see if these topics were also relevant to GCP-goers, and second, to further develop the explanations that had been proposed by Holmes and Warner (2005) during the bathhouse project.

Formal Interviews

After the completion of the questionnaires, formal interviews took place. During this process, participants, first, completed the same self-directed questionnaire that was administered at the two GCPs, and then they took part in a taped, in depth, semi-structured interview, which lasted approximately one hour. This interview process continued until no new interview material was provided – that is, until data saturation occurred. The participants that were chosen to take part in this data collection method were selected according to the degree of information they were willing to share, their socioeconomic status, educational background, et cetera; in addition to this, an attempt was made to include ethnic diversity in the sample. The interviews themselves were conducted using open-ended questions. This method has been accused of having two major shortcomings: (1) that the researcher answers questions asked by the interviewees and (2) that the personal opinions of the researcher interfere with the research process. However, it has also been argued that these two pitfalls are, in fact, major benefits of this method because answering interviewee questions, instead of stealthily attempting to evade them, increases the degree of rapport and trust between the interviewer and interviewee (Fontana and Frey 2004). Since an interview is an interaction between two individuals, and the purpose of the semi-structured interview is to gain a better understanding of the subject, the interviewer and the interviewee must communicate openly.

Analysis Techniques

Self-Administered Questionnaire

The collected survey data were subjected to univariate analysis using SPSS: indices of central tendency (means, medians, and modes). Such information was useful in describing the sociodemographic background of GCP attendees and in providing an overview of their self-reported sexual practices; this may facilitate a better understanding of the target population in future public health initiatives within the context of GCPs.

Semi-Structured Interviews

Constant comparative analysis structured the analytical process, and was employed after every interview to guide the questions for subsequent interviews. To accomplish this task, each interview was transcribed and coded based on an analysis of the interview content; that is, codes were assigned based on the content of the statements, the overall meaning of the interview, the language and sentence structures employed by the interviewee, and the general positioning of these within the larger political structure. This analysis included a line-by-line reading of the text, and a second reading to identify metaphors and content (Silverman 2003). The metaphorical reading included a language and content analysis, which was performed within the aforementioned theoretical framework. Once this was completed, the metaphors were linked together using the same theoretical framework. Because the research data were organized according to the perceptible characteristics of each participant as well the context of the interaction, the interview transcripts were first scrutinized separately, and then in combination (Ryan and Bernard 2003).

Skeeting: Understanding a 'Location-Specific' Spectacle and its Participants

In total, two parties were attended, during which non-probability sampling methods created a convenience sample through self-selection. During these two parties, 209 questionnaires were completed; 66.5 per cent (n=139/209) of these were collected during the first party. In addition, 20 semi-structured interviews were completed, each of which lasted approximately one hour.

Self-Directed Survey: Demographics

Regarding participant demographics, information was gathered about age, language preference, sexual preference, education level, gross income, and self-defined ethnicity. Please refer to Table 5.1 for more details.

Sexual Practices

Regarding sexual practices, participants identified their oral and anal sexual practices, and how they handle the resultant ejaculate. Please refer to Table 5.2 for more information.

Table 5.1   Demographic information

Category		Number
Age		**32.96 +/- 8.57**
Language	French	130 (62.2%)
	English	79 (37.8%)
Sexual Preference	Exclusively men	182 (87.1%)
	Men & Women	20 (9.6%)
	Exclusively women	7 (3.3%)
Education	High School	36 (17.2%)
	College / Bachelor	123 (58.8%)
	Master's / Doctorate	44 (21.1%)
Income	< $29 999	54 (25.9%)
	$30 000–$59 999	77 (37.4%)
	$60 000–$99 999	37 (18%)
	> $100 000	30 (14.4%)
Ethnicity	Caucasian	180 (86.1%)
	African Canadian	11 (5.3%)
	Asian	6 (2.9%)
	Latin	4 (1.9%)
	Aboriginal	2 (1%)
	Other	7 (3.3%)

The mean age of participants was 33 years, with, 62.2 per cent (n=130/209) having completed French questionnaires. The majority of the sample (87.1 per cent; n=182/209) reported exclusively having sexual contacts with men, and 79.9 per cent (n=167) have completed post-secondary education. As for ethnicity, the majority was Caucasian (86.1 per cent; n=180/209).

Table 5.2   Sexual practices

Category		Number	
Oral Sex	Give with condom	4	(1.9%)
	Give without condom	97	(46.4%)
	Get with condom	11	(5.3%)
	Get without condom	83	(39.7%)
Anal Sex	Top with condom	94	(45.0%)
	Top without condom	21	(10.0%)
	Bottom with condom	71	(34.0%)
	Bottom without condom	18	(8.6%)
Ejaculate	Take in Mouth	26	(12.4%)
	Take on Face	27	(12.9%)
	Take on Chest	60	(28.7%)
	Take in Anus	12	(5.7%)
	Give in Mouth	35	(16.7%)
	Give on Face	40	(19.1%)
	Give on Chest	58	(27.8%)
	Give in Anus	17	(8.1%)

Self-reporting of sexual practices indicated that unprotected oral sex and protected anal sex were the most common forms of sexual contact. Regarding anal sex, 'top' indicates being the penetrative partner, while 'bottom' signifies being the receptive partner. In addition, while these two penetrative forms of sexual contact were most common, the process of dealing with ejaculation was external to the mouth and anus.

Semi-Structured Interviews

In contrast to mainstream biological interpretations of sexual activity that position ejaculation for the purpose of species propagation as the underlying physiological drive behind all sexual contact, other authors such as Gagnon and Simon (2005) posit that the process of experiencing an orgasm is more complex than simply the expulsion of semen. One example of such a counter-procreative sexual process is *skeeting*, which stands in direct contrast to the biological view of sexuality because it is a practice in which semen is deposited externally to all sexual partners. In this activity, individuals desire to ejaculate on a partner, rather than inside of them. Analysis of this research project confirmed that the location of ejaculation, in addition to the seminal fluid itself, is important for some individuals. At this point, the qualitative data that lead to this statement will be presented.

Skeeting – Erotic Ejaculation as Location Specific

The first identified theme related to *skeeting* is that the pleasurable sensations of an orgasm are related to the act of ejaculation as a sexual performance. This perception of ejaculation transforms the physiological expulsion of semen into an erotic spectacle in which it is not only the physical sensation of ejaculation (and its corresponding orgasm) that is sought, but also the visible display of ejaculation as a theatrical act. Witness the following participant's description of ejaculation as a 'show':

> I think that most guys will pull out because it's more of a show. Like when you
> cum inside someone, especially with a condom on, you don't see anything – you
> don't see any sort of physical reaction. But if you pull out and you see a guy
> ejaculate and it's like, 'ok, you've sort of seen the end result of it'. (Ott-2)

For the above participant, witnessing the physical act of ejaculation is an important interrelated aspect of the orgasm process. However, further exploration (with the below participant) of the idea stated above reveals that for him, while orgasm and ejaculation are intertwined, it is the actual process of ejaculation (not orgasm) that provides the desired result of a sexual performance. It is the visualization of the ejaculate (i.e., the sexual substance) that causes desire. Even in cases of penetrative anal sexual acts performed using a condom, the preference is for a non-penetrative, but visualized, ejaculation without a condom. For example:

Will you cum inside the person with the condom on?
I prefer to pull out.
Do you pull out and cum in the condom or do you cum on the person?
It all depends.
Do you have a preference for that?
I'd rather shoot without the condom.
As in shooting on the person?
On the person, over the person, it depends. (TO-1)

As evidenced by this second quotation (TO-1), protected anal penetration followed by *skeeting* (that is, removing the condom to visibly ejaculate) conflicts with the idea that unprotected ejaculation occurs because condoms might be related to a potential decrease in stimulation. In fact, *skeeting* is about 'showing off', about 'shoot[ing] without the condom' (TO-1), about it being 'more of a show' (Ott-2). Thus, for the two participants cited above, the eroticism involved in ejaculation does not necessarily equate to a desire for skin-to-skin contact. Indeed, their desire for condom-less ejaculation should not be interpreted as a desire for unprotected anal penetration. Rather, these men prefer an erotic exhibition – an uninhibited display of ejaculating semen onto themselves or someone else. The following participant echoes this practice of penetrative anal sex followed by the removal of condoms ('people cum inside me with condoms on, but most guys pull out and … cum') as shown below:

Now, does the person cum inside you with a condom on?
It depends. They have, but most people pull out. I have had people cum inside me with condoms on, but most guys will pull out and either cum on themselves or cum on me (Ott-2).

The above participant relates that he engages in protected penetration, followed by conspicuous ejaculation. While this participant discusses these sexual practices in relation to penetrative sexual contact, the following participant states that, at times, his desire to witness an orgasm and its resulting ejaculation supplants the need for direct sexual stimulation. He states:

Yeah, maybe as a kid working in night clubs and you know working at stripper's club and stuff like that, where depending on who the gentlemen was or whatever, if you're on the pole, a hundred bucks and he wants to watch you cum. I'd be sitting here, he'd be two feet away, you know cheering on. I'd shoot and I'd smack him right in the head two feet away (TO-1).

According to this participant, ejaculation is also an erotic spectacle for any witnesses to the act – this includes individuals who are not having or causing an orgasm. It is not just the process of ejaculating on a person, but rather, the process of being able to see the ejaculation which this participant describes as being sexually stimulating and sought after (e.g., 'a hundred bucks and he wants to watch you cum'). The following participant also illustrates this same point:

Well, for guys that I suck it seems more and more that I'd be willing to do that [be ejaculated on], and seems, for a lot of guys that they want that. It seems to be a turn on for some guys. They want to blow in your mouth. Other times, I'll suck them until they're ready to cum, and I like watching them blow. I like a really nice blowjob, or an ejaculation. I like watching a nice ejaculation, too. That's a turn on as well (Ott-1).

The above participant precisely states that his desire is for a visual orgasm: 'I'll suck them until they're ready to cum, and I like watching them blow' and 'I like watching a nice ejaculation'. Even the non-ejaculating partner receives sexual satisfaction from witnessing another individual's expulsion of semen. Furthermore, the eroticism of *skeeting* is affecting not only the individual ejaculating, but also the one who is causing it. In fact, in contrast to passively watching, participation in the act heightens the eroticism for the individual not having an orgasm. Thus, the discharged substance is important.

In addition, the below cited participant indicates that the inherent physical properties of semen provide a method by which the non-ejaculating partner experiences heightened pleasure. Being ejaculated on further promotes a connection between the two partners involved. The following participant highlights:

> **Is there much with facials, or with people cumming on each other?**
> It's feeling the heat on your chest, on your face. If it hits your face okay, but once
> it starts getting in your eyes and you know burning, then it doesn't really do that
> much for me (Ott-1).

The heat of semen on the recipient's body is also an erotic component of the experience. For the above participant, it is the sharing of semen and the transgression of the boundaries that separate the two individuals that enhances the eroticism of this sexual act ('It is feeling the heat on your chest, on your face'). Nevertheless, there exists a repulsion/attraction to semen: 'If it hits your face okay, but once it starts getting in your eyes … then it doesn't really do that much for me'. This participant acknowledges that when semen lands in his eye, the erotic nature of it dissipates, because it has transgressed its appropriate boundaries. Location is important.

Skeeting – The Importance of Semen

In addition to the importance of location during ejaculation, as a second theme, seminal fluid also played an important role for the participants in this research study. For example, without prompting, the participant quoted below describes in detail the length and distance of his ejaculations. This signifies how ejaculating on someone may represent feelings of domination, intimacy, masculinity, or eroticism, but that ultimately, ejaculation and ejaculate are of central importance during the sexual experience.

> But seeing the person shoot and if they can shoot really far and stuff like that.
> Like you know, if I get worked up and if I hold my cock in the right way, like not
> jerking it, but in holding it down at the base as it's building up, then I can shoot
> way over my head. On occasion there are unbelievable streams of cum (Ott-1).

Moreover, the following quotation also emphasizes that this participant's perception of visible ejaculation (skeeting) as a measure of masculinity enhances the eroticism of *skeeting* – the further one can skeet the more masculine one is:

> A good friend of mine used to have jack-off parties, and we'd lay tape measures
> on the floor to see who can cum the farthest. I can hit the four foot level repeatedly

and he's like "Jesus man, you're never going to get them in". Maybe it's seeing it, and maybe the look on people's faces (TO-1).

The eroticism that is intertwined with *skeeting* is directly related to its magnitude as a spectacle: the more impressive the *skeet*, the more erotic it becomes. Thus, *skeeting* is a visual display of manhood through powerful ejaculation, which in turn serves to enhance its erotic nature. The following excerpt highlights this:

> Sometimes you just hardly cum at all, you just dribble, like you just cum out a little bit. You ooze all over the place. But, I definitely like it when a guy can really blow a lot.
>
> **What do you like about that?**
>
> Well, I guess it's the power, of seeing it blow.
>
> **Is it knowing that you've made this person cum?**
>
> Well, it's one thing that you've made them cum, you've made them do that, but it's just a turn on to see someone ejaculate and shoot really, really far.
>
> **So it's also the act in itself?**
>
> Yes, it's just the act of them shooting that far. So it's maybe it's subconsciously it's like a power-macho thing. Like guys with bigger dicks are like more, there's some draw to that. Guys that can ejaculate farther, there's something erotic with that (Ott-1).

As with previous participants, the above participant reports that it is not exclusively the orgasm that he seeks. Rather, it is a specific type of ejaculation which involves great distances and large quantities. Similar to the sporting event after which it was named, *skeeting* (rather than skeet shooting) is a form of male competition, in which men vie to achieve the furthest and largest ejaculation. Thus, for the above participant, the process of ejaculation is a macho display of sexuality which culminates in further eroticism.

Discussion

As noted above, the initial form of data collection in this project occurred in the form of self-directed questionnaires which revealed that, in general, the anal sex activities of only a few research participants in this study culminated in unprotected internal ejaculation: 8.1 per cent deposit semen rectally, and 5.7 per cent receive semen rectally. Based on the levels of anal sex that were reported (42.6 per cent and 55.0 per cent of the sample reported engaging in receptive and penetrative anal sex, respectively), the foregoing levels of internal unprotected ejaculation that was recorded could have been a surprising result. However, as was predicted by the findings of Holmes and Warner's (2005) research project, semen exchange in the form of *skeeting* was found to be a fairly common practice amongst the group of men involved in this project. Indeed, 12.9 per cent of the participants reported having their faces *skeeted* on and 28.7 per cent reported having their chests *skeeted* on, while 19.1 per cent reported *skeeting* on their sexual partners' faces and 27.8 per cent reported *skeeting* on their sexual partners' chests. This signifies that nearly one-third of the participants reportedly engage in *skeeting*, thus both aligning with the findings of Holmes and Warner (2005) and also signalling the need for this practice to be further explored as an important area of public and sexual health.

From the interview data, two different findings about *skeeting* arose. The first, which came to light during the preliminary analysis of the interview data, suggested that *skeeting* was a sexual practice that the research participants undertook using a false logic about the precise mechanisms of microbial and viral transmission via genital fluids (see CDC 2006, PHAC 2006). In other words, due to the fact that semen exchange is not necessary for STI/HIV transmission, at first glance, it seemed as though the interview participants were undertaking sexual practices which they incorrectly believed would not allow them to either acquire or transmit STIs and HIV. While less fluid exchange may equal less chance for STI/HIV transmission, the problem was that, first, there is no definite evidence supporting this practice, and second, the participants seemed to believe that infectious agents only existed within the semen. This belief thus seemed to transform semen into *the* infectious agent, not one of many transport mediums for STIs/HIV.

Despite this initial suspicion, however, further exploration dispelled this finding: the true significance of *skeeting* had nothing to do with safer sex practices. Instead, the participants described it as a highly ritualized and erotic act: the visual culmination of the pulsations, swellings, movements and throbbings of their bodies that simultaneously drew in and repelled its participants. This eroticism, notwithstanding its association with seminal fluid, was not solely related to the substance of semen itself, but rather, was associated with the visible display of ejaculate onto an appropriate context – not inside a person, not in the anus or the eyes, but outside and onto the body. Because of these stipulations, a concurrent desire and repulsion toward semen, based on the location of a seminal deposit, became evident. That is, while semen exchanged was desired, it had to be done in a certain fashion for this desirability not to transform into anxiety or repulsion.

As previously noted by Holmes and Warner (2005), the desirable component of semen arose from individuals feeling that this substance is the natural culmination of sex, or an agent which enhances intimacy and connection. While such findings were repeated in this study, within this project semen was also identified as a readily perceivable substance that once outside the body is also feared because of its being a bodily fluid capable of infection transmission (PHAC 2006). This thus positions semen as both a desirable component of the sexual act, and a factor involved in 'messy' outcomes, such as, increased likelihood of STI/HIV transmission (Carlisle 2001).

In response to these potentially detrimental, or 'messy', effects of coming into contact with another's bodily fluids, including semen, public health strategies have created acceptable environments within which semen can exist. These include: outside the body, within condoms, or within monogamous sexual partnerships in which other precautions, such as, relevant STI/HIV testing has occurred (PHAC 2006). However, the results of this research, in addition to a plethora of previously undertaken studies, reveal that these public health messages are not always being followed – semen, and other bodily fluids, are still being exchanged without a condom in casual or anonymous sexual partnerships (Halkitis, Parsons and Bimbi 2005, Holmes and Warner 2005, Suarez and Miller 2001).

In light of this evidence, it is imperative that new theoretical approaches are used to comprehend the subjective importance that bodily fluid transmission, such as *skeeting*, has for some people. One possible alternative for understanding these practices is the concept of abjection (Kristeva 1982, McAfee 2004). Indeed, such an approach can be used here to provide a sound theoretical understanding of the simultaneous attraction and repulsion that the research participants described in relation to their own and others' expelled semen. As such, it can be used to move beyond traditional public health strategies about semen which seem to have been based on the assumption that semen is inherently dangerous. Moreover, this concept can also be employed to help shed light on why the external segregation of other's semen from oneself must be both figurative and literal, with sexual contacts being separated by protective barriers/boundaries, and with semen remaining spatially confined inside these spaces.

Most readily, Kristeva's (1982) concept of abjection identifies that semen is not inherently a substance that produces either anxiety or fear. Rather, as Kristeva (1982) argues, the emotional responses associated with the abject are context related. It is about keeping the 'unclean' away from the 'clean' self, and thus, it is only when the boundaries between these two places are breached that anxiety, fear, or repulsion ensues. The research participants in this study reported such precise reactions in relation to semen when this bodily fluid ended up in/on locations capable of STI/HIV transmission. Provided that other's semen remained external to their bodies, and thus away from any porous membranes, the research participants quite contently continued to view semen as an erotic substance.

What this means is that *skeeting* could be considered a practice which carefully navigates the delicate balance between the eroticism and the repulsion that the research participants ascribed to semen. It is an action which mitigates the undesired aspects of the abject substance by ensuring that semen remains within public health approved locations. However, despite this suggestion, it is important to mention that the interview participants never overtly mentioned *skeeting* in relation to STIs/HIV transmission. Nevertheless, analysis of the research results indicates that the participants' engagement in this practice does, in fact, constitute an unintentional harm reduction strategy. Such an assertion can be made because, as the participants described *skeeting*, this practice involves a visual climax in which the main deposit of bodily fluids that occurs during sex does not occur in/on locations which permit STI/HIV transmission. The semen of one individual does not come into contact with any permeable membranes of an other/others. While it is important to acknowledge that semen is not required for STI/HIV transmission, a decrease in the quantity of bodily fluids that are exchanged could correspond with a decrease in the quantity of bacteria or virus that can be transmitted. For HIV, this would amount to a theoretical reduction in the quantity of virus that could be transmitted – particularly in relation to men when high HIV viral loads in their semen.

Therefore, it could be argued that the participants in this study unintentionally follow relevant public health STI/HIV suggestions by engaging in a sexual practice which maintains the eroticism they desire, but which nevertheless reduces the likelihood of infectious disease transmission. It is a practice that maintains the naturalness and enhanced connection that Holmes and Warner's (2005) research participants reported desiring, but which does so with a possibly lessened likelihood of infectious disease transmission. Thus, the individual who wishes to engage in semen exchange, but who is aware of STI/HIV transmission, may decrease personal anxieties associated with the abject object (semen) by forcing it onto surfaces that are virtually incapable of infection transmission (i.e., face, chest, buttocks, floor, bed, etc.). In this way, these individuals have adopted a method of dealing with an abject substance, which, for some of them, is a highly important and ritualized aspect of a sexual encounter (Douglas 2005, Holmes and Warner 2005). Further supporting the harm reduction nature of the *skeeting* practices of this study's participants is that they primarily reported using condoms during penetration, thus dramatically reducing their contact with their sexual partners' other (that is, non-seminal) bodily fluids. This leaves the only bodily fluid exchange being the splattering of semen onto their sexual partner.

To summarize the above bluntly, *skeeting* is an eroticization of the withdrawal technique; a means by which those who wish to indulge in the abject, but who also wish to ensure that semen remains within its appropriate boundaries, can achieve both these goals. This means that when *skeeting* is approached from the theoretical perspective of abjection, it is no longer a second-rate method for dealing with infectious disease transmission. It is not a practice driven by ignorance and carelessness. Put differently, despite public health authorities often categorically caution against the withdrawal technique, when semen is comprehended using the concept of abjection, *skeeting* (that is, eroticized withdrawal) becomes a fairly sound strategy for navigating the pulls of desire and the repulsions of fear related to semen and STIs/HIV. As such, Kristeva's (1982) concept of abjection helps re-position this *skeeting* as an excellent (and already sexually desired) harm reduction strategy that diminishes the likelihood of semen being deposited within other's bodies. It is a method for simultaneously maximizing the desirably components of semen, while also minimizing the fear and repulsion that it produces when it comes into contact with permeable membranes of the human body. As such, this practice is one that public health workers need to further explore in an effort to better understand how individuals who report that semen exchange is an important aspect of their sexuality can continue to indulge in their desires, but within minimized probability of STI/HIV acquisition and transmission.

Conclusion

As can be seen, when engaging in health initiatives, it is important to acquire an understanding of the target health practice and its meaning for specific populations. At times, a message may unintentionally produce unexpected outcomes, including those that the intervention was aimed to reduce. Furthermore, it is also important to constructively address potentially negative outcomes of population-based messaging. In the domain of sexual health, the total-condom discourse has positioned semen as a dangerous substance, but by proscribing this substance, public health workers may have produced an increase in its erotic value for some individuals. Consequently, public health workers may wish to capitalize on the already-existent eroticism of *skeeting* when they design future health initiatives. In doing so, they should also return to the harm reduction aspect of *skeeting* by encouraging, or at least suggesting, this sexual practice as a means by which individuals who engage in protected penetrative sexual contacts can satisfy their potentially repressed desires for semen exchange.

References

Abbott, E. 2000. *A History of Celibacy*. Cambridge: De Capo Press.

Bataille, G. 1992. *Death and Sensuality: A Study of Eroticism and the Taboo*. New Hampshire: Ayer Company.

Bennett, P. and Hodgson, R. 1995. Psychology and health promotion, in *Health Promotion: Disciplines and Diversity*, edited by R. Bunton and G. Macdonald. New York: Routledge, 23–41.

Boulos, D., Yan, P., Schanzer, D., Remis, R.S., and Archibald, C.P. 2006. Estimates of HIV prevalence and incidence in Canada, 2005. *Canada Communicable Disease Report*, 32(15), 165–74.

Carlisle, C. 2001. HIV and AIDS, in *Stigma and Social Exclusion in Healthcare*, edited by T. Mason, C. Carlisle, C. Watkins, and W. Whitehead. New York: Routledge, 117–25.

CDC. 2006. Sexually Transmitted Diseases Treatment Guidelines, *Morbidity and Mortality Weekly Report*, 55, RR-11.

Douglas, M. 2004. *Purity and Danger*. New York: Routledge.

Douglas, M. 2005. *Risk and Blame: Essays in Cultural Theory*. New York: Routledge.

Ekstrand, M.L., Coates, T.J., Guydish, J.R., Hauck W.W., Collette, L. and Hulley, S.B. 1994. Are bisexually identified men in San Francisco a common vector for spreading HIV infection to women? *American Journal of Public Health*, 84(6), 915–9.

Elford, J. 2006. Changing patterns of sexual behaviour in the era of highly active antiretroviral therapy. *Current Opinion in Infectious Diseases*, 19, 26–32.

Emmons, K.M. 2001. Health behaviours in a social context, in *Social Epidemiology*, edited by L.F. Berkman and I. Kawachi. New York: Cambridge University Press, 242–66.

Evans, D. 2001. The stigma of 'sexuality': concealability and course, in *Stigma and Social Exclusion in Healthcare*, edited by T. Mason, C. Carlisle, C. Watkins, and W. Whitehead. New York: Routledge, 104–16.

Fontana, A. and Frey, J. 2004. Interviewing: the art of science, in *The Landscape of Qualitative Research: Theories and Issues, 2nd Edition*, edited by N. Denzin and Y. Lincoln. Thousand Oaks: Sage, 47–78.

Gagnon, J.H. and Simon, W. 2005. *Sexual Conduct: The Social Sources of Human Sexuality, Second Edition*. New Jersey: AldineTransaction.

Glass, T.A. 2001. Psychosocial interventions, in *Social Epidemiology*, edited by L.F. Berkman and I. Kawachi. New York: Cambridge University Press, 267–305.

Halkitis, P.N., Parsons, J.T., and Bimbi, D.S. 2001. Intentional unsafe sex (barebacking) among gay men who seek sexual partners on the Internet. Personal Communication – Unpublished manuscript.

Hammersley, M. and Atkinson, P. 2005. *Ethnography: Principles in Practice. Second Edition.* London: Routledge.

Holmes, D., Gastaldo, D., O'Byrne, P., and Lombardo, A. 2008. Bareback sex: a conflation of risk and masculinity. *International Journal of Men's Health*, 7(2), 171–91.

Holmes, D., O'Byrne, P, and Gastaldo, D. 2007. Setting the space for sex: architecture, desire, and health issues in gay bathhouses. *International Journal of Nursing Studies*, 44, 273–84.

Holmes, D., O'Byrne, P., and Gastaldo, D. 2006. Raw sex as limit experience: a Foucauldian analysis of unsafe anal sex between men. *Social Theory & Health*, 4(4), 319–33.

Holmes, D. and Warner, D. 2005. The anatomy of a forbidden desire: men, penetration, and semen exchange. *Nursing Inquiry*, 12(1), 10–20.

Kristeva, J. 1982. *Powers of Horror: An Essay on Abjection*. New York: Columbia University Press.

Last, J.M. 2001. *A Dictionary of Epidemiology*. New York: Oxford University Press.

Lupton, D. 1997. *The Imperative of Health: Public Health and the Regulated Body*. London: Sage.

Lupton, D. 1999. Introduction: risk and sociocultural theory, in *Risk and Sociocultural Theory: New Directions and Perspectives*, edited by D. Lupton. Cambridge: Cambridge University Press, 1–11.

Lupton, D. 2004. *Risk*. London: Routledge.

MacIntyre, S. and Ellaway, A. 2001. Ecological approaches: rediscovering the role of the physical and social environment, in *Social Epidemiology*, edited by L.F. Berkman and I. Kawachi. New York: Cambridge University Press, 332–48.

McAfee, N. 2004. *Julia Kristeva*. New York: Routledge.

Public Health Agency of Canada. [PHAC]. 2005. *HIV/Aids Epi updates* (No. H121-5/2005E), Ottawa, ON: Surveillance and Risk Assessment Division, Centre for Infectious Disease Prevention and Control, Public Health Agency of Canada.

Public Health Agency of Canada. [PHAC]. 2006. *Canadian Guidelines on Sexually Transmitted Infections, 2006 Edition.* Ottawa: Queen's Printer.

Ryan, G.W. and Bernard, R.H. 2003. Techniques to identify themes. *Field Methods,* 15(1), 85–109.

Shah, C. 2003. *Public Health and Preventative Medicine in Canada, 5th Edition.* Toronto: Elsevier Saunders.

Silverman, D. 2003. Analyzing talk and text, in *Collecting and Interpreting Qualitative Materials, 2nd Edition*, edited by N. Denzin and Y. Lincoln. Thousand Oaks: Sage, 310–39.

Suarez, T., and Miller, J. 2001. Negotiating risks in context: a perspective on unprotected anal intercourse and barebacking among men who have sex with men – where do we go from here? *Archives of Sexual Behaviour*, 30(3), 287–300.

PART II
Abject Positioning

Chapter 6

Spoiled Identities: Women's Experiences After Mastectomy

Roanne Thomas-MacLean

Introduction

Breast cancer can disrupt the taken-for-granted nature of embodiment, leaving women with much uncertainty throughout diagnosis, acute care and beyond. Upon receiving a diagnosis of breast cancer, the body becomes suspect. Further, dominant discourses provide women with a limited repertoire with which to understand and make sense of negative aspects of breast cancer and embodiment. This chapter explores the experiences of women who have had breast cancer in order to further understanding of 'spoiled identities' resulting from this illness. Data were gathered in a qualitative study. Interpretation specific to this chapter focuses on issues of embodiment, using Julia Kristeva's work as a starting point. Exploring the ways in which the body becomes abjectly experienced may illuminate previously unexamined elements of breast cancer survivorship, thus furthering knowledge about the meaning of illness for women.

Background

In writing critically of the legacy of breast cancer, I do not wish to 'spoil' the identities of those women who would be most apt to cast themselves as 'survivors' or 'heroines'. Rather, the intent is to write about, and perhaps for, those women who find aspects of their stories missing from the popular, pink ribbon-esque discourse that implies that all women should survive breast cancer and survive well – with elegance, poise and grace. For instance, Lantz and Booth (1998: 907) argue that 'the portrayal of the breast cancer epidemic in the US popular press reflects a strong social desire to create order and control over a frightening disease'. Yet, not all is well with all women after breast cancer. Negative aspects of illness remain unvoiced, despite the abundance of positively cast research and biographies which function very prescriptively (Carter 1993, Ferrans 1994, Loveys and Klaich 1991, Lugton 1997, Pelusi 1997, Timpson 1999, Utley 1999, Wyatt, Kurtz and Liken 1993). I would argue that there is an ethical imperative to understanding these aspects of experience and that this might be considered congruent with Kristeva's view of ethics as 'an open system … always in process, on trial, under revision' (Oliver 1993: 17). We have an ethical obligation to seek out and understand that which is missing from breast cancer discourse and popular narratives in order to influence health care practices and policies. Understanding what is currently invisible may also further understanding of the importance of stories and qualitative research.

In other work, I have discussed the ways in which narratives are shaped by and continue to shape culture and experiences (Thomas-MacLean 2004a, 2004b). Herein, I focus more on embodiment (see for example, Barral 1969, Butler 1988, Crossley 1994, Ledermann 1982, Merleau-Ponty 1974, O'Loughlin 1998, Rehorick 1986, Toombs 1992, Turner 1995) as a starting point from which to examine the ways in which women understand their own 'spoiled identities'. In writing about that which might be perceived as negative, I do not mean to suggest that women cannot live positively after breast cancer, but I do suggest that neglecting 'spoiled identities' makes the possibility of fully understanding life after breast cancer more remote than if the wide variety of experiences were addressed. Without exception, all of the women who have shared with me their own stories of breast cancer have been admirably strong, and active with work, family, community engagement, physical activity and hobbies. However, also without exception, all women have shared with me another side of their lives and what might be considered the abject aspects of illness and embodiment.

My own interest in embodiment stems from the work of Merleau-Ponty (1974), along with other contemporary phenomenological writers (Bentz and Shapiro 1998, Rehorick 1986, van Manen 1997, 1998). I have also drawn upon the work of feminist scholars (Birke 1998, Bordo 1987, Bungay and Keddy 1996, Darling-Wolf 2000, Holmes 1989, Kasper 1995, Lennon 1998, Martin 1990, Maticka-Tyndale and Bicher 1996). Adding consideration of abjection to these theoretical lenses opens the door to new reflections of the subtleties of illness. For instance, it is commonplace now to recognize that cancer and the body may be referred to as 'it' thereby reflecting some of the objectifying language of medicine. But, one might also understand this type of language usage through the concept of abjection – meaning a type of rejection or distancing of self from that which is viewed as repulsive or negative, or otherwise disturbing, yet an integral part of self.

In their research with cancer patients in palliative care, Waskul and van der Riet (2002) describe the abject body as 'messy, polluted, sick, and damaged' (487) and state that their research participants 'experienced their bodies as permeable, vulnerable, and out of control' (Waskul and van der Riet 2002: 487). Waskul and van der Riet (2002) draw upon well known work in sociology and stigma, that of Erving Goffman. More recently, Ellis (1998) has written about stigma, thereby extending the reach of sociology in this area. Waskul and van der Riet (2002) note that the 'abject embodiment of cancer patients is complex, multifaceted, and layered. Patients negotiate a self that is pinched between the institution of medicine and the abject body itself' (Waskul and van der Reit 2002: 491). While this is congruent with my own work with women who have had breast cancer,

I would assert that abjection continues beyond the completion of treatment and outside of the realm of medical care, while being inextricably connected to medical encounters. Further, while Waskul and van der Reit's (2002) conceptualizations of the diseased, grotesque and painful body may be located within my own interviews with women who have had breast cancer, my emphasis here is upon exploring the ways in which identity and self are continually experienced as abject, even after women have left the health care system. I have written about some of the nuances of the biomedical legacy (Thomas-MacLean 2004a) elsewhere, but this chapter represents a new interpretation of my data as approached from an understanding of abjection.

My reading of Kristeva shows that she writes about abjection in a very psychoanalytical way; for instance, she speaks of the separation from 'the Mother'. In this chapter, I work with a more sociological reading of her work and its subsequent explorations by others, with a focus on the applicability of the concept of abjection for understanding breast cancer experiences:

> Indeed, much of recent critical thought deploying the term *abjection* [emphasis hers] has gone straight for a theory of the political significance of abjection in order to figure out the deep forces of oppressive social and political relations (Butler 1993 is an obvious case in point). In these kinds of debate, abjection is a scarcely visible dynamic of aggressivity that is used to shore up identities that institute and maintain existing power relations (Beardsworth 2004: 80).

Further, drawing out more sociological aspects of Kristeva's work means that abjection may be thought of as 'the threat it poses to relations with others and the social bond' (Beardsworth 2004: 80). Kristeva herself writes of the abject as 'the place where meaning collapses' (Kristeva 1982: 2). Breast cancer may be considered an abject place or experience, as it reflects the politics of everyday life and represents a threat to relationships, as well as a complex positioning of self wherein meaning may be transformed.

Using an interpretive lens informed by the concept of abjection to examine interview transcripts from women with breast cancer led to the emergence of three interrelated themes which illuminate the idea of 'spoiled identity': looking and not looking, self and other, and that which is foreign. The first theme refers to women's experiences after surgery when they were both drawn to examining the site of their surgery but also repulsed by it. This is very much connected to new negotiations between the participants and others around embodiment – the second theme of this chapter. The third theme examines the idea of breast cancer and its associated treatments as foreign. I discuss each of these themes and the participants' experiences as they are connected to various understandings of abjection and spoiled identities. However, before turning to these themes, I outline the methodological approach utilized in my work.

Methods

My original approach has been outlined in detail elsewhere (Thomas-MacLean 2004a, 2004b, 2005). Very briefly, my approach to data gathering and interpretation built upon my interests in phenomenological and feminist research and was informed by critical perspectives in sociology. In terms of methods, I first facilitated one focus group discussion with five women, who had experienced breast cancer, in the province of New Brunswick, Canada. This discussion was followed by interviews with twelve breast cancer survivors throughout the province of New Brunswick. Each participant was interviewed twice and each individual interview lasted from one to two hours. Participants were selected using snowball and purposive sampling techniques.

Participants' ages ranged from 42 to 77. Only two of the participants were working outside of the home at the time of our interviews. The sample was ethnically homogenous and was therefore reflective of the nature of the New Brunswick population. Ten of the twelve women had children. Most were married; two were widowed. The number of years that had passed since their diagnoses ranged from one to 24. Breast cancer treatments included mastectomy, radiation and chemotherapy as well as combinations of these three modalities. All of the participants said that they had undergone a mastectomy. Seven women received adjuvant treatment (i.e., Tamoxifen).

Initial interviews built upon my understanding of narrative research and the importance of understanding the women's stories of breast cancer, beginning with diagnosis and moving toward the present. At the second interview, I reviewed key themes emerging from the initial interviews with each participant in order to establish some confirmation of my interpretations. This overview was followed by questions arising from the initial transcripts. These questions were specific to each participant. Next, I asked approximately 30 open-ended questions pertaining to sleep patterns, clothing, use of breast prostheses, and diet. At the end of each interview, participants were encouraged to clarify or enhance their discussion of any topic they wished. All of the participants were assigned pseudonyms and all interviews were audiotaped and transcribed verbatim.

As mentioned previously, earlier interpretations of this data have been published elsewhere. The interpretation which now follows concentrates on the concept of abjection and the idea of an identity which has been spoiled by illness. I must acknowledge, however, that any attempt to understand abjection is both 'hazardous' and an 'adventure' (Beardsworth 2004: 93). Nonetheless, attention to the idea of a 'spoiled identity' is missing from both the academic literature and from popular discourse, but is vital to further understanding of what it means to have breast cancer.

Looking and Not Looking

Women show it is not concern about the appearance of the breast (or maintaining a stereotypically feminine body type), but the possibility of repulsion that induces fear and anxiety. Kristeva notes that abjection involves 'repugnance' (1982: 2). Beth speaks of this repugnance when she talks about seeing her surgical scar for the first time: 'It was ugly. This big scar goes clear across my chest. I remember. I remember putting a nightgown on and looking three cornered…At first I thought it was gross.' Diane's discussion of her scar echoes that of Beth's, but Diane provides more detail:

> Seeing it [her chest] with the bandage off – there's a scar there and it looked awful, but other than that, I knew that there was going to be scars there and there wouldn't be a breast there anymore. I guess the extent of the scar and maybe the fact, I don't know what I was anticipating and what it was going to look like…but it didn't look like whatever I might have expected. It just, I don't know if whether I expected there might still be a little bit of a curve there or what. But the extent of the scar sort of from the breastbone through right under the arm was greater than I anticipated. I thought they could just do a little hole and take it all out. Because when I had the biopsy, the scar was just a small scar from the side and I guess I was thinking maybe something like that. It didn't particularly distress me. It's just different than I thought it would be. It's bigger, it's ugly, but it's there, you know. The scar itself is no big deal now, just there.

Diane's words imply that there is some element of temporality associated with abjection. She says that her scar 'looked awful' and that it was not what she anticipated. However, she continues and states that, even though 'it's ugly'; it is 'just there'. Diane describes abjection through words that carry negative connotations, but, in speaking of the present, she acknowledges that the scar is simply there. Marie speaks of her scar in a similar way:

> But mine is quite neat and the fact that I didn't have a big breast so there's not a whole lot of tissue there and I think they fold it underneath in case you want to have reconstructive surgery so there's not a whole lot of skin there, you can be a little neater. And it keeps getting better, at first it was raw looking but it gets better all the time.

One might interpret Diane and Marie's descriptions to mean that the passage of time can alleviate some of the experience of abjection. Healing may play a role in the diminishing of abjection, but it is also possible that the passage of time removes some feelings of repugnance.

It is also important to note that before providing the description above, Diane prefaced those remarks with a statement that indicated that she wondered whether or not she would be able to look at herself after surgery. Martha's experience differs slightly from Beth's, cited above, in that Martha said she avoided the viewing of her scar, but she does capture some of the uncertainty expressed by Diane. Rather than a direct experience of repugnance, Martha conveys the fear associated with abjection and the possibility of being repulsed by one's own body:

> The first three or four times I showered, I kept my eyes closed. I was afraid to look. And then gradually I would open my eyes and look down and ah…I thought it was going to look worse than it did. I guess I had envisioned something far worse, so it did not affect me that badly.

Martha's fear of repugnance is remembered as more challenging than actually viewing the site of her surgery. Thus, there are differing viewpoints about seeing and trying not to see, but the four women all shared some difficulties with this part of abject embodiment after surgery.

Simultaneously, the relationship between abjection and breast cancer surgery can be explored in other ways. Kristeva writes that 'the abject simultaneously beseeches and pulverises the subject' (1982: 5). Nowhere is this aspect of abjection – pulverisation – more clearly expressed than in Arlene's account of the time immediately following her breast cancer surgery, but Arlene also shares Martha's fear of repugnance initially:

> My mother was with me the night that they took the stitches out after the operation and it was a bloody looking mess. There's no way to describe it. I was black and blue, I was swollen but Mom stood there and held me and then I got up the nerve to look at it and they were taking stitches out and after that, it never bothered me. As a matter of fact, I watched them. They put staples in. I wanted to see what the staples looked like.

While the exact experiences of repugnance and pulverisation vary, Martha, Beth and Arlene share some notion of alterations to the body – anticipated or real – that are perceived as negative. These include bruising, scarring and sutures. These injuries represent a particularity or specificity about the abject body which is connected to repugnance, and these elements of experience are not present in breast cancer discourse. The concepts of abjection and spoiled identity provide a new way of discerning what some women found disturbing about the post-surgical period. Connected to these aspects of abjection and spoiled identity, is the desire to protect others from these experiences. In other words, self-repulsion and repugnance are linked to the possibility of others being repulsed.

Self and Other

The women I interviewed expressed some desire to protect other people from the abject body. Oliver notes: 'Kristeva brought the speaking body back into language by putting language into the body [and] she brings the subject into the place of the other by putting the other into the subject' (Oliver 1993: 13). Catherine expresses this aspect of abjection very poignantly when asked about viewing the site of her surgery for the first time:

> Uhm … hmm … [I looked at it] very reluctantly. I didn't want to look and I finally – I sort of didn't look and my neighbour came over and she's very open and she was doing a lot, helping me a lot and she said, "Do you mind if I see your incision?" And I said, "Well, okay". And she said, "You haven't looked at it have you?" And I said, "No". And she said "Well look at it. It's alright". So I did and it was okay.

Catherine's words relate back to the first theme in which the possibility of abjection was described, but this quotation also introduces a new element of abjection and that is the blurring of boundaries between self-other. In writing of Kristeva's 'demassification of the problematic of *difference*', Oliver (1993) asserts that '[t]he subject can understand the other, sympathize with the other, and moreover, take the place of the other, because the subject is other … the subject can relate to an other as other because she is an other to herself' (13). A connection between self-other developed between Catherine and her neighbour because the latter was able to sense Catherine's discomfort with self. The neighbour transgressed the boundary of self-other by positioning her self in Catherine's place and working toward a new, unbounded position of empathy.

Catherine continues:

> My husband – I wasn't even aware of it – but one night he said, "Why do you turn away from me when you're getting dressed?" And I said, "Oh. Am I?" And he said, "Yes, let me see you." And I really didn't want him to but he seemed to be okay with it, he didn't – he said, "It's fine." So it's traumatic, you know. You've lost a piece of yourself and you don't look the same.

Catherine's words show how the boundaries between herself and her partner were blurred through her resistance to allowing him to see her scar. It is interesting to note that Catherine's husband wanted to see her, but that she felt she had to protect him from abjection. Arlene's feelings about this situation are similar to Catherine's and the reaction of Arlene's partner was similar to Catherine's as well:

> He never once looked at it with disgust, but it took me a long time to let him look. It took a long time for me to get undressed and dressed in front of him but there's none of that now. It was me more than him. I didn't want him to see me that way.

Lynn was also surprised by her husband's positive response and stated that she 'really appreciated' his willingness to look at her scar, even while she was still in the hospital.

Another participant, Beth, also said that it took months before she would let her husband see her naked, but that he did not show any sign of being repulsed by her scar. These experiences contrast with Susan's discussion about her husband's reaction:

> He never looked at it for a long time and he still won't actually look at it you know [four years later]. He does kind of, but he doesn't, like he'd rather not because it just kind of freaks him out…he thinks a lot of the cancer coming back.

Beardsworth (2004) writes that '[a]t the psychoanalytic level of Kristeva's thinking, abjection is the most unstable moment in the maturation of the subject because it is a struggle with the instability of the inside/outside border' (81). The instability of the border between self-other is revealed through participants' accounts. As England writes, 'human bodies…are abject in that they are not bounded entities' (2006: 356), despite how the dominant discourses of western philosophy would contend. Women feared a negative response from their partners and, in Susan's case, it appears that her fear was justified. However, for Catherine, Beth and Arlene, the reluctance to allow their partners to see them appears to be linked to the idea of repugnance or repulsion. Their words seem to indicate that they are afraid of seeing that type of rejection, and that they did perceive their identities as women to be spoiled in some significant way.

Susan's partner was reluctant to look, but not out of any sense of repulsion. His unwillingness to see her scar is linked to his fear of recurrence and fits with Beardsworth's (2004) thoughts on abjection: '[It] captures a condition of the subject that is sent to its boundaries, where there is, as such, neither subject nor object, only the abject' (83). The scar poses as a reminder of the difficulties associated with illness, but also points to a blurring of boundaries between the familiar and the foreign, another aspect of an identity spoiled by illness.

That Which is Foreign?

Breast cancer can involve many foreign elements, including the perceived invasion of disease, hospitalisation and being in unfamiliar territory, and the insertion of ports for the administration of chemotherapy. The origins of the word foreign illustrate the connections between this aspect of abjection and ideas related to looking/not and self-other. Foreign derives from various words associated with 'out of doors' (ferren), 'on the outside' (foranus) and simply 'outside' (foris) (Harper 2001). Abjection contains these conceptualisations of the foreign, as England (2006: 354) notes: 'Horror occurs when boundaries are transgressed, when what is seen as normal suddenly becomes inverted – when bodies just will not die, when monsters appear, when there is no sanctuary and nothing is familiar'. As stated previously, England (2006) is writing of horror films, but there is much about breast cancer that could be considered horrific, as Janice shows when she speaks of a port-a-cath and the pain associated with it:

> But the nurse came in and explained. There's a foreign substance in there, so like it wasn't just the incision I was feeling, it was the foreign substance in there rubbing on everything on the inside. Like the inside was raw where they had like put it in there and any time you moved or anything, until that got situated, it was just like something rubbing on an open sore ... When I woke up, I tried to turn over. It was just like this foreign substance in my chest, so it just seemed like it ripped ... I thought, "This is worse than the mastectomy."

Janice's pain and her frequent use of the word 'foreign' indicate that this aspect of abjection resonates with some experiences of breast cancer. She shows how '[a]bject bodies elide boundaries and disturb categories. When these bodies breach the boundaries between good/evil; interior/exterior; self/Other, they show the vulnerability of these socially constructed dualisms' (England 2006: 358). This breaching of boundaries constitutes part of the spoiled identity.

Other participants also showed that breast cancer is considered foreign and comprises a breaching of boundaries as they use particular words and phrases to refer to the illness. Susan repeatedly uses the word 'it' to describe her tumour: 'Once I knew it was there, it was quite a size [two inches in diameter]...but it just really puzzles me that I didn't notice it'. Marie uses the word 'suspicious' to describe the process of diagnosis:

> Well it was that first mammogram that revealed there was a suspicious mass and so I got called for a recall ... So [the doctor recommended a] partial mastectomy, just to remove the suspicious tissue. It wasn't very long after that, probably the next week that I had a quadrant, the upper left quadrant of my left breast removed.

Judith describes the possibility of reconstructive surgery in a way that invokes foreign aspects of abjection: 'A friend had implants put in and I would never have that because that to me is something foreign in your body'. It is Arlene's words, however, that provide illustrations of the most dramatic connections between abjection and the foreign:

> And both my husband and I told the surgeon that we didn't want a biopsy. We wanted the whole breast to go. My biopsy came back cancerous so we made the appointment for the second surgery and, again, we told them we wanted everything gone ...All I wanted was for it to be gone ... I was supposed to go the next day for my sixth chemotherapy treatment and I asked the doctor what

he felt about it and he reassured me that the five treatments would have killed
everything for me to have got down so low.

Arlene says she wanted 'everything gone' and uses 'go, gone' repeatedly, implying
that there is movement associated with the foreign, that her desire was to make the
illness leave. She then violently describes chemotherapy as 'killing everything'.
The use of the word 'everything' suggests that she experienced breast cancer as a
foreign invasion that was all encompassing, even though she had no metastasis.
This might be considered illustrative of the spoiled self in that the body or a certain
part of the body was not abjectified, but her self in its entirety. This engulfment
may be congruent with Beth's reflections on the possibility of a recurrence: 'If
there's an unusual pain or something within my own body, then I wonder, until I
find out what it is'. Beth's words are congruent with Kristeva's thoughts in this
respect: 'In the symptom, the abject permeates me, I become abject' (Kristeva
1982: 11) and show the links between pain, recurrence, abjection and the self.

Phyllis carries the foreign aspect of abjection further when she talks about
potential environmental causes of breast cancer and wonders whether or not
stress played a part: 'I think that's half of what triggered me, when my husband
died'. Participants' words clearly convey various aspects of abjection, including
the blurring of boundaries between that which is foreign and the self, between
self-other, as well as the associated act of viewing one's body after breast cancer
surgery and anticipating the reactions of others. Reading their words within
the context of an understanding of abjection suggests there is room for further
study and innovations in health care for women with breast cancer, particularly if
attention is paid to the idea of a spoiled identity.

Implications for What Counts as an Episode of Care

Despite the lack of discussion about abjection in breast cancer discourse, women
in this study still anticipated the experience of an abject body, and the related
spoiling of self. Women were afraid to look at their surgical sites or thought that
scars would look differently than they did. This suggests an opening for health
care professionals. What might be the benefits of seeing images of breast cancer
surgical scars in advance? Would this demystify the process? Or, is it possible
that, presented with such images, women might become more fearful of the
abject? While the women's accounts of abject bodies suggest this is an area to be
addressed, it is not clear what the best approach might be, or if there could indeed
be a common approach to preparing women for the experience of abjection.
Introducing this concept into breast cancer discourse, however, might be a first
step toward innovations in supportive care.

Also invisible in dominant breast cancer discourse is the context of abjection.
Although England (2006) is writing of horror films when she describes abject
spaces, her description might also apply to hospitals, or even the shower – a

place that is reminiscent of horror movies, but that was also a site of discomfort associated with the spoiled identity of one participant. England (2006) states: 'Abject spaces are considered dangerous and frightening because they are places of uncertainty' (355). Hospitals are the site of potential experiences of uncertainty for those with breast cancer and hospitalisation may involve abject bodily expressions, such as leaking fluids, infection and scarring as participants show. Yet, participants may also encounter the abject in more personal settings, such as the shower. The implications of abjection and place are not explored in the literature surrounding breast cancer and suggest possible sites for enhancing supportive health care.

Abjection may also be linked to anxiety and fears associated with recurrence are not adequately addressed within the current confines of the health care system. Moreover, one of the participants, Susan, shows fear of recurrence is not experienced only by 'the patient', but by family members as well. Anxieties about recurrence can be triggered almost every day by the viewing of the breast cancer surgical scar. How well are patients' families informed about life after breast cancer and the possibilities of recurrence? The fact that viewing the abject body might induce anxiety also suggests a possible site for intervention or supportive care, for as Kristeva notes, the abject exists outside the 'rules of the game' but 'does not cease challenging its master' (Kristeva 1982: 2). As I noted in earlier work (Thomas-MacLean 2004b), the experience of breast cancer, and now by extension, a spoiled identity, does not end with the conclusion of acute care – a point missed by health workers in many areas whose view steadfastly remains 'fixed' and limited to an episode of care. Such containment signals the failure of treatments to take account of the long term effects of treatment – they are extra mural, figured as outside of the tight controls of the event. But as we know, the abject awaits.

Conclusion

The women's accounts of breast cancer show that abjection and a spoiled identity may last well beyond treatment. Their experiences of an identity spoiled by illness shows that many of the boundaries that are taken for granted (self/other; familiar/foreign; inside/outside) are rather fragile. Despite the impact of a spoiled identity on a woman's everyday life, abjection has received little attention in popular discourse which tends to emphasize positive and heroic narratives of survivorship. Reading the study participants' words through the lens of abjection suggests the gaps in the literature are indeed vast and that changes to supportive care are warranted. Epistemologically, the tensions between dominant breast cancer discourse and the conceptualisation of spoiled identity indicate that this area of dissonance may also be worthy of additional attention from those engaged in qualitative health research.

References

Barral, M.R. 1969. Merleau-Ponty on the body. *Southern Journal of Philosophy*, 7 (Summer), 171–179.

Beardsworth, S. 2004. *Julia Kristeva: Psychoanalysis and Modernity*. Albany: State University of New York Press.

Bentz, V.M. and Shapiro, J.J. 1998. *Mindful Inquiry in Social Research*. Thousand Oaks: Sage.

Birke, L. 1998. Biological sciences, in *A Companion to Feminist Philosophy*, edited by A.M. Jaggar and I.M. Young. Malden: Blackwell Publishers Inc., 194–203.

Bordo, S. 1987. *The Flight to Objectivity: Essays on Cartesianism and Culture*. Albany: State University of New York Press.

Bungay, V. and Keddy, B.C. 1996. Experiential analysis as a feminist methodology for health professionals. *Qualitative Health Research*, 6(3), 442–452.

Butler, J. 1988. Performative acts and gender constitution: an essay in phenomenology and feminism. *Theatre Journal*, 40, 519–531.

Butler, J. 1993. *Bodies that Matter: On the Discursive Limits of Sex*. New York: Routledge.

Carter, B.J. 1993. Long-term survivors of breast cancer: a qualitative descriptive study. *Cancer Nursing*, 16, 354–361.

Crossley, N. 1994. *The Politics of Subjectivity: Between Foucault and Merleau-Ponty*. Brookfield: Ashgate.

Darling-Wolf, F. 2000. From airbrushing to liposuction: the technological reconstruction of the female body, in *Women's Bodies/Women's Lives: Health, Well-Being and Body Image*, edited by B. Miedema, V. Anderson and J.M. Stoppard. Toronto: Sumach Press, 277–293.

Ellis, C. 1998. 'I hate my voice': coming to terms with minor bodily stigmas. *Sociological Quarterly*, 39(4), 517–537.

England, M. 2006. Breached bodies and home invasions: horrific representations of the feminized body and home. *Gender, Place and Culture*, 13(4), 353–363.

Ferrans, C.E. 1994. Quality of life through the eyes of survivors of breast cancer. *Oncology Nursing Forum*, 21(10), 1645–1651.

Harper, D. 2001. Online Etymology Dictionary. Available at: http://www.etymonline.com [accessed: 5 September 2007].

Holmes, H.B. 1989. A call to heal medicine. *Hypatia*, 4(2), 1–8.

Kasper, A.S. 1995. The social construction of breast loss and reconstruction. *Women's Health: Research on Gender, Behavior, and Policy*, 1(3), 197–219.

Kristeva, J. 1982. *Powers of Horror: An Essay on Abjection*. New York: Columbia University Press.

Lantz, P.M. and Booth, K.M. 1998. The social construction of the breast cancer epidemic. *Social Science and Medicine*, 46(7), 907–918.

Ledermann, E.K. 1982. Conscience and bodily awareness: disagreements with Merleau-Ponty. *Journal of the British Society for Phenomenology*, 13, 286–295.

Lennon, K. 1998. Natural sciences, in *A Companion to Feminist Philosophy*, edited by A.M. Jaggar and I.M. Young. Malden: Blackwell Publishers, 185–193.

Loveys, B.J., and Klaich, K. 1991. Breast cancer: Demands of illness. *Oncology Nursing Forum*, 18(1), 75–80.

Lugton, J. 1997. The nature of social support as experienced by women treated for breast cancer. *Journal of Advanced Nursing*, 25(6), 1184–1191.

Martin, E. 1990. Science and women's bodies: forms of anthropological knowledge, in *Body Politics: Women, Literature, and the Discourse of Science*, edited by M. Jacobus, E.F. Keller and S. Shuttleworth. New York: Routledge, 47–68.

Maticka-Tyndale, E., and Bicher, M. 1996. The impact of medicalization on women, in *Social Control in Canada*, edited by B. Schissel and L. Mahood. Toronto: Oxford University Press, 149–173.

Merleau-Ponty, M. 1974. *Phenomenology, Language and Sociology: Selected Essays of Maurice Merleau-Ponty.* London: Heinemann Educational Books.

O'Loughlin, M. 1998. Overcoming the problems of 'difference' in education: empathy as 'intercorporeality'. *Studies in Philosophy and Education*, 17(4), 283–293.

Oliver, K. (ed.) 1993. *Ethics, Politics, and Difference in Julia Kristeva's Writing* (1st ed.). New York: Routledge.

Pelusi, J. 1997. The lived experience of surviving breast cancer. *Oncology Nursing Forum*, 24(8), 1343–1353.

Rehorick, D.A. 1986. Shaking the foundations of lifeworld: a phenomenological account of an earthquake experience. *Human Studies*, 9, 379–391.

Thomas-MacLean, R.L. 2004a. Memories of treatment: The immediacy of breast cancer. *Qualitative Health Research*, 14(5), 628–643.

Thomas-MacLean, R.L. 2004b. Understanding breast cancer stories via Frank's narrative types. *Social Science & Medicine*, 58, 1647–1657.

Thomas-MacLean, R.L. 2005. Beyond dichotomies of health and illness: life after breast cancer. *Nursing Inquiry*, 12(3), 200–209.

Timpson, J.R. 1999. Disability and impairment in breast cancer: towards an understanding of altered body functioning and a standard of care for nursing practice. *European Journal of Oncology Nursing*, 3(1), 14–24.

Toombs, S.K. 1992. *The Meaning of Illness: A Phenomenological Account of the Different Perspectives of Physician and Patient.* Dordrecht: Kluwer.

Turner, B.S. 1995. *Medical Power and Social Knowledge.* London: Sage Publications.

Utley, R. 1999. The evolving meaning of cancer for long-term survivors of breast cancer. *Oncology Nursing Forum*, 26(9), 1519–1523.

van Manen, M. 1997. From meaning to method. *Qualitative Health Research*, 7(3), 345–369.

van Manen, M. 1998. Modalities of body experience in illness and health. *Qualitative Health Research*, 8(1), 7–24.

Waskul, D.D. and van der Riet, P. 2002. The abject embodiment of cancer patients: dignity, selfhood, and the grotesque body. *Symbolic Interaction*, 25(4), 487–513.

Wyatt, G., Kurtz, M.E. and Liken, M. 1993. Breast cancer survivors: an exploration of quality of life issues. *Cancer Nursing*, 16, 440–448.

Chapter 7

'Betwixt and Between Nothingness': Abjection and Blood Stem Cell Transplantation

Beverleigh Quested

Introduction

Blood Stem Cell Transplantation (BSCT) is a miracle of modernist science allowing people with leukaemia to be rescued from their imminent death. Cutting edge science, technology, medical science and blood discourses intersect in BSCT. The evolution of BSCT from nuclear weapon research and development further imbues BSCT with an aura of complexity, technology and of man conquering nature. The medical term for this process is Haemopoietic Stem Cell Transplantation but such a term subjugates the social and cultural understandings surrounding blood. Blood Stem Cell Transplantation is deliberately used in this work to include wider understandings of blood stem cell transplantation.

A critical ethnography exploring the multiplicities of BSCT in a BSCT unit along with nine allogeneic recipients'[1] experiences of the complex technical environment of BSCT is the basis of this work. This ethnography followed the transitions as individuals became patients, patients became BSCT recipients and then to survivors (or not[2]). BSCT is a life saving technology that takes recipients to the edges of survival. The transplantation of (an)other's blood stem cells adds to this process, challenging the borders of I/other, flesh and blood, and inside/outside. This work shows how BSCT reduces an individual to an abject state of *empty* and then with the transplantation blood of an 'other' to a recipient. This works describes how incorporating (an)other's blood system in BSCT unravels identity and necessitates a rewriting of flesh and blood. The transplanting of blood stem

---

1   Allogeneic refers to a Blood Stem Cells Transplant where the blood stem cells come from another person either a relative or a Matched Unrelated Donor where blood stem cells are donated by a stranger with similar genetic typing located through a transplant registry. The nine people undergoing BSCT were interviewed during their transplant and for 12–18 months afterwards or their deaths. They were given pseudonyms Adam, Bernard, Charles, David, Emily, Francis, Gary, Harry and Ian.

2   During this research Bernard, Charles, David and Ian died as a result of their disease or complications associated with BSCT.

cells involves more than the mechanistic replacement of aberrant body parts and is mediated through medical science and through blood.

The Social Realms of Blood

Blood possesses multiple cultural meanings, and Table 7.1 lists some of the terms and discourses related to blood.

Physiologically blood's functions include oxygen transporter, clotting and coagulant, and bearer of immunity and identity. For millennia blood has inextricably signified death as the red fluid flowed from mortal wounds. The horror felt as a blood clot congeals and transforms into other, the self unbounded. Menstrual blood signals the onset of fertility and represents a world of primordial viscerality out of which a child is conceived and grows, a world that pre-empts 'I' and starts with (an)other's flesh and blood.

Before genetics blood was the mechanism that linked individuals to families through history with bloodlines providing powerful declarations of belonging. The persistence of bloodlines is crucial to for family continuity. Becoming blood brothers creates a permanent link of kinship that is beyond friendship. Blood is thicker than water physically and metaphorically. Blood as a signifier of kindred also denotes class, country and character. Royal blood is described as blue, denoting stratification of society on not only class lines but on innate 'biological superiority'.

> The aristocracy had affirmed the specificity of their bodies; nobility is first a vital, corporeal characteristic... where sovereignty was transmitted through bloodlines; where the orders of society are hereditary castes (Lingis 1999: 299).

A 'red blooded Aussie' epitomizes a certain character, strength and vigour. Racial purity is defined in terms of full blood, half blood. In World War Two non-Aryans were excluded from donating blood for transfusion in Germany and the United States of America segregated blood transfusion supplies on racial lines (Starr 1999: xii), thereby, reflecting beliefs that blood carried more than the replacement blood cells and plasma needed, blood carried race and religion. Blood could pass on hereditary traits and character.

In Ancient Greece and modern day Japan blood is linked with personality type. Anger can make your blood boil and a stubborn individual is bloody minded. Tempestuous and volatile individuals are called hot blooded. Cold blooded individuals are reserved and calculating, the viscera disappearing as reason and consciousness dominate. Bad blood signifies bitterness and acrimony. Bad bloodlines can pass on hereditary diseases such as Haemophilia[3] or Huntington's

---

3   Haemophilia is an inherited clotting disorder.

Table 7.1   Blood terms and discourses – social cultural and scientific

Blood brothers	Blood lines	Blood ties	Blood oath
Bloodstock	Mixed Blood	Half blood	Full blood
Red blooded	Blue blood	Blood money	Your flesh and blood
Blood cells	Blood test	Blood Stem Cell	Blood Counts
Blood group	Blood donor	Blood transfusion	Bone Marrow
Blood letting	Blood bank	Plasma	Tainted Blood
Hot blooded	Cold blooded	Blood clot	Bloodless
Bad Blood	Blood Curdling	Flesh and Blood	Bloody minded
Red Blood cells	White blood Cells	Blasts	Platelets
Bloodshed	Life blood	Blood thirsty	Diseased Blood
Blood Rules	Blood sport	Blood bath	Blood, sweat and tears
Blood Cancer	Blood sucker	Blood on your hands	To the marrow of one's bones
My blood ran cold	Make your blood boil	Runs in the blood	More than flesh and blood can stand
The scent of blood	Contaminated Blood	Red blooded Aussie	Give one's blood for one's country
French Blood	Haemopoiesis	Anaemia	Blood donation -the gift of life
Jewish Blood	Leukeamia	Haematology	Blood is thicker than water

chorea[4]. Tainted blood can carry HIV[5]. Blood can be infiltrated with leukaemia, cancerous white blood cells that leave the body unable to adequately defend against infection.

Blood transfusion epitomizes the medical model of replacing parts of the machine. Blood is fluid human tissue transplanted into another, pre-empting transplantation of solid organs such as heart, lungs, kidneys, skin or cornea. Separating blood into components such as red cells, platelets and plasma[6] provides further evidence of the replacement of lacking or malfunctioning body parts. Haematology is the medical specialisation related to blood with a scientific structural framework for the growth and development of blood cells referred to as haemopoiesis. Blood cells are produced and mature in the bone marrow to then flow through the body's blood vessels. The phrase 'to the marrow of one's bones' disclosing a deep interiority of the body and a central core of self.

Flesh and blood are inextricably intertwined as Shylock in the Merchant of Venice (IV, 1: 321–29) discovers when he is thwarted in obtaining his pound of flesh as he was not entitled to the blood. Flesh is conceptually recognized as embodiment, surface and perception whereas blood is the interior, invisible and unperceived organs (Leder 1990, Merleau Ponty 1968). The 'and' is unexpungeable simultaneously linking embodied perception and 'other', the unseen silent interiority of viscera. The relations between self and other, body and the world, visible and invisible, visceral and corporeal are mediated through flesh and blood. 'I know the entirety of my perceptual world rests upon the unperceived coursing of my blood, if it were to cease, all else would cease as well' (Leder 1999: 207). Such disappearance is never complete; when flesh is ruptured blood becomes visible, as it clots becoming a solidified 'other'. As the boundaries between self and 'other' are threatened feelings of abjection arise (Kristeva 1982). Furthermore, when blood becomes visible the 'and' is expunged, flesh and blood disconnect as does the construction of embodied self and other. The visibility of blood ruptures the constructions of self and other.

Transplantation is accepted as a routine aspect of medical care premised on a mechanistic understanding of the body in which parts can be interchanged and are therapeutic tools (Barnard and Sandelowski 2001). However the inclusion of (an)other's body within your own is not found solely within the realms of medicine's mechanistic body. In the act of Holy Communion one metaphorically eats the body and blood of Christ which was shed for you, this ingestion a sacred act contributing to sublime transcendence. For vampires receiving of (an)other's

---

4 Huntington's Chorea is a hereditary disease of the brain that progresses to a total incapacitation and death.

5 HIV– Human Immunodeficiency Virus also known as AIDS – a virus transmitted by blood that can be fatal.

6 Component therapy involves transfusing only the specific component of blood that an individual lacks such as red cells to carry oxygen or platelets to help form a clot or plasma that contains clotting factors.

blood is a depraved act driven by a monstrous desire. Social taboos prevent the ingestion of human body parts with cannibalism seen as aberrant and deviant. However, to receive a blood transfusion for a physiological need is to 'receive one of life's best gifts' (Australian Red Cross Blood Service: www.transfusion.com. au) as the result of donor's altruistic act. Yet both the transfusion recipient and the vampire end up with (an)other's blood within their bodies. The divide between the sublime and the monstrous enacted through blood for transfusion and vampires. Medicine constructs their replacement and inclusion of body parts within a plane of sacred space, where science replicates the work of nature or god.

Identity comes from a sense of sameness, of continuity over time that can reply to 'who am I?' (Ricoeur 1992: 116). The replacement of blood effects change, an 'other' settles in. How much can a body be changed when (an)other's blood is in your veins and marrow in your bones? How much can be replaced before you stop being you, before you become something else? How do you respond to a body that now has to include two distinct genetic identities and a medically created chimera? How do you respond to being flesh, blood and other's blood? The following discussion shows how BSCT changes the understandings of flesh and blood to become *blood and flesh.* Where blood becomes visible while flesh as embodiment and self is hidden. It also shows the how identity is challenged.

Blood Stem Cell Transplantation

Blood Stem Cell Transplantation processes involve locating a donor, harvesting blood stem cells, eradicating bone marrow by chemotherapy and/or radiotherapy, transplanting blood stem cells via an IV infusion into the patient's vein where they establish in the bone marrow and eventually the blood stem cells engraft[7]. It takes around five to seven days to eradicate the bone marrow and then 14–21 days for the cells to engraft. BSCT is a highly specialized and technological process requiring numerous events to be undertaken in a specific sequence. But, the basic premise is simple, mimicking as it does agrarian practices to control nature by tilling the soil, planting seed and waiting for the crop to grow. For some patients, BSCT offers the only option of cure for a life threatening disease. It is not offered lightly as patients can and do die during the BSCT process (Hoffbrand et al. 2001: 98). BSCT treatment takes patients to extreme limits of biological life; lethal doses of chemotherapy and or radiation are knowingly administered as part of the treatment plan. Once the chemotherapy/ radiotherapy has begun there is no turning back, with a destroyed bone marrow the individual would die within a short time.

The chemotherapy/radiotherapy destroys aberrant cells and creates a 'space' in which the infused stem cells will be able to grow (Santos 1983: 617). The chemotherapy drugs have numerous side effects that can be quite severe initially

---

7   Engraftment refers to the transplant 'taking', settling into the bone marrow and new blood cells growing.

and persist for months. Infusing blood stem cells into the recipient's body is a technically simple but crucial step and is called Day Zero[8]. Days in BSCT are counted in a minus and plus fashion around the infusion of stem cells, such as Day –1 or Day +3. Infusing blood stem cells changes the patient to a recipient.

While the stem cells engraft to produce new blood and immune system the recipient is unable to fight infections. To minimize infections they are cared for in an isolated room, eats a low bacteria diet[9], and close physical contact with family is discouraged. Nursing and medical staff closely observe to detect signs of infections, bleeding or other problems. Supportive measures such as nutritional supplementation and analgesia for ulcerated mouth pain are introduced to ameliorate side effects from the chemotherapy. Engraftment is indicated by rising white blood cell and platelet counts.

Every aspect of the person undergoing BSCT life is affected. Loach (1997) used the term catastrophic to describe her experience of BSCT. The experience of BSCT is acknowledged as traumatic and daunting (Haberman 1988, Steeves 1992, Shuster et al. 1996, Thain and Gibbon 1996, McQuellon et al. 1998, Jones 2000, Saleh and Brockopp 2001). Such a process is not the linear trajectory or smooth transition for recipients alluded to within nursing and medical scientific literature.

Creating the Chimera: The In-Between

The presence of 'foreign' cells in recipient's blood is referred to as chimerism and was first used in animal experiments that preceded transplantation in humans (Santos 1983: 611). Chimerism comes from the term chimera, the monstrous three-headed beast in Ancient Greek mythology with a lion's, serpent's and a goat's head. The recipient is chimerical in that they have original self, donor and the hybrid mix of both. The newly implanted blood stem cells will produce blood of the donor's type while the recipient's other body cells such as skin will continue to be the recipient, DNA testing will show two different DNA types (the donor and recipient) until the transplanted graft fails or death. The recipient's body has two genetic identities permanently intertwined with the resulting hybrid creating an ill-defined monster; the monstrous co-opted by the medical world.

---

8   Counting time in this manner reflects influences from atomic research in BSCT, in a nuclear blast ground zero is the point from which all effects were measured.

9   To reduce exposure to bacteria and acquiring certain infections, certain foods have to be avoided and food has to be prepared and cooked in certain ways; this is referred to as a Low Bacteria Diet.

Becoming a BSCT Recipient: Reconfiguring Bodies and Identity

A person diagnosed with leukaemia becomes a patient. The borders that defined and ordered the person are dissolved and are redrawn as patient and then recipient. Flesh and blood is reordered to be *blood and flesh* and self and other becomes *self, other and both*. The ensuing discussion shows how such a transition occurs for the people undergoing BSCT.

Becoming Unwell: The Appearance of the Invisible

Blood is normally silent and invisible, but such silence can have fatal consequences. Blood diseases are menacingly quiet; anaemia eventually shows in tiredness, extremely high white cell counts make bone aches and bruising may occur only when platelet levels are life threateningly low. A salient feature of the BSCT patients' diagnosis stories was a precipitous pathway into serious illness. When Francis was first diagnosed he felt only slightly unwell but was dangerously ill. Francis expected that his body would tell him if he was seriously ill, but it had remained silent. When he was recovering he felt extremely tired and unwell, yet medically was progressing well. The lived body and the sense of feeling well (or not) could not be relied upon. How could Francis or the other recipients know if they were sick or well? They could not trust their bodies to tell them.

In medicine the physiological body with organs is placed in the foreground, and makes the hidden visible with concrete measures such as blood counts. The lived body cannot be trusted but the blood counts[10] provide evidence. As such the recipients came not to trust how they felt but what their counts were telling them.

> I've got a whiteboard on the front here, so they give you the counts, the blood count, your haemoglobin, platelets, and white cells and neutrophils and that's the real excitement of the day 'cos you can see …what's happening you know? Otherwise you sit here, you really don't know if what they're giving you is working. Or not (Francis Day – 1).

Adam was asked how he was going, he nodded to toward the white board with his counts written on it and said getting there (Adam Day +14)

The blood counts told the recipients objectively what they could not trust their bodies to do; it showed how they were going for better or worse. The medically objectified body on the white boards took precedence over the perceptions of the lived body, providing a tangible reassurance to the ambiguity of perception. The 'and' had been disrupted as blood came to be visible and perception subjugated. The subject had become the object, the relationship altering flesh and blood

---

10   Blood Counts refer to the level of haemoglobin, platelets, and white cells that were watched as markers of treatment effect and bone marrow recovery.

(self and other) to become blood. In such a change the subject (self) disappears from the plane of abjection in which subject is declared (Kristeva 1982).

Choosing to Undergo BSCT

A diagnosis enables medical science to forecast the patient's anticipated lifetime with and without treatment. The nature of the recipients' disease predicted a sooner than intended death, and without medical treatment they would not survive very long. BSCT is not without risk, dying in the process a possibility. BSCT it is not undertaken lightly by the transplant unit in offering treatment or the recipients in choosing to undergo it in the hope they will be cured. The recipients described their choice, 'I haven't got any choice' (Bernard), Adam saw 'only one way to go' and it would give Charles 'a chance in life'. Transplant gave the recipients a choice of a possible cure, the alternative was living with the uncertainty of how many more months of life their disease would allow them.

They are key steps in BSCT that have to be completed in the correct order, failing to undertake a step can be fatal. Recipients had to comply totally with treatment demands and did so willingly in order to survive. In the resulting political landscape recipients subjugated their autonomy and power to the dictates of the transplant unit, justifying their subjugation for the possibility of living longer. The recipients handed over their autonomy and possible future as they entered the transplant program, in doing so relinquishing control and power.

Becoming a Patient

Admission to hospital involves becoming a patient, and is accomplished by a number of steps. New forms of identity are added when you are admitted to hospital in the form of a hospital identification number[11] and a wristband with your name and identification number. The identification number ensures two people with the same name aren't mixed. A wristband is added because at times the patient may not be able to confirm their own identity. The wristband signify's the person as a patient who may be incapable and the identification number simultaneously indicates uniqueness with the number but sameness as other have the same name.

On admission a patients is assigned to bed in the medical specialty's ward. The assignment of particular beds in hospital wards has a long tradition in nursing, from the Nightingale (1969) era when the sickest patients were placed closest to the nursing office to the isolation of the infectious patients. In BSCT, recipients are admitted to a room on their own that physically separates them from the outside world which is seen as a threat to their survival as it contains infectious risks to their very fragile immune systems. Protectively the world is shrunk to create a clean and contagion free area. Furthermore in this space the hospital now controls

---

11   These numbers are also known as Unit record numbers, Medical record numbers, or Patient identity numbers.

when and if visitors were allowed. However, nursing and medical staff could enter the room anytime and the private domains of an individual's life became public. Segregation from the outside world had begun, the recipient's world had shrunk, and space they occupied was regulated and always public.

Patients are assigned to a medical specialty who oversees care. The person becomes named and objectified as a medical 'case', reduced to a collection of body systems, dissected into objects, diagnosis of a particular aberrant cell type (Latimer 2000: 20). A clinical bio-medical gaze (re)presents through x-ray or pathology slides the patient's corporeal body that can be read and interpreted in absentia (Atkinson 1995: 62). The person recedes as objectification proceeds to a body, to a disease, to aberrant cells and genetic code. Blood is already a hidden fluid and the bio-medical gaze further distances the person and their body. David complained that doctors 'still act like I'm not here' when they discussed him at the end of his bed but did not include him in the discussions. This reflected his awareness of decisions made when he was not actually present, as well as not being acknowledged. In this instance the actual person in the bed was invisible; David was visible as a case but had been reduced by medical science to a non entity.

Patients are complicit in this process acquiescing to become a patient (Sakalys 2000). Furthermore,

> When patients enter the hospital or clinic, they enter the medical world, in which they must conform to a set of rigid rules and routines with which they are unfamiliar. The hospital is almost a total institution like a prison, in which patients have little or no control at all over when they eat or sleep, the clothes they wear, the level of noise or light to which they are exposed, and the manner in which they defecate or urinate (Lupton 1994: 94).

Patients are complicit in their subjugation so they can obtain the care and treatment they require. As the recipients stated 'they had no choice'. As part of the sick role the social self is subordinated as they relinquish their social roles and power (Frank 1995: 172). All of the participants gave up aspects of their social role and identity, stopping being partners, wage earners and put their lives on hold. BSCT recipients sold their business (Adam), reluctantly handed over control (Charles), were not being a husband or a wife (Adam and Emily) or left their country home to move to the transplant centre (Francis and Gary), and described putting their lives on hold (Francis). Bernard obtained a new uniform, buying a number of pairs of identical pyjamas to the replace the suit and tie he wore as businessman referring to them as 'same PJ's again, the uniform'. The edges of how a person would define himself or herself had started to unravel – they were no longer defined by their work, and no longer could control the subsistence of their lives. The release from normal social obligations transformed them culturally into a patient. In the status change from person to patient part of their identity had been stripped away.

Learning a New Language

Common meanings for such technical or haematological terms do not exist there are no synonyms for leukaemia. Patients can only enter into discussions about their disease by learning and using the haematological discourse. The recipients learnt the foreign language of haematology and transplant care. 'Haematologist took a bone marrow biopsy, showed up that I was 36 per cent blast cells' (Francis Day – 1). Ian referred to his sisters' tissue typing and their blood groups 'they were good matches, Mary's O-positive, and Helen and I are A-positive and I had Helen's'. David knew a previous heart problem 'perio-car'[12] was important information to pass on to the doctors and the investigations he would require. He had learnt medical language, investigation and decision making practices. He had learnt some of the language and culture of medicine. David did not have exactly the right term; he had learnt some of the language but was unable to fully engage with all the medical discourse.

Recipients learnt to understand the transplant schedule[13] that individually listed the sequence of events for their transplant, to count time around day zero, the names of drugs they were receiving and the side effects. None of the participants came from a medical background and this was language not used in their daily lives. Furthermore, using the medical terms meant adopting the medical objectification of their bodies. Francis refers to himself as '*I* was 36% blast cells', objectifying his own body and using the concreteness of numbers and medical categorisation to define himself. Constructing themselves as object to deal with the unseen interiority of their bodies, making the invisible visible to themselves.

Enculturation into BSCT

Routines of the wards and the transplant process were learnt by recipients; when the mealtimes were, when nurses would check their temperature or administer medications, when the doctors visited on rounds all impacted on their day to day activities. The recipients learnt the rules as a means to have some control over their lives to avoid 'surprises' (Charles) and to 'plan their day' (Bernard).

The treatment regimen, low bacteria diet and numerous intravenous medications meant recipients were able to exert little control over a number of aspects of their daily life such as what they could do, when they could do it and where they could go or even what they could eat. Usually, we protect access to our bodies, determine

---

12   David had Pericarditis, irritation of the membrane sac around his heart.

13   Transplant schedule: The transplant schedule is a map of the BSCT process for that patient. BSCT requires numerous steps to be completed in a specific sequence. To ensure care occurs in the right order the unit prepared for each patient a discrete listing the major steps arranged in a chronological order from minus days pre-transplant to care up 12–18 months after the transplant.

who is allowed to have close personal contact, and defend our personal space. In BSCT frequent access to the body and at least daily surveillance of the body were part of the routine care and medical and nursing staff had intimate access to recipients' bodies. The taking of blood specimens, the observation of temperature, blood pressure, pulse and respiration, and the monitoring of the patient's skin for bruising and infections aid in rendering a body passive to observation and control (Kelly et al. 2000: 956).

BSCT recipients had central venous catheters (CVC) inserted into their upper chest/shoulder area to enable the numerous drugs to be given, the blood tests taken and blood stem cells administered. Metaphorically the CVC could be likened to an umbilical cord providing a conduit for sustenance, blood and life. Adapting to the demands of time connected to intravenous lines for treatment came with limitations to mobility and restrictions in space. CVCs require ongoing cleaning, dressing and observation by nurses. Furthermore, the recipients had to dress so that the catheter was easily accessible for nursing staff.

> In all cultures, dress is more than simply a means of bodily protection: it is, manifestly, a means of symbolic display, a way of giving external form to narratives of self identity (Giddens 1991: 62).

Clothing was a visual signifier of the shift to patient as normal outer layers were track pants and t-shirts but moved to pyjamas and eventually anonymous hospital gowns as the transplant proceeded. The narratives of personal identity writ large upon their clothing, as they recovered after the stem cell infusion pyjamas and track pants reappeared.

Entering the transplant process and being admitted to the ward disrupted every aspect of a person's life, no aspect was left unaltered. The person was reconstructed to become a case for medicine, located within a network of normal and disease, learnt their body could not be trusted, became subject to the dictates of the hospital and sequestered in a hospital bed, lived in a public space, had to dress in a certain manner, learnt a new language, and gave up social roles. The transition from person into a patient enacted through the reconfiguration of body, blood, space, time, identity and politically through the control and power exercized by the institution and the transplant process.

Their bodies penetrated by central lines, the medical gaze bringing bloody organs to the fore, language that constructed them as bodies with parts, and their social identity left behind, people were eroded down to patients. People became patients through the subtle shifts of power, language, reconfiguring of their bodies and the actions of the nurses, medicine and the institution. Blood and flesh had become the dominant way of being challenging the self, perception and the trust of their embodiment. Ultimately, the recipient becomes visible to all while eroding inwardly in on themselves as their identity was stripped progressively away.

Infusion of the Cells – Creating the Chimera and Recipient

Blood and What Else

A clinical detachment in the actual infusion of cells pervades the literature related to infusion of Blood Stem Cells. However, infusing (an)other's blood stem cells bring all of the shifting meanings of blood as source of life and death as well as identity to the fore (see Table 7.1). Recipients and their families thought more than just physiological blood stem cells were being infused. Bernard's wife wondered if 'maybe he'll get some of his brother's characteristics. He is a little quieter and that would be nice sometimes'. Personality and character might also come with the cells. Bernard reassured himself that his determined character would come with their cells 'things go wrong and then have to put it right but they do put it right' (Bernard).

Equally, there was concern that unwanted effects may come with the cells. David sought reassurance his unknown donor was male, 'I hope I've got a male donor cos you know I wouldn't want to change [gesturing in an effeminate manner]'. David was worried that female blood stem cells might make him less masculine. What else might the transplanted blood cells affect? Francis worried about his unknown blood stem cells donor;

> Comes tomorrow, yeah. It's an unrelated, so I don't know who or what … being an
> unrelated, they don't tell you who or where or what – what from (Francis Day – 1).

Blood stem cells have the uncertainty of being, the *it* and *what* emphasizing they were beyond just blood cells; who they came from was unknown, where they were from and what else they carried was also unknown. The *it* reinforcing again the shifting subjectivity coming from the blood stem cells and transplant. The cells had a substantive history and identity; they were not just replacement parts. Francis was linked by blood to an unknown individual, blood ties but with no known links apart from genetic matching. However, recipients knew their survival depended on the generosity of an 'other' and were very grateful that the blood stem cells were so altruistically being given. The twin sides of sublime connectedness and abject isolation reflected in the donor and recipient relationship.

Before the Infusion

The recipients' were waiting for the cells to be infused and their empty marrow ready to receive the new stem cells. They had no choice but to proceed. The reality of receiving (an)other's cells, the possibility of death during transplant and having to place their life in other people's hands was overwhelming for the recipients. They no longer had control over their selves or their lives. The future extended only as far as later that day when the blood stem cells will be infused that would inextricably bind them to an 'Other'. Their future depended on the infusion of a small bag of 100 ml or so of another's blood stem cells. Adam described, 'it's not just a drip it's the future'. The cells needed to replenish not only their marrow and blood cells but their futures.

All of the participants had a period of angst prior to the infusion of the blood stem cells. The recipients were unsure what (an)other's cells would do to them and how they would change. In confronting their mortality recipients questioned who they were and what they believed and describe a vacuum in which they were unsure of where to place themselves. Some recipients had difficulty describing how they felt. For some there were tears and silences, or a few words hesitantly expressed 'empty, stressed out, or fragile' (Emma, Harry, Francis respectively). Unusually, for Bernard normally articulate and verbose he did not have the words to make sense of or describe the experience, it remained unsaid. David was asked how he felt and what did he expect of the transplant prior to the cells going in; David responded with uncertainty, he took a long while answering – he closed his eyes for around a minute or more and when he opened them tears came out. 'Empty' was the only reply that verbally came. He couldn't describe his feelings.

They were unable to eat, sleep, or read. They were distressed, apprehensive, irritable and fidgety. Others expressed an ambivalence and uncertainty 'I really didn't want to go ahead even though I did' (Emma). Emma admitted to being scared of the unknown and how she was to start the next part of her journey.

Adam described himself as 'I'm empty it's up to grace of god and medicine'. Powerless to change the situation, Adam waited reliant on god and medicine to take him forward. He had gone through all the emotions and now empty was just waiting. He had looked at God, he had looked at medical science but there remained the unease of exactly where he was, empty, waiting for god and medicine to intervene.

Ian had researched and understood the process of infusing the stem cells as a simple and an anti-climax but felt a dissonance between what he knew and what he felt 'you know it's not you. But you've got to do it'. The ambivalent feelings of self and other, *its not you but you've got to do it.* Ian was quite emotional and had tears in his eyes as he eloquently described 'I feel betwixt and between nothingness', an apt and evocative description of the uncomfortable space of abjection.

They were stripped down to bare physiological life, their power, identity and autonomy overwhelmed and overtaken by the transplant process as they confronted their mortality. The transplant eroded away aspects of their identity, their place in the world, their trust in their bodies to tell them if they were sick or well and located them in the present with a contingent future. They waited in an extremely uncomfortable space uncertain of who or what they may become, what else might come with the blood and how the 'other' would change their bodies, their bloodlines, their self or their future. Kristeva would recognize such a space as abjection that is 'above all ambiguity' (1982: 9). The distress they felt was emotional and spiritual; an existential crisis. Their bone marrow was empty and so were they. They didn't have the words to describe the unnameable abject place; they were in the abyss of abjection the 'nothingness of the self becomes the existential 'crisis' of the self' (Ricoeur 1992: 168).

Infusing Cells

The medical literature refers to the infusion of another cells is like a 'simple blood transfusion'. This perspective fails to account for the emotional sentient experience. All the recipients ensured family were present when the cells went in, some took photos to record the event. Adam viewed the infusions as 'It's not just a drip it's the future', aware the stem cells were the key to future survival. Even while administering the stem cells notions of what else came with the blood were mentioned 'our blood is so thick and rich' one noted as their brother's blood stem cells were administered. While technically a 'non event' some used humour to deflect their discomfort. Bernard combined his and his brother's names to reflect his new status. Francis found the dissonance between volume and impact confounding and amusing, 'well you think, this is going to change your life. It's only 100 ml [laughs]'.

After the event a mellowness and slight withdrawal into themselves took place. They became less articulate, retreating into themselves, as Ian said, 'batten down the hatches'. In the days after transplant the recipients described the infusion as, anti climax (Adam), a non event (Francis), 'an anticlimax and a non event, well not a non event but ... [long silence]' (Bernard). Harry said he was 'fine now … I was unsure how I was going to react'. A few days later Ian's distress had been rewritten over, 'I was pretty sleepy at the time however, it [administration of the cells] was and wasn't a non event'. Once the physical administration of the cells occurred it became a non-event, the unknown had been faced, fear and uncertainty relegated to a distant memory with a rewriting of their history and redrawn boundaries of their self. They had moved on to waiting for their cells to grow.

Conclusion

Blood diseases are menacingly quiet and the slide into bloody illness becomes audible only when mortality is precariously threatened. Blood sits within a multiplicity of cultural meanings and the significance of BSCT is that it challenges many of these understandings such as past bloodlines – disrupted as another's cells are infused, linked only by genetic similarity. The creation of this new blood line, within an individual, disturbs the contained sense of one's singular identity and belonging.

In BSCT recipients' bodies and identity are disturbed and disrupted. BSCT changes recipients, as they learn the language of haematology, confront their mortality, are 'emptied', accept (an)other, deal with another's blood running through their veins for the rest of their existence, as well as then having to renegotiate with their social world. Fundamental ontological questioning by patients of who am

I, and what do I believe occurs as embodied individuals confront death, identity, shattering of independence, altered social roles and physical symptoms of the blood stem cell transplant process.

Abjection is an un-nameable sensation when conscious self-awareness is lost and the self dissolves. When 'I/me' (self and other) were declared the primordial, abject way of being in the world is submerged. In BSCT, the chaos of disease, the addition of (an)other's blood, and the creation of the chimera fractures understandings of the self continuously returning recipients to an abject state. Abjection occurs as boundaries between self and other are met, crossed, transplanted and purposely manipulated. At the moment of transplantation, the abject awaits while science struggles for success of its experiments, remaking the new 'you', medical science so often offers is not the you of old – a chimeric identity emerges – self-other-hybrid. If successful, out of the fractured self a new potentiality emerges where individual character endures even though parts of the body machine have been replaced.

References

Atkinson, P. 1995. *Medical Talk and Medical Work: The Liturgy of the Clinic.* London: Sage Publications.

Australian Red Cross Blood Service, 2006. Transfusion Medicine Service [online]. Available at: www.transfusion.com.au/resoucelibrary/coi_ch01_intro.asp [accessed: 15 October 2006].

Barnard, A. and Sandelowski, M. 2001. Technology and humane nursing care: (ir) reconcilable or invented difference? *Journal of Advanced Nursing*, 34(3), 367–375.

Frank, A. 1995. *The Wounded Storyteller: Body, Illness and Ethics.* Chicago: University of Chicago.

Giddens, A. 1991. *Modernity and Self Identity: Self and Society in the Late Modern Age.* Cambridge: Polity Press.

Haberman, M. 1988. Psychosocial aspects of bone marrow transplantation. *Seminars in Oncology Nursing*, 4(1), 55–59.

Hoffbrand, A., Pettit, J. and Moss, P. 2001. *Essential Haematology.* Oxford: Blackwell Science.

Jones, C. and Chapman, Y. 2000. The Lived Experience of seven people treated with autologous bone marrow/peripheral blood stem cell transplant. *International Journal of Nursing Practice*, 6, 153–159.

Kelly, D., Ross, S., Gray, B. and Smith, P. 2000. Death, dying and emotional labour: problematic dimensions of the bone marrow transplant nursing role. *Journal of Advanced Nursing*, 32(4), 952–960.

Kristeva, J. 1982. *The Powers of Horror. An Essay on Abjection.* New York: Columbia University Press.

Latimer, J. 2000. *The Conduct of Care: Understanding Nursing Practice.* Oxford: Blackwell Science.

Leder, D. 1990. *The Absent Body.* Chicago: The University of Chicago Press.

Leder, D. 1999. Flesh and blood: a proposed supplement to Merleau-Ponty, in *The Body: Classic and Contemporary Readings* edited by D. Welton. Malden, Massachusetts: Blackwell, 200–210.

Lingis, A. 1999. The subjectification of the body, in *The Body: Classic and Contemporary Readings,* edited by D. Welton. Malden, Massachusetts: Blackwell, 286–306.

Loach, L. 1997. Blue Days. *Nursing Times*, 93(32), 30–31.

Lupton, D. 1994. *Medicine as Culture: Illness, Disease and the Body in Western Societies.* London: Sage.

McQuellon, R., Russell, G., Rambo, T., Craven, B., Radford, J., Perry, J., Cruz, J. and Hurd, D. 1998. Quality of life and psychological distress of bone marrow transplant recipients: the 'time trajectory' to recovery over the first year. *Bone Marrow Transplantation*, 21(5), 477–486.

Merleau-Ponty, M. 1968. *The Visible and the Invisible.* Evanston: Northwestern University Press.

Nightingale, F. 1969. *Notes on Nursing.* Toronto: Dover Publications.

Ricoeur, P. 1992. *Oneself as Another.* London: The University of Chicago Press.

Sakalys, J. 2000. The political role of illness narratives. *Journal of Advanced Nursing*, 31(6), 1469–1475.

Saleh, U. and Brockopp, D. 2001. quality of life one year following bone marrow transplantation: psychometric evaluation of the quality of life in bone marrow transplant survivors tool. *Oncology Nursing Forum*, 28(9), 1457–1464.

Santos, G.W. 1983. History of Bone Marrow Transplantation. *Clinics in Haematology*, 12, 611–639.

Shakespeare, W. 1984. *The Merchant of Venice.* Rydalmere: Hodder Education.

Shuster, G., Steeves, R. and Richardson, B. 1996. Coping patterns among bone marrow transplant patients: a hermeneutical inquiry. *Cancer Nursing*, 19(4), 290–297.

Starr, D. 1999. *Blood. An Epic History of Medicine and Commerce.* London: Little, Brown and Company.

Steeves, R. 1992. Patients who have undergone bone marrow transplantation: their quest for meaning. *Oncology Nursing Forum*, 19(6), 899–905.

Thain, C.W. and Gibbon, B. 1996. An exploratory study of recipients' perceptions of bone marrow transplantation. *Journal of Advanced Nursing*, 23, 528–535.

Chapter 8

Managing the Other within the Self: Bodily Experiences of HIV/AIDS

Marilou Gagnon

Introduction

Based on the work of Julia Kristeva (1982), the concept of abjection allows us to explore the experience of illness and the way it is socially and culturally enacted through the human body and its bodily functions. The expulsion of bodily products – or the rejection of what is not of the body – is a highly ambivalent process through which the integrity of the body and the self are (re)affirmed by the ill individual. As suggested by Holmes and his colleagues (2006: 308), the ill individual 'needs to reject subhuman matter in order to strengthen his or her subjectivity and preserve a *Self propre* (clean, proper, self-controlled) but in doing so is continuously facing doubts about personal integrity and autonomy'. In order to function effectively as a social being, the same individual will need to wash away (expel) the signs of illness before entering a clean and ordered symbolic state (Cregan 2006).

The manifestations of illness threaten the locus of control over the self by revealing the uncertainty of the clean and proper body. As the lines that differentiate the inside from the outside of the body shift and fluctuate, one's own sense of subjectivity is destabilized because the abject can necessarily be found inside and outside the surface of the skin (Holmes et al. 2006). Consequently, the ill individual whose integrity is breached must face his own feelings of abjection and his new status as an object of social abjection – the recipient of social disgust. Based on Kristeva's work (1982), we now understand that illness and its physical manifestations irrupt into and disrupt the symbolic order of our society (Cregan 2006). From this perspective, the individual body becomes an object to be read and deciphered during the social encounter in order to ensure the permeability of boundaries. The individual body is, therefore, presumed to be uncontaminated and harmless in the absence of deviant physical manifestations (signs and symptoms of illness).

There is a definite need to explore the personal and social experience of abjection as it is lived by individuals who bear the symbols of illness, which according to Persson (2005: 238), is the object of a broad range of social, moral and cultural meanings around 'corporeality, selfhood, suffering and mortality'. The purpose of this chapter is to introduce the theoretical work of Julia Kristeva

(1982) and other authors in order to examine the relationship between the body and HIV/AIDS. The main objective of this theoretical piece is to introduce the key findings of an interpretive analysis which includes several qualitative studies on the bodily experiences of HIV/AIDS. The rationale for conducting an interpretive analysis was supported by the incessant need to further our understanding of the relationship between the body and HIV/AIDS in the post-Highly Active Antiretroviral Therapy[1] (HAART) era, a period of tremendous paradoxes for people living with HIV/AIDS.

Revisiting the Literature: The Body and HIV/AIDS

In order to localize qualitative studies that examined the relationship between the body and HIV/AIDS, we performed a conventional literary search (CINAHL, Medline, PsychInfo) using keywords such as body, body image, HIV, AIDS, lipodystrophy. The selected articles needed to report the findings of a qualitative study, be published after 1990 and in either English or French. The inclusion criteria for this paper aimed at broadening the inquiry to incorporate studies that were published prior to and after the advent of HAART. The quality of each retrieved publication was appraised according to the criteria provided by Walsh and Downe (2006), but did not constitute an exclusion factor due to the potential richness of findings that would be otherwise refuted. In doing so, the objective was that a novel, integrative and substantive interpretation of findings will be produce and will then exceed the individual value of each qualitative investigation.

Every study was examined by the author in order to identify the content, the intention and the signification of the findings; key ideas, metaphors, concepts and phrases were retrieved and synthesized along with the intention of the participants and the initial interpretation of the researcher(s). The goal of this process was to create a group of concepts that would be used in comparing and contrasting the qualitative studies. This 'compare and contrast' procedure was done simultaneously with the reciprocal translation or the sequential integration of study findings into a unique conceptual combination. Throughout the analysis, the researcher intended to preserve the hermeneutic and the dialectical aspect of each qualitative inquiry; thus, the ultimate goal was to portray individual constructions while comparing and contrasting them in order to generate a new construction on which to build on. The final step of the analytical process consisted of integrating the work of different authors in order to theorize the bodily experience of HIV/AIDS.

In order to achieve rigour while conducting the interpretive analysis, the author ensured that the phenomenon of interest was described in a credible and

---

1   Highly Active Antiretroviral Therapy (HAART) is a combination of three (or more) different antiretroviral agents. This treatment is taken daily to suppress the replication of the virus (HIV) and reduce the amount of circulating virus in the blood. The objective of HAART is to slow down the progression of HIV infection.

consistent manner, that the analytical process was rooted in the original data and was faithful to the description and interpretation of the phenomenon (truth-value), that the criterion could corroborate with outer settings while being grounded in its original context (fittingness), that the analytical process was auditable and was externally (theoretical literature) and internally (verbatim) validated and that the conformability and the applicability of findings could be established (Jensen and Allen 1996).

The Construction of the HIV-infected Body

The HIV-positive body (and its bodily fluids) is the focal point of the HIV/AIDS epidemic where it acts as 'a site of death and contagion, of prejudice and moral penalties' (Murphy 1995: 66). Since the beginning of the HIV/AIDS epidemic, scholars have argued that the social, cultural, medical and scientific construction of the HIV-positive body each serve a clear function in shaping the experience of people living with HIV/AIDS. As such, there is a need to explore how the HIV-positive body is generally constructed in order to understand how people who live with the illness (HIV/AIDS) relate to their own physicality. Most importantly, there is need to expand on this particular phenomenon and expose its compatibility with Kristeva's concept of abjection. According to Murphy (1995: 13), 'the [human immunodeficiency virus] enters the social world on two primary levels: as a biological event that infects our bodies and as a social event to which a variety of meanings is attached by the choices we make in response to [HIV/AIDS]'. Since the beginning of the HIV/AIDS epidemic, one of the strongest socio-cultural responses has been to construct the HIV-positive body as the object of abjection. The early images of AIDS were those of wasted bodies (cadaver-like bodies) which evoked thoughts of terror and death – 'the utmost portrayal of the abject' (Holmes et al. 2006: 308). Photographs of the HIV-infected body were disturbing to the observer because it embodied the unbreakable relationship between life and death as well as the dangerousness of AIDS. As such, the physical manifestations of AIDS (fat wasting, Kaposi sarcoma, skin lesions) became crucial markers of those who were 'contaminated' by the virus. In the first few years of the epidemic, Sontag (1989) explained that HIV-positive individuals were branded with the ravages of the illness. Their bodies displaying 'a plethora of disabling; disfiguring and humiliating signs and symptoms' (Sontag 1989: 21). At that time, the body was commonly constructed as a symbol of imminent physical and social death, a process that concurred with a progressive decline of the immune system and the emergence of AIDS-related pathologies.

Based on the work of Elizabeth Chapman (2000), it is understood that the HIV-infected body is constructed as a contaminated entity, one that transgresses the proper and clean self. People not only become infected with the human immunodeficiency virus, they also become infectious by embodying the risk of contamination. Consequently, the HIV-infected body (as the object of abjection) produces 'a severe dismemberment of the social body' (Murphy 1995: 13) by raising issues of touch. According to Chapman (2000: 853), 'people with HIV [become] aware of the virus coursing through their veins, and they live with the knowledge that other people are fearful of coming in contact with their blood or bodily fluids'. They also come to reject their own bodily fluids, a process that is 'both manifest (concrete), a physical product of the subject and imaginary (symbolic), existing metaphorically because of the cognitive process taking place in which the abject evokes filth and is associated with pollution of the body and mind' (Holmes et al. 2006: 307). Therefore, the HIV-infected body is constructed as a site of abjection where the uncertainty of boundaries evokes disgust, fear and rejection of the physical contact.

In the medical and scientific communities, the HIV-infected body is described as being invaded by a foreign agent (the viral agent), one that disturbs its system, its order and its rules. Through the biomedical lens, the body becomes physically situated in space in order to create tangible targets and internal pathways for the application of localized therapy (Persson 2004). In 1996, the introduction of HAART resulted in the construction of an HIV-infected body as mechanistic and extrinsic to mind or self, one that is grounded in a medical (objective) language. Hypothetically, HAART symbolized the end of abjection by its ability to contain and conceal the physical manifestations of HIV/AIDS and most importantly, the risk of contamination. The HIV-infected body was to become a silent entity, one that rendered the physical and social manifestations of the illness to a period of latency, hidden within the body. Yet, the emergence of the lipodystrophy syndrome – HAART-related body changes – led the illness (HIV/AIDS) to become 're-detectable' by 'forcing it out onto the surface of the skin and into the collective view through a new, conspicuous corporeality' (Persson 2005: 253).

First described by Carr and his colleagues in 1998, the lipodystrophy syndrome is characterized by an intricate combination of local (external) and systemic (internal) symptoms that are caused by HAART. It is now recognized that the physical manifestations of lipodystrophy often result from a combination of lipoatrophy (loss of adipose or fat tissue) and lipoaccumulation (accumulation of adipose or fat tissue) including symptoms such as, subcutaneous lipoatrophy of the face, limbs and buttocks, and fat accumulation in the abdomen, breasts, and dorsocervical spine (Grinspoon and Carr 2005). The post-HAART era calls for a better understanding of the bodily experiences of HIV/AIDS and lipodystrophy as they both transform the lives of people living with HIV/AIDS. Faced with the new reality of the HIV/AIDS illness (HAART-related lipodystrophy), there is a definite need to examine how the HIV-infected body is (re)constructed as the object of abjection. As such, our findings stand as a form of resistance against the dominant scientific discourse in the field of HIV/AIDS, one that conceptualizes HIV/AIDS and the lipodystrophy syndrome as disembodied phenomena.

Re-embodying HIV/AIDS in the Post-HAART Era

Key findings of this interpretive analysis were regrouped in four main themes (the self, the other, embodiment and sequel of experiences) that were then conceptualized and theorized within a hypothetic model of interaction (Figure 8.1). This interpretative schema illustrates how the body is experienced in relation to the HIV/AIDS illness.

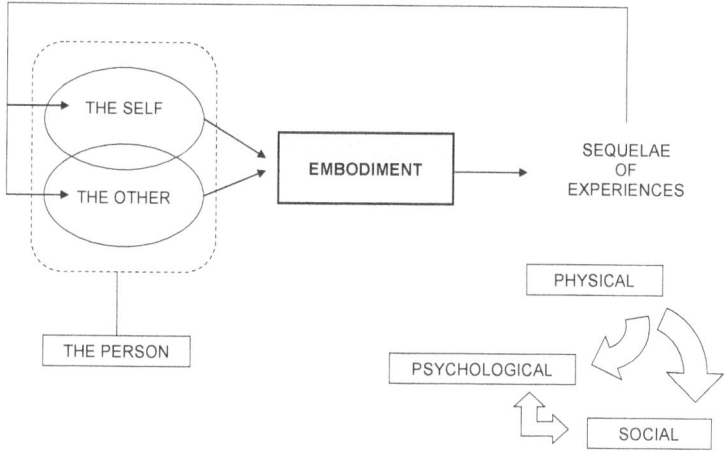

Figure 8.1   The bodily experience of HIV/AIDS

The Self

It is recognized that 'illness threatens a person's sense of integrity of self in relation to the body and to the social world' (Charmaz 1995: 657). According to Charmaz (1995), there is a definite need to expose this process since it has an impact on the way illness is embodied and lived within modern society. The contaminated or unhealthy body influences the definition and perception of one's identity within the public and private realms by creating a tension between the self and the body (Charmaz 1995). Gadow (1982) suggests that illness is a disruptive process that interrupts and terminates a state of unity (self-body), one that characterizes healthy individuals. This author argues that illness, as a disruptive event, creates a distance between the body and the self (Gadow 1982). As such, the bodily manifestations of illness result in the opposition of the body and the self which can eventually lead to the 'reconceptualization' of one's identity (Wendell 1996: 169). Furthermore, the 'onset of illness destroys the absence of the body consciousness and renders a conscious responses to new, often acute, awareness of the body' (Wendell 1996: 178). From this perspective, illness symbolizes the end of an unconscious alliance between the body and the self, one that can no longer be maintained in the presence of illness. As suggested by Shildrick (2002: 50), 'to be a self is above all to be distinguished from the other, to be ordered and discrete, secure within the well-defined boundaries of the body'. In the presence of illness, the body is no longer clean, proper or silent, nor is it absent for the consciousness (Leder 1990). It is disruptively real and visible. Consequently, the body cannot be studied in the absence of disease, damage or fragmentation because it is the disruptive condition that is of interest, not the state of unity that characterizes healthy individuals.

In the field of HIV/AIDS, qualitative studies that examine the body were published between 2000 and 2006 as a response to a change in momentum; people living with HIV/AIDS in industrialized countries gained access to treatment (HAART), prolonged their life expectancy and most importantly, developed a body altering syndrome called the lipodystophy syndrome. In the post-HAART era, people living with HIV/AIDS describe the self to be equally distorted as the ill body in which they reside. This phenomenon is exemplified in the following verbatim excerpt: 'With HIV I am not normal, I become deformed in all ways. My face, body, everything. Obviously, when your face and body deforms, your mind starts to deform because it starts to affect you … ' (Varas-Diaz et al. 2005: 135). According to Charmaz (1995), the manifestations of illness threaten the integrity of the body as well as the integrity of the self. The physical boundaries are visibly disrupted and broken down. As a result, the boundaries of the self can longer be maintained. For people living with HIV/AIDS, the boundaries become blurred by the estranged transformation of a body that is no longer compatible with the self. This particular phenomenon is described in this citation: 'How horrible is it to have your body change in such a way…I had three opportunistic infections… almost went blind. I could handle that, because it was still me. I could still relate to my physical being, and now I can't' (Reynolds et al. 2006: 666). One could argue that the post-HAART era is particularly disruptive because the body has become a space of alienation for people living with HIV/AIDS; a space where the self cannot be separated from its physical becoming. As the most visible boundary of all, the outer layer of the body is the physical limit of the self and a site where 'any compromise of the organic unity and self-completion of the skin, may indicate the abjection of the self' (Shildrick 2002: 51). The skin is a blank canvas where inscriptions and symbols are featured for everyone to read and deciphered. Therefore, it is central to how we relate to ourselves and to others (as suggested by Marc Lafrance, see Chapter 9).

People living with HIV/AIDS describe their bodies to be grotesque, deformed and damaged by the manifestations of illness as exemplified by the following verbatims: 'I felt like a freak, um, because my body wasn't mine any more…' (Reynolds 2006: 668); "I'm that weird looking deformed guy with the big neck' (Collins et al. 2000); 'The main effect for me has been an enormous abdomen, and certainly initially I lost weight in general but gained a great deal abdominal size. And I suppose this was put down to, in my mind at least, lipodystrophy. On the whole I'm left a bit freakish...' (Power et al. 2003: 138). While the body is transformed by the illness into an estranged entity, the self is equally defined as an estranged entity and internalized by the person, who then assimilates a new identity. As suggested by Leder (1990: 91), 'the body is no longer alien-as-forgotten, but precisely as re-membered, a sharp searing presence threatening the self'. Through their physicality, people living with HIV/AIDS embark in a journey of becoming, a process that generates an alter ego that will be known as the *Other*.

The Other

The body is a site of transcription, communication and signification for deviant representations (signs and symptoms of illness). It could be argued, then, that the inscription of illness onto the body generates a new dimension of the self which we will refer to as the Other. Such a phenomenon is well described by people living with HIV/AIDS who consider their bodies as being central to the experience of illness: the body becomes an object that is regulated by external forces (virus, illness, medications, treatments) and an unwanted presence that cannot be controlled. Therefore, the illness challenges the locus of control over one's body, identity and self – a process that is reported in every qualitative study: 'I feel that my body changes are out of my control, and its concurrent with feeling my life is out of control' (Collins et al. 2000: 548); 'Yeah, I think that it's [unhappiness with his body] linked in generally with being HIV-positive, that your body is not doing what it should do...' (Tate and George 2001: 166). The body also becomes a symbol of the illness. It is perceived to be the mapping of deviance, imperfection, failure and vulnerability – the symbol of Otherness. Through such a process, the body is re-conceptualized in relation to the self and emerges as the representation of disruptions that are externally and internally imposed on the ill individual. Not only are people living with HIV/AIDS labelled as Others in the collective realm, but the same process is experienced in the private realm: '...I would look at myself in the mirror and not see the same person I used to be' (Varas-Diaz et al. 2005: 134); ' ... I don't see my body as before. If I look at myself in the mirror I see it old, it's wasting' (Varas-Diaz et al. 2005: 135); ' ... almost alienated from my body there's this inbuilt distance between who you are now and what you're seeing ... ' (Tate and George 2001: 167).

The qualitative studies describe how the ill individual becomes alienated from his own body and his own self. With no sense of integrity, the individual can no longer live 'normally' or consider himself 'normal'. This is particularly true when the illness forces itself into the defining features of the individual (both internally and externally): 'It's something you have (HIV). It's like a little spot on a white sheet. You take a white sheet and let a black spot fall on it. Even if you wash it, the spot stays there' (Varas-Diaz et al. 2005: 135). This verbatim exemplifies how the body and the self are portrayed as immaculate entities and how they are spoiled by the presence of a foreign agent, an intrusive virus that stains the body and the self permanently. It also suggests that people living with HIV/AIDS go through a process of becoming – becoming somebody else; somebody who is defined by the illness. Somebody who is no longer 'normal' in terms of embodiment and social status: 'With HIV I am not normal, I become deformed in all ways; my face, body, everything ... ' (Varas-Diaz et al. 2005: 135). Through their physicality, people living with HIV/AIDS are reminded of the social meanings, myths and stereotypes that are associated with their illness and in some cases, internalized these perceptions as defining attributes of their bodily experiences; people living with HIV/AIDS become Others prior to their entrance into the social sphere.

Embodiment

Gadow (1982) argues that 'human existence essentially means embodiment and that the self is inseparable from the body'. It is generally understood that humans are social beings who materialize their existence in a process of becoming, one that transforms the body and the self into perceptible entities. In fact, Cregan (2006: 3) states that 'embodiment – the physical and mental experience of existence – is the condition of possibility for our relating to other people and to the world'. Our physicality is the very means by which we define our existence as social beings because the body is a symbolic vehicle that delineates how meaning is shaped, presented and represented in society (Cregan 2006). Within the social sphere, 'we relate to each other through our embodied being and the fact of our social interrelationships shapes the way we constitute our embodied being' (Cregan 2006: 5). The body is, therefore, an object of communication and a technical mean that carry the self (and *the Other*) into the social sphere. Therefore, the body penetrates the perceptible realm through a process of becoming and a process of retroaction; while becoming a social being (embodiment), one is exposed to bodily experiences that transform positively or negatively the self and the other.

As suggested by Alonzo and Reynolds (1995), stigmatization is a significant feature of the experience of HIV/AIDS. The bodily manifestation of illness, on the other hand, intensifies the social burden reported by people living with HIV/AIDS: '[talking about facial lipoatrophy] When you see a person today and the next day, you can see the bones and skin in his face, specifically in the face. I would say that the face ...it's the biggest stigma faced by patients today' (Varas-Diaz et al. 2005: 133); '[talking about lipodystrophy] It's just a new version of letting people know what you have. I think that's the biggest problem. Cause in a way, you are kind of wearing a sign that say, hey, you're positive. It's out there' (Reynolds et al. 2006: 668); 'I always felt quite well but now you know, I mean I just feel like I have AIDS stamped on my forehead' (Power et al. 2003: 140); 'People in my community can tell that I'm HIV-positive from just looking at my face' (Collins et al. 2000: 549). Overall, people living with HIV/AIDS indicate that visibility is an important issue when entering the social sphere. As such, stigmatization is typically described as an experience of visibility: being visibly different, being visibly 'sick' and/or being visibly HIV-positive.

As a symbol of illness, the body is branded with deviant representations (signs and symptoms of illness) which serve to cast a 'discrediting attribute' onto the stigmatized individual (Goffman 1963). The stigma 'allows the identification of differentness, the construction of stereotypes, the separation of labelled persons into distinct categories, and the full execution of disapproval, rejection, exclusion and discrimination' (Link and Phelan 2001: 364). When asked to describe their relationship with the physical dimension of illness, people living with HIV/AIDS identify stigma as being a core component of their socialization. Persson (2005) suggests that this phenomenon is directly related to the 'visual embodiment of HIV/AIDS'. More specifically, Goffman (1963) considers that the visibility of the stigmatizing attribute is a crucial factor in the social experience of the self and the other (embodiment). The individual who is defined by this attribute is nonetheless visible and vulnerable. Because they are and feel visible to others, people living with HIV/AIDS are and feel vulnerable. They describe how being exposed creates a feeling of insecurity and invasion: '[talking about lipodystrophy] Our privacy is being invaded' (Reynolds et al. 2006: 668).

Gadow (1982) proposes that human existence essentially means embodiment and that the self is inseparable from the body. As such, the experience of the body cannot be separated from the experience of self in society. It is important to understand that a visible stigma will necessarily damage or spoil the identity of people living with HIV/AIDS (Goffman 1963). Through embodiment, the *Other* becomes an intricate component of the self, one that will transform the psychological, social and physical trajectory of the ill individual.

Squeal of Experiences

The qualitative studies that have examined the bodily experiences of HIV/AIDS have done so within a perspective of disruption. While there was one research done in the context of weight loss (fat wasting), the qualitative studies were otherwise conducted in relation to lipodystrophy – a condition that is characterized by the abnormal redistribution of adipose tissue. The qualitative studies concerned with the experience of HAART-related body changes (the physical experience) reported numerous psychological and social repercussions. According to our analysis, these experiences were directly related to a process of embodiment – one that introduces the Self and the Other into the social sphere by using the body as its vehicle. The experiences were part of a retroactive process that influenced positively or negatively the construction of the self and the other (see Figure 8.1).

Physical experience   The physical experience of people living with HIV/AIDS is discussed according to two dimensions of the illness-treatment alliance: the bodily manifestations and the bodily functions. In most studies, HAART-induced body changes are described as part of a mandatory passage in the experience of

HIV/AIDS: 'I have been living with this thing for 15 years, so well I am just grateful every day that I am still alive and I know without these pills I certainly probably would be dead, so its striking the balance' (Varas-Diaz et al. 2005: 139); 'On the one hand, the drugs are doing a great job … so what kind of side effects do you put up with?' (Reynolds et al. 2006: 667); 'I think the biggest issue is trying to figure out where these changes belong … are they part of the disease process or part of the side effects of the medications?' (Reynolds et al. 2006: 667). Across studies, the physicality of the illness-treatment alliance is considered a key feature of the bodily experience of HIV/AIDS. Interestingly, this particular dimension of the HIV/AIDS experience is described in terms of the internal disruptions (impaired bodily functions) and external disruptions (impaired bodily manifestations) of the body.

Psychological experience   The psychological experience of people living with HIV/AIDS is discussed in relation to the detrimental impact of the altered body onto the self. The body which is distorted, visible, estranged and unfamiliar is associated with psychological difficulties that transform the perception of the self and motivate the perception of the Other. These psychological repercussions are very distressing to people living with HIV/AIDS: 'Through my whole experience living with this disease, that [lipodystrophy] is probably the worse thing emotionally and mentally. I never felt so unattractive in my life' (Reynolds et al. 2006: 667). As demonstrated by the qualitative findings, negative repercussions such as altered body image, altered self-confidence, self-hatred, depression and suicidal ideation are part of the bodily experience of HIV/AIDS.

The negative repercussions described above shape the way people living with HIV/AIDS relate to themselves: they are distanced from themselves and distancing themselves from the interpersonal encounter. Furthermore, the psychological burden reported by ill-looking individuals explains why so many others are delaying, modifying or discontinuing antiretroviral therapy: 'I'll lay in bed at night, and I'll think, well you idiot, why did you event get on these drugs?' (Reynolds et al. 2006: 669); 'I've actually even started thinking about if this keeps up, especially in the face thing…I'd consider even, like discontinuing the regimens or taking a break' (Reynolds et al. 2006: 669); 'I have fear now that of getting off the drugs. I'll stop my drugs and be dead in a year …Do I want to look like a cartoon character or be dead?' (Reynolds et al. 2006: 669). While the psychological experience originates from the physicality of HIV/AIDS (the physical experience), the qualitative findings signal important relationships between the psychological experience and the social experience.

Social experience   The social experience of people living with HIV/AIDS is discussed in relation to the process of embodiment and the subsequent projection of the self and the Other into the social sphere. The body is described as a symbol of socio-cultural meanings and representations that are engraved on the surface of the skin. People living with HIV/AIDS express the sensation of being branded with the corporal sign of their illness and as such they describe how the body acts as an indicator of their serological status: '[talking about facial lipoatrophy] my face tells the story' (Reynolds et al. 2006: 668). The stigmatization is said to originate from the self and from the social encounter; this process entertains a strong relationship with the psychological experience of the altered body. Furthermore, the embodiment is described as a process of becoming stigmatized. Such a phenomenon is closely related to the physical experience and the psychological experience of HIV/AIDS.

People living with HIV/AIDS report being excluded and excluding themselves from the collective realm in order to avoid interpersonal interactions or the unpleasant reminder of their awkwardness: 'I don't want to be around them because I don't want to have to go through the process explaining to them or having to deal with issue of running from them or feeling uncomfortable… so I just avoid them' (Reynolds et al. 2006: 668). Qualitative findings report that involuntary disclosure is a common phenomenon for people who cannot hide their bodies: 'It is no secret what this face means. I have been open about my status, but I prefer to announce it myself' (Collins et al. 2000: 549). The social burden of the bodily experience of HIV/AIDS appears to explain some of the psychological suffering that results from the process of embodiment or the presence of the Self and the *Other* within the collective realm. Not only do people living with HIV/AIDS internalize their own detrimental discourse, but they also integrate a social identity that is spoiled by their ill-looking body. Therefore, the social experience transforms the perception of the self and motivates the construction of the *Other*.

Final Remarks

The present interpretive analysis has allowed the author to construct a hypothetical model that illustrates how the body is experienced in relation to the HIV/AIDS illness. This interpretive schema was based on the work of Julia Kristeva and other authors, which facilitated the conceptualization, and the theorization of a phenomenon that has not (to our knowledge) been explored in the literature. In the post-HAART era, lipodystrophy has become the utmost portrayal of the abject by blurring the lines between body and self, self and other, sick and healthy, concealed and exposed, visibility and (in)visibility.

Based on the work of Julia Kristeva (1982), we understand that 'it is not lack of cleanliness or health that causes abjection but what disturbs identity, system, order [and] what does not respect borders, positions, rules' – 'the in-between, the ambiguous, the composite' (1982: 4). The lipodystrophy syndrome (as the symbol of HIV/AIDS) disturbs the construction of self by engraving itself onto the surface of the skin, thus making it impossible to erase, expel or reject – impossible to maintain a '*Self propre*' (Holmes et al. 2006). In addition, the physical manifestations of HAART causes a dismemberment of the social body by making HIV/AIDS visible and consequently, by reiterating the dangerousness of the social encounter. As such, lipodystrophy defies the normative boundaries that govern the way bodies are presented and represented in society.

The lines between the sick and the healthy are no longer existent because contrarily to the pre-HAART era, the physical manifestations of HIV/AIDS are now symbolic of an optimal control of the virus. Therefore, people living with HIV/AIDS find themselves in an in-between position because their health is contained within a sick body, one that disrupts the rules that dictate the position of the sick and the healthy in society. Furthermore, the presence of lipodystrophy reveals the 'ambiguous capacity' (Persson 2004: 46) of antiretroviral agents or the 'capacity to be beneficial and detrimental to the same person at the same time' (Persson 2004: 49). It also demonstrates how the incorporation of biotechnologies (medications) is an ambiguous process – 'lipodystrophy is a striking example of a particular biotechnical inscription being processed and redistributed by a body in unintended ways' (Persson 2004: 54). In light of this interpretive analysis, it is argued that the physical manifestations of HAART transform the body and the Self by constructing the *Other*, an object of abjection which is internalized and embodied by people living with HIV/AIDS – thus, managing the *Other* within the self appears to be the only way to regain a sense of integrity and autonomy.

References

Ahmed, S. 1998. Animated borders: skin, colour and tanning, in *Vital Signs: Feminist Reconfiguration of the Biological Body*, edited by M. Shildrick and J. Price. Edinburgh: Edinburgh University Press, 45–65.

Alonzo, A.A. and Reynolds, R.N. 1995. Stigma, HIV and AIDS: an exploration and elaboration of a stigma trajectory. *Social Science & Medicine*, 41(3), 303–315.

Carr, A. et al. 1998. A syndrome of peripheral lipodystrophy, hyperlipidaemia and insulin resistance in patients receiving HIV protease inhibitors. *AIDS*, 12(7), F51–F58.

Chapman, E. 2000. Conceptualization of the body for people living with HIV: issues of touch and contamination. *Sociology of Health & Illness*, 22(6), 840–857.

Charmaz, K. 1995. The body, identity, and self: adapting to impairment. *The Sociological Quarterly*, 36(4), 657–680.

Collins, E., Wagner, C. and Waimsley, S. 2000. Psychosocial impact of the lipodystrophy syndrome in HIV. *AIDS Read*, 10(9), 546–551.

Cregan, K. 2006. *The Sociology of the Body*. London: Sage Publications.

Gadow, S. 1982. Body and Self, in *The Humanity of the Ill: Phenomenological Perspectives*, edited by V. Kestenbaum. Knoxville: The University of Tennessee Press, 86–100.

Gagnon, M. and Holmes, D. 2008. Moving beyond the biomedical standpoint: broadening our understanding of the experience of lipodystrophy in people living with HIV/AIDS. *Research and Theory for Nursing Practice*, 22(4), 228–240.

Goffman, E. 1963. *Stigma: Notes on the Management of Spoiled Identity*. New Jersey: Prentice-Hall Inc.

Grinspoon, S. and Carr, A. 2005. Cardiovascular risk and body-fat abnormalities in HIV-infected adults. *New England Journal of Medicine*, 352, 48–62.

Holmes, D., Perron, A. and O'Byrne, P. 2006. Understanding disgust in nursing: abjection, self and the Other. *Research and Theory for Nursing Practice*, 20(4), 305–316.

Jensen, A.L. and Allen, N.M. 1996. Meta-synthesis of qualitative findings. *Qualitative Health Research*, 6(4), 553–560.

Kristeva, J. 1982. *Powers of Horror: An Essay on Abjection*. New York: Columbia University Press.

Leder, D. 1990. *The Absent Body*. Chicago: The Chicago University Press.

Link, B.G. and Phelan, J.C. 2001. Conceptualizing stigma. *Annual Review of Sociology*, 27, 363–85.

Murphy, S.J. 1995. *The Constructed Body: AIDS, Reproductive Technology, and Ethics*. New York: State University of New York Press.

Persson, A. 2004. Incorporating pharmakon: HIV, medicine, and body shape change. *Body & Society*, 10(4), 45–67.

Persson, A. 2005. Facing HIV: body shape change and the (in)visibility of illness. *Medical Anthropology*, 24, 237–264.

Power, R., Tate, L.H. and Taylor, C. 2003. A qualitative study of the psychosocial implications of lipodystrophy syndrome on HIV positive individuals. *Sexually Transmitted Infections*, 79, 137–141.

Reynolds, N.R. et al. 2006. Balancing disfigurement and fear of disease progression: patient perceptions of HIV body fat redistribution. *AIDS Care*, 18(7), 663–673.

Shildrick, M. 2002. *Embodying the Monster: Encounters with the Vulnerable Self*. London: Sage Publications.

Sontag, S. 1989. *AIDS and Its Metaphors*. New York: Farrar, Strauss & Giroux.

Tate, H. and George, R. 2001. The effect of weight loss on body image in HIV-positive gay men. *AIDS Care*, 13(2), 163–169.

Varas-Diaz, N., Toro-Alfonso, J. and Serrano-García, I. 2005. My body, my stigma: body interpretations in a sample of people living with HIV/AIDS in Puerto Rico. *The Qualitative Report*, 10(1), 122–142.

Walsh, D. and Downe, S. 2006. Appraising the quality of qualitative research. *Midwifery*, 22, 108–119.

Wendell, S. 1996. *The Rejected Body. Feminist Philosophical Reflections on Disability*. New York: Routledge.

Chapter 9

'She Exists Within Me': Subjectivity, Embodiment and the World's First Facial Transplant

Marc Lafrance

Introduction

On 27 November 2005, the first partial face transplant was carried out on 38-year-old French woman Isabelle Dinoire. Disfigured by a dog bite, Dinoire underwent the 15-hour operation in the city of Amiens under the care of doctors Bernard Devauchelle and Jean-Michel Dubernard. While the circumstances surrounding Dinoire's operation were widely reported by news outlets around the world, the most authoritative account of them is presented in Noëlle Châtelet's 300-page book *Le baiser d'Isabelle: L'aventure de la première greffe du visage*. Based on interviews with the patient and the many specialists who treated her, *Le baiser d'Isabelle* tells Dinoire's surgical story. In what follows, I conduct a close reading of this story by considering the events that took place before, during and after Dinoire's formidable facial reconstruction. Drawing on a variety of social and cultural theories, I examine how Dinoire's 'personal troubles' are bound up with a number of 'public issues' relating to subjectivity, embodiment and the medical management of health (Mills 1959). In the end, I argue that to fully understand the implications of Dinoire's face transplant, we must be prepared to rethink and refigure what it means to be human in an age of advanced biotechnology.

The Events Leading up to the First Facial Transplant

As the first book to chronicle Isabelle Dinoire's facial transplant operation, *Le baiser d'Isabelle* has been widely read and reviewed across the world. Often invoking images reminiscent of Homer's *Odyssey* and Ovid's *Metamorphoses*, Châtelet's prose has an epic feel to it. Indeed, for Châtelet, the first facial transplant operation can be seen as a stately ship setting sail for the first time in waters as deep as they are dangerous. And while *Le baiser d'Isabelle* is, without a doubt, a sentimental story of Dinoire's surgical trajectory, both the grandeur and the gravitas that characterize it are to some extent understandable. After all, facial transplants have major implications: on the one hand, they have the potential to dramatically improve the lives of those who suffer from facial disfigurement; on the other hand, however, they threaten to reshape our relationships to our bodies and the bodies of others in ways we cannot predict or control. Put slightly differently, facial transplants force both the individual and the collective to reflect on the subjective stakes bound up in bodily parts and processes – to reflect, in other words, on who owns these parts and processes, on what they represent and on how they ought to be managed by those in the fields of medicine and science.

As I have already mentioned, Isabelle Dinoire was disfigured when she was brought to hospital in the summer of 2005. She had been mauled by her dog and, as a result, no longer had a nose, a mouth or a chin. At a press conference in February 2006, Dinoire – as she is cited by Chatelêt (2007) – explains the circumstances surrounding the mauling:

> The 27th of May, after a very difficult week, with many personal worries, I took some medication to forget. Then, I fainted and fell on the ground against a piece of furniture. When I woke up, I tried to light a cigarette and I did not understand why it was not staying between my lips. It was then that I saw the pool of blood and the dog beside it! I went to see myself in the mirror, and then, I could not believe what I was seeing. It was too horrible (14–15)[1].

What Dinoire saw in the mirror that night was, to put it crudely, a head without a face. Though her forehead and her eyes were still intact, her other facial features were gone. What she was left with was, according to Dinoire, 'the head of a dead person' and 'the face of a monster' (36). Dinoire was in critical condition – both physically and mentally. And while the physical threats to her survival were real, it was the mental threats that appear to have preoccupied her most profoundly. Alone and confined in the discomfiting quiet of her hospital room, Dinoire describes her state of mind as follows: 'I was so in another world. Without a doubt, I had lost my sense of time, of things, of reality. I no longer knew who I was. […] I cried in despair. I saw no exit.' (37)

Dinoire was at this point in her life 'a dissocialized woman': her cognitive functioning was limited, her linguistic capacities were minimal and her ability to interact with others had all but disappeared (210). In brief, Dinoire's 'psychic machine' had stopped (42). While Dinoire was surely suffering from some form of traumatic shock in the days and weeks following her admission to hospital, her large-scale incapacitation suggests nevertheless that crises of embodiment are closely connected to crises of subjectivity. In fact, the mental disintegration that followed Dinoire's physical disfigurement indicates that human beings not only rely on but require a special kind of corporeal coherence in order to function happily and healthily. This coherence is, according to Anzieu (1995), Dolto (1984), Lacan (1977), Merleau-Ponty (1945) and Schilder (1978), derived from

---

1   Unless otherwise specified, all citations by Isabelle Dinoire are from *Le baiser d'Isabelle*. All translations are my own.

what has come to be known as the body image. Poised somewhere between mind and body, the body image is crucially constitutive of how we view, understand and quite literally 'make sense' of ourselves. Not only does it enable us to marshal the many perceptions and sensations that impinge on our bodies, but it serves as what Anzieu calls the 'bedrock' or 'foundation' of our minds (61). The body image is, therefore, the sensory-perceptual apparatus in and through which the workings of cognition, language and memory are established and secured.

With this in view, it could be argued that Dinoire's inability to think, speak and interact in the period following her disfigurement was caused – at least in part – by the spectacular collapse of her body image. That said, the question remains as to why her disfigurement caused such a collapse. To answer this question, it is worth looking more closely at Schilder's (1978) work. For Schilder, the body image can be understood as an internal map of the body's parts and processes as they are lived and experienced. Not unlike the 'cortical homunculus' (Grosz 1993: 33–5), the body image consists primarily of the parts and processes to which the subject is most exposed and in which he or she is most invested; for this reason, genitals, hands and faces tend to be among its most prominent features.[2] The face in particular is a psychically-charged part of the soma insofar as it is almost always on show and is vitally bound up with the acts of eating, speaking and – as the title of Châtelet's book suggests – kissing. It is surprising, then, that Châtelet makes no mention of the body image when she is describing Dinoire's early days in the Amiens hospital.[3]

Above and beyond what it says about body image, the mental disintegration that followed Dinoire's physical disfigurement tells us that a continuous skin surface is central to how we relate to both our own faces and the faces of others. As brought into relief by Anzieu's (1995) model of the skin ego and Lacan's (1977) notion of the mirror phase, the continuity of the skin's surface is vital to the subject's sense of wholeness – even if, as Lacan argues, this wholeness is illusory. Indeed, the fact that Dinoire fell to pieces after she was bitten by her dog suggests that our deep dependence on the skin's continuity is only revealed to us when this continuity fails. For Leder (1990), failures of this sort are emblematic of what he calls 'bodily dysappearance'; that is, a state in which our awareness of our bodies becomes acute and excessive. We experience bodily dysappearance as 'that which stands in the way, an obstinate force interfering with our projects' (84). No longer an embodied subject, Dinoire was – in her pre-operative state – 'just a body' (Davis 2003: 16).

After weeks of isolation, Dinoire was approached by the hospital's maxilla-facial microsurgeon Bernard Devauchelle. Devauchelle explained to Dinoire that the standard medical protocol in cases like these consists of skin

---

2   See Grosz (1993: 33–6, 62–86) for a discussion of how notions like the body image and the cortical homunculus are both implicitly and explicitly gendered.

3   Interestingly, the clinical literature on acquired disfigurement is similarly inattentive to questions of body image (Pruzinsky 2004).

graft surgeries. To carry out such surgeries, the doctors harvest coetaneous tissue from other parts of the body in an attempt to rebuild something resembling a face. The operations are long, painful and, above all, numerous. Dinoire could expect, according to Devauchelle, a minimum of ten operations and a result that would likely be deeply disappointing. There was, however, another surgical procedure – one yet to be performed – that Dinoire could consider: a partial facial transplant. Owing to both her age and the particularities of her wounds, she was – according to Devauchelle – the perfect candidate. Dinoire accepted, arguing that the facial transplant was her only hope for a normal life. Indeed, according to Chatelêt, Dinoire was 'effervescent' about the operation and was fully aware of the risks associated with it (87).

There is no good reason to doubt that Dinoire consented fully and freely to the transplant. That said, however, there is something slightly disturbing about the frequency with which *Le baiser d'Isabelle* presents us with statements like 'There was no other solution' (51) and 'She did not have a choice' (59). In my view, the frequency of such statements raises a number of questions about the conditions under which Dinoire consented to the operation. Shildrick (2008a) raises similar questions in her discussion of the world's first heart transplant recipient Louis Washkansky. More specifically, Shildrick wonders about the extent to which Washkansky – who survived for a mere 18 days after his operation – understood himself in the same way his surgeons did: that is, as a research subject. While it seems fairly clear that Dinoire was aware of the fact that she was and still is a research subject, ethical questions remain. For instance, was the prospect of living differently – that is, with a disfigured face – presented to her as a legitimate course of action? What sort of medical care was she promised if she agreed to the transplant and how did it compare to the care she would have received if she had opted for a more conventional form of facial reconstruction? And, finally, how did her well-documented depression and the feelings of worthlessness that accompanied it play into her decision to move forward with the operation – an operation that was likely presented to her as a courageous act that would secure for her a place in medical history? On all of these questions, *Le baiser d'Isabelle* is silent.

Over the course of the period leading up to her transplant surgery, Dinoire attempted to reintegrate herself into society. This reintegration was thwarted, however, by the fact that she now occupied what Châtelet describes as a space between the human and the inhuman. While Dinoire was, of course, human in the days and weeks preceding the operation, her interactions with those around her made her feel otherwise. That is, without a recognisably human face, she lost her ability to live as a recognisably human subject. The constant stares, the punishing gazes and the manifestations of fear and disgust were enough to make Dinoire feel like she was living without – rather than within – the social world. While over time she learned to, as Goffman (1959) puts it, manage the impressions of those around her by wearing a surgical mask, this too had its problems insofar as she was now viewed as a source of infection, contagion and contamination. Assumed to have the avian flu or foot and mouth disease, shopkeepers disinfected their shops after she left them and parents urged their children to stay away. With the mask or without it, Dinoire's claim to the category of the human was no longer guaranteed.

The difficulties Dinoire encountered as she attempted to reintegrate herself into society beg the question: why did Dinoire's facial disfigurement cause her to be viewed as inhuman or, as she herself puts it, monstrous? For Shildrick (2002), monstrous bodies are 'those which in their gross failure to approximate corporeal norms are radically excluded' (2). Following Shildrick, Dinoire's dog bite can be seen to have 'transmogrified' her; that is, to have effected a 'strange and grotesque transformation' (Sullivan 2007: 552) that made her unbearable to those around her. Yet the question remains as to why, exactly, the transmogrification was as unbearable as it was. Kristeva's (1982) work on abjection is relevant here. The centrepiece of her developmental model, abjection refers to the process in and through which the infant separates itself from its mother and her body. Before this separation, the infant experiences itself as one and the same as its mother and, as a result, has only the most schematic sense of its own borders and boundaries. To consolidate these borders and boundaries, it must abject its mother and, in doing so, reject its communion with, dependence on and vulnerability to her and her body. 'The abject confronts us', explains Kristeva, '[…] with our earliest attempts to release the hold of the maternal entity even before ex-isting outside of her, thanks to the autonomy of language. It is a violent, clumsy breaking away, with the constant risk of falling back under the sway of a power as securing as it is stifling.'(13) As Kristeva's explanation makes clear, the abject relates to that which threatens the boundaries of inside and outside, self and other, subject and object. As she herself puts it: 'It is […] not lack of cleanliness or health that causes abjection but what disturbs identity, system, order. What does not respect borders, positions, rules. The in-between, the ambiguous, the composite.'(4) Kristeva's work on abjection allows us to gain some insight into why Dinoire's disfigured body was, both to herself and those around her, a monstrous body. Indeed, Dinoire's messy, leaky and – above all – flayed face was monstrous because it was abject; or, put slightly differently, because it did not conform to the requirements of normative embodiment which – as Shildrick (2002) points out – are predicated on containment and protection. Shildrick explains:

> Against an ideal of bodily closure that relies on the singular, the unified and the replicable, monstrosity, in the form of either excess, lack or displacement, offers gross insult. For the most part, inevitably, such monstrosity is manifest as surface phenomena in which the skin itself as putative boundary of the self's clean and proper body … may be compromised both in form and structure (162).

For Shildrick, monstrosity is characterized first and foremost by the abject – that is, by that which disrupts the notions of separation and distinction that underlie Western understandings of the autonomous self. Like Shildrick, I argue that Dinoire's disfigurement was disturbing because it exposed her body – and, by extension, all bodies – as open and vulnerable to the other. In fact, Dinoire's disfigurement revealed the extent to which all bodies are 'animal, mortal, material' and that 'there are no clear or impenetrable or unbreached borders between what [they] are and what [they] reject, between what [they] expel and what [they] contain' (Covino 2004: 4). Hence, insofar as it called into question the sovereignty of the subject, Dinoire's flayed face made clear that we are all bound up in both our own abjection and the abjection of the other.

The persistence with which Châtelet portrays Dinoire's transplant as a kind of 'rehumanization' raises other questions about what we understand – both individually and collectively – by the term human. As Dinoire's pre-operative experiences show, and as Butler (2004) argues, qualifying as a human in our society requires more than physical aliveness. Instead, it requires a range of fairly specific physical traits including, but not limited to, a continuous skin surface and a finite number of facial features. When these traits are not present in the way subjects and societies expect them to be, the humanness of the human is called into question. While, for many of us, feeling human is part and parcel of what Garfinkel (1967) calls the 'natural attitude', the anxiety awakened by our encounters with monstrosity suggests that we have, at the very least, an unconscious awareness of our own potential for it. Indeed, because Dinoire's disfigurement was confined to her face – leaving the rest of her body intact – it very vividly revealed this potential. It could be argued, then, that it was the intimate inmixing of the 'monstrous' and the 'human' that made Dinoire's disfigurement especially excruciating for those around her. Shildrick (2002) explains:

> So long as the monstrous remains the absolute other in its corporeal difference it poses few problems; in other words, it is so distanced in its difference that it can clearly be put into an oppositional category or not-me. Once, however, it begins to resemble those of us who lay claim to the primary term of identity, or to reflect back aspects of ourselves that are repressed, then its indeterminate status – neither wholly self nor wholly other – becomes deeply disturbing (2–3).

While Dinoire was slowly starting to resume her life, Devauchelle had assembled an enormous team of surgeons, immunologists, haematologists, dermatologists, anaesthesiologists, prosthesiologists, endocrinologists, physiotherapists and psychiatrists. Yet before Devauchelle's team could proceed with the transplant, it needed to gain permission from the state's *Agence de la biomédicine*. Of course, this approval was not guaranteed; after all, as Châtelet makes clear, facial transplants represent a sort of double transgression in contemporary Western societies: that is, a transgression not only of conventional medical practices, but of our most basic understandings of and relationships to the human self and the human body. Given the admittedly high stakes of the operation, Devauchelle's team and, perhaps most importantly, Devauchelle's patient, had to be beyond reproach. It is, therefore, not surprising that a scandal erupted when the press began probing the circumstances surrounding Dinoire's disfigurement. Important questions started to emerge: Why did Dinoire take as many pills as she did on the night her dog mauled her? Was she trying to commit suicide? And if she was trying to commit suicide, how could any state-sponsored ethics committee recommend a psychologically unstable woman for an operation that promises to be an epic challenge on physical, psychological and social levels? Though neither the book nor the media reports elucidate exactly how these questions were handled by Devauchelle and his team, it is – in my view – not insignificant that Dinoire's psychiatrist refused to frame her patient's state of mind in suicidal terms. Châtelet explains:

> For the psychiatrist, the term "suicidal" is to be used with caution. She prefers the term "voluntary medicinal intoxication." Medicinal intoxication relates to those patients who, feeling bad at a certain moment, abused medication prescribed to them by their doctor (antianxielytics, antidepressants) to feel better. Maybe they are searching more for an artificially prolonged sleep than for an absolute death. This is how she interprets Isabelle's act – the one on which we have long dwelled (41).

Regardless of whether this framing of Dinoire's psychological state was accurate, it was – without a doubt – crucial for those hoping to perform the transplant operation. In fact, when Devauchelle and his colleagues were faced with repeated questions about whether Dinoire had intended to commit suicide on the night she was injured, they all steadfastly denied it and, in doing so, adopted the same framing as the psychiatrist. Interestingly, however, when Dinoire herself is given the chance to speak, she is emphatic about the fact that suicide was not far from her mind on the night of the life-altering incident. For instance, when Dinoire finds out – shortly after the surgery – that the brain-dead woman whose face she received had herself committed suicide, she clearly and compellingly identifies her own trajectory with that of the deceased. Though Châtelet does not at any point admit that Dinoire was suicidal on the night of the accident, the first-person testimonies she includes in *Le baiser d'Isabelle* suggest that this was very much the case. Dinoire explains: 'I found out from the journalists that she had committed suicide. It was one month after the transplant. Somewhere, we were connecting. Two attempts saved one of us. It is strange to know that she wanted to die like me. Strange to know that it is she who saved me.' (261) Following Foucault (1963), then, the state's framing of Dinoire's psychological profile can be seen as a concrete instance of the medical apparatus producing human subjectivity in a particular way in order to organize certain kinds of bodies and authorize certain forms of knowledge production and clinical practice.

The *Agence de la biomédecine* approved the surgery on four conditions: first, the removal of the facial graft must not interfere with the removal of other organs; second, the brain-dead donor's face must be reconstructed after the graft is removed; third, the patient and the donor's family must receive psychological follow-up; and fourth, all of the doctors involved in the operation be involved freely and voluntarily. On the one hand, these conditions bear out Foucault's

(1976) claim that the modern-day medical apparatus is more productive than repressive – or, put slightly differently, that it exercises power over its subjects by managing life rather than by threatening death. On the other hand, however, these conditions suggest that the state is – at the very least – uncomfortable with its role in facial transplant surgeries. More specifically, these conditions show that the state is anxious to make the evidence of the grafting process disappear as well as to ensure that it is not endangering the mental or physical lives of anyone connected to the transplant operation – be they the patient, the donor's family or the doctors performing the operation. Implicit in these conditions, then, is the recognition that what is being removed from one body and put in another is not just a 'spare part'; it is, instead, a substantive being with a history and, perhaps more importantly, an identity of its own.

The World's First Facial Transplant

Having found a donor with a skin tone that resembled Dinoire's, and satisfied that they could live up to all of the ethical conditions, the medical team went to work. Not surprisingly, the transplant procedure was multifaceted and involved a number of enormously intricate parts. To start, the surgical team harvested bone marrow cells from the donor and injected them into the recipient in order to both acquaint the recipient's body with the immunological make-up of the donor's body and reduce the chance that the graft would be refused. Shortly thereafter, the team removed the donor's facial skin, nose, lips and chin. With the graft quite literally in hand, it was put in a sterile bag, kept in a sub-zero container and transported to the hospital where Dinoire would be undergoing her operation. Before leaving the donor, however, the team's prosthesiologists reconstructed her face so that there would be no visible traces of the harvest. Once the donor's bodily integrity had been restored – or rather, once the donor's bodily integrity appeared to have been restored – Dinoire's operation could proceed. And proceed it did: after over 15 hours of surgery, Devauchelle and his team had successfully transplanted the donor's face on to Dinoire's.

Though those who knew her before the incident claimed that she was entirely recognizable, there can be no doubt that her face changed in and through the operation. Her original face had a wide, tilted nose, a prominent chin and thin lips. The donated face, however, has given her a straight and narrow nose, a neater chin and a fuller mouth. When she appeared in public shortly after the operation, it was clear that Dinoire had partial control over the transplanted muscles. Though she could speak, she was unable – at this point – to close her mouth fully. One year following the transplant, Dinoire could eat, drink and speak with ease; she could close her mouth and smile; and, as Devauchelle points out in several interviews, her scar was less prominent. Owing perhaps to the fact that it represents the border between old face and new face, Dinoire's transplant scar appears to have preoccupied many – including Châtelet – a great deal. Emphasizing the

near-perfect skin-tone match between donor and patient, Châtelet seems to want
to subdue the anxieties Dinoire's scar awakens; after all, the transplant scar is a
stunning testament not only to the abject meeting of two bodies but to the hybrid
alterity that such a meeting represents. In my view, these anxieties may account
for why Châtelet insists – again and again – on the fact that the continuity between
the two skin tones is 'stupefying' and 'magnificent' (200).

The operation was, of course, heralded as a great success. That said, however,
Châtelet's portrayal of this success is paradoxical. At times, she portrays it as a
triumph of surgical medicine and its specialized division of labour while, at others,
she portrays it as a miracle. That these paradoxical portrayals run alongside one
another, not only in the book but in a large number of media reports, suggests that
modern Western societies are not content to view Dinoire's operation in strictly
scientific terms. Instead, it suggests that these societies long for what Weber (1978)
calls an 'enchantment of the life-world' – that is, a life-world in which magic and
mystery persist alongside scientific rationality. Indeed, Châtelet's concomitant and
contradictory invocation of both science and magic is brought into relief not only
by her representations of Dinoire, but by those of the donor. Consider, for instance,
her description of how the prosthesiologist reconstructs the donor's face so that,
even after the graft is harvested, she will look like herself:

> Dumbstruck, everyone looks at face that Anthony has made manifest. It is a
> face, it is the face of the donor. It is... the face just as it was before! Anthony is
> himself moved by this little miracle of which he is the creator. With the silicone,
> he fills the hole of the tube in the crux of the neck. He would also be ready, if
> asked, to erase all of the gashes on the body with the rest of his silicon, in order
> to give back to the donor the appearance of dignity so necessary to her dignity.
> The bringing into being of this restored face is an act of giving life, yes. He
> experiences it as a gratifying birth (182–183).

As with many other representations of surgical medicine (Blum 2003), then,
those associated with Dinoire's facial reconstruction suggest that modern Western
societies remain attached to and invested in the notions of magic, miracle and
mystery even as they contemplate the immensely intellectualized initiative that is
the facial transplant operation.[4]

The Events Following the First Face Transplant

Now in possession of a complete face that – with skilfully applied make-up
– betrayed only the most minor traces of surgical intervention, Dinoire seemed
well-placed to resume a normal life. Yet despite the fact that the operation was

4   See Corning (2003), Gura (2002) and Rosenberg (1990) for examples of other
studies that use the rhetoric of magic and the language of science simultaneously.

intended, at least in the long-term, to give Dinoire a normal life, in the short-term it did anything but this. Though she was no longer as disfigured as she had been before the surgery, there was now another formidable force interfering with her ability to assimilate back into everyday social life: the news and tabloid media. In fact, the media were so aggressive in their pursuit of Dinoire that she, once again, had to remain secluded in hospital. To remedy the situation, Devauchelle decided to hold a press conference, for it became clear that such a conference would be the only way of subduing the frenzy that had been created by the operation. According to Châtelet, Devauchelle and his colleagues were uncomfortable with the press conference as it compromised the confidentiality so central to transplant protocols. Unlike those who treated her, however, Dinoire was resigned to the fact that she would have to go public: 'Over time I realized that it would no longer be anonymous' explains Dinoire, 'that we would no longer have the choice, because of the media'(141). That Dinoire and Devauchelle felt that they had no choice but to involve the media in this process once again bears out Foucault's (1976) claim that we live in a society that demands of its subjects extensive confessions relating to the body – confessions that constitute, in the collective imagination at least, a kind of master-key to the so-called truth of the human being. Similarly, Dinoire's intuitive sense that she had no choice but to show herself to media forces and allow them to participate in her recovery process suggests, as Heyes (2007) does, that these forces are playing an increasingly significant role in how subjects understand, relate to and produce themselves as embodied subjects (89–111). Indeed, unlike the Washkansky case discussed by Shildrick (2008a), the lack of confidentiality in the Dinoire case was driven not by medical forces but by media forces – forces which appear, in the early postmillennium, to have an increasingly insatiable appetite for surgical spectacles (Brooks 2004, Tait 2007).

At this point, it was not only the media that prevented Dinoire from resuming the normal life of which she had dreamed for months: there was the constant physical therapy aimed at reanimating facial muscles, the taxing life-long immunosuppressant medication required for the graft to survive and, perhaps most importantly, the vexatious question of who she was now that she had the skin and bones of another within herself. Though she was urged by the team of psychologists and psychiatrists assigned to her case to 'appropriate' these new body parts – that is, to integrate them straightforwardly into her sense of self – Dinoire was ambivalent about doing so. Interestingly, Châtelet does not reflect in any meaningful way on the implications of this ambivalence – opting instead to focus on the benefits of the procedure and how they have enabled Dinoire to resume a more fulfilling life. The fact that Châtelet chooses not to reflect on Dinoire's ambivalence is, however, unsurprising given that she too appears to be ambivalent about Dinoire's new face. While, in some instances, she is eager to reassure us that the operation was a perfectly rational scientific pursuit necessitated by dire events, in others, she cannot help but dwell on the 'strangeness' of the operation and the hybrid human being it has created (20). Regardless of Chatelêt's framing, there is a wealth of material in *Le baiser d'Isabelle* that – when read critically – provides some insight into the sorts of crises of subjectivity that can and often do ensue when the body of the other is surgically introduced into the body of the self. Consider, for instance, Dinoire's early experiences with her new mouth:

> And then inside, there was a sensation. It did not belong to me. It was soft. It was atrocious. It was, I do not know whether it is right to say this, it was disgusting. When I think about it, the hardest thing to accept, was this: having the inside of the mouth of someone else. ... I had said it to Sylvie: "It is all soft!" "That is normal," she responded. It was as though it had no life. It really was a foreign body. To touch that with the tongue ... (239).

Here Dinoire makes clear that her new mouth is, at least in the beginning, abject to her. Interestingly, Dinoire attributes this abjection to precisely the sorts of disconcerting combinations described by Kristeva and her interlocutors; namely, those of self and other, fluidity and solidity, animate flesh and inanimate flesh. It is, moreover, not surprising that the mouth is the first and foremost site of Dinoire's abjection. After all, the mouth is – to use Shildrick's (2002) term – a vulnerable space insofar as it is an orifice that opens us up to others. Similarly, the mouth is – as Freud (2001) claims – a cathected space insofar as it bears the traces of early infantile dependence and erogeneity. And finally, the mouth is – as Dinoire herself points out – an identity-defining space insofar as it serves as the seat of speech and personal expression. As the most intimate and immediate point of exchange between the 'me' and the 'not-me', Dinoire's experiences of abject orality can be seen to crystallize the kinds of corporeal complexities bound up with facial transplant surgeries.

Like the inside of her new mouth, the hair that grows out of her new chin is cause for consternation on Dinoire's part. Given that it is – quite literally – a living memory of the other and her body, it too blurs the boundaries between the subjective and the objective. Dinoire explains: 'I had never had a hair grow out of my chin. I knew it was mine but at the same time "she" is there. I am making her live, but that hair is hers.'(Allen 2007: 1) Dinoire makes similar remarks about her new nose which, as she puts it, is not really 'her nose' but rather 'a nose' (248). Yet despite these occasional references to her new chin and her new nose, it is her new mouth that appears to pain and perplex her most. Could this pain and perplexity be part of why Dinoire continued, against the advice of each and every doctor, to 'smoke cigarette after cigarette in hiding' (Allen 2007: 1)? Dinoire was, as Devauchelle makes clear, well-aware of the awesome risks associated with such a habit. And yet she smoked anyway. While Devauchelle links her smoking to stress, I would argue that it can be linked it to something else – something more along the lines of an intricate negotiation between new self and old self. In fact, if like Abraham (1927) and Klein (1986) we view aggression exercized in and through the mouth as one of the most elemental forms of sadism, then Dinoire's smoking can be seen as the old self resisting – even punishing – the new self. Alternatively, Dinoire's smoking can be seen as an attempt to unite the new self and the old self;

that is, to make the new self one with the old self by forcing the former to engage in the latter's habit. Either way, it strikes me that Dinoire's decision to continue smoking cannot be reduced to stress-related issues; instead, it must be viewed as psychically complex and somatically fraught.

If at moments Dinoire appears to be anxious about her new facial features, at others she appears to be calm and contemplative about them. That is, it is when Dinoire abandons the spare parts model and acknowledges her hybridity that she seems most at peace with her transplant. 'I appropriated it insofar as it is I who manage to make it move,' explains Dinoire. 'Forget it, no. I don't want to and I won't. She exists in me. She will always be in me and she will always be a part of me. She is my saviour, like a twin sister. Yes, it can only be this way.' (261–2) Dinoire's insistence that she now has a hybrid body was criticized by those in her medical entourage. Some viewed it as primitive, simplistic and ultimately untenable, while others saw it as injurious to her mental health. As she herself suggests, the doctors would have much preferred that she adopt the spare parts model and, by extension, understand her new face as hers and hers alone. According to the doctors, this sort of understanding would pre-empt psychological confusion and better allow Dinoire to orient herself psychically, somatically and socially. Dinoire declares:

> For me, it is something obvious. They would have preferred that I forget it, yes. For them, the doctors, all of them, it is easier. But me, I know that her part is there. It will never be my nose and my mouth. […] For the doctors, it should be integrated, but it remains a part that is not mine. I don't know. It's hard to explain. What I know, is that I don't want anyone to damage it, given the donation the donor offered me. It is something too big. Now I am fighting for two! (264–265).

That Dinoire felt pressured to embrace the spare parts model is evidenced by the fact that when she is at the press conference – surrounded by the specialists who treated her – she adopts a rhetorical tone that departs considerably from the one that characterizes the excerpts presented above. 'No, there is no comparison between the face I have today and the one I had before' explains Dinoire, 'but this face belongs to me. […] What did I say when I saw my reconstructed face? Thank you.'(22) Unlike this last excerpt, those presented earlier make clear that Dinoire was neither willing nor able to straightforwardly adopt the spare parts model. Nor was she willing to relinquish the knowledge that her new body parts had their own history and their own identity. Instead, Dinoire chose to welcome the other into herself; an other whom she would protect, defend and, most importantly, remember. By refusing to abject this other, Dinoire brings to life not only the radically intercorporeal being described by Merleau-Ponty (1945) but the radically concorporeal being described by Shildrick (2002).

The dualist epistemology characteristic of Western medicine in particular and Western society in general has trained many, if not most, of us to think that it would be easier for Dinoire to live her new life if she could manage to forget about her donor and, by extension, repress the abject parts of herself. Yet new research at the intersection of cultural theory and critical health theory suggests otherwise. Consider, for instance, recent work by Shildrick (2008a, 2008b) on heart transplants and the patients who undergo them. On the basis of anecdotal evidence, Shildrick suggests that heart transplant patients who adopt the spare parts model might have a different prognosis than those who do not. More specifically, she argues that for the patients who do adopt this model, recovery can start off quick but end up lethal. Like Shildrick's work on heart transplants, my work on face transplants suggests that dominant conceptions of subjectivity and embodiment are not altogether adequate for making sense of what takes place when organs are taken from one and given to another. To make sense of this phenomenon, our understandings of the human being must call into question the rigid boundaries between self and other which continue to define and delimit our most fundamental sense of who we are. Indeed, to gain a wide-ranging understanding of facial transplants and their many implications, we need far-reaching conceptual tools that enable us to see the self as crucially constituted by the other. What is more, we need to dispense with the idea that the mind is the seat of the self and the body is a set of exchangeable and replaceable parts. While the spare parts model continues to dominate present-day surgical paradigms, the fears, fantasies and anxieties that pervade Chatelêt's *Le baiser d'Isabelle* suggest that this model is insufficient for making sense of what happens – both privately and publicly – when one's body parts are replaced with those of an other.

References

Abraham, K. 1927. *Selected Papers*. London: Hogarth.

Allen, P. 2007. Isabelle Dinoire may never kiss again. *The Daily Telegraph* [Online, 1 October 2007] Available at: http://www.telegraph.co.uk/news/main. jhtml?xml=/news/2007/10/01/wface101.xml). [accessed: 4 August 2009].

Anzieu, D. 1995. *Le moi-peau.* 2nd edition. Paris: Dunod.

Blum, V. 2003. *Flesh Wounds: The Culture of Cosmetic Surgery*. Los Angeles: University of California Press.

Brooks, A. 2004. Under the knife and proud of it: an analysis of the normalization of cosmetic surgery. *Critical Sociology*, 30(2), 207–39.

Butler, J. 2004. Doing justice to someone: sex reassignment and allegories of transsexuality, in *Undoing Gender*. New York: Routledge, 57–75.

Châtelet, N. 2007. *Le baiser d'Isabelle: L'aventure de la première greffe du visage*. Paris: Seuil.

Corning, P. 2003. *Nature's Magic: Synergy in Evolution and Fate of Humankind.* Cambridge: Cambridge University Press.

Covino, D.C. 2004. *Amending the Abject Body: Aesthetic Makeovers in Medicine and Culture*. Albany, NY: State University of New York Press.

Davis, K. 2003. *Dubious Equalities and Embodied Differences: Cultural Studies on Cosmetic Surgery*. Lanham, MD: Roman and Littlefield.

Dolto, F. 1984. *L'image inconscient du corps*. Paris: Seuil.

Foucault, M. 1963. *Naissance de la clinique*. Paris: Gallimard.

Foucault, M. 1976. *La volonté de savoir: L'histoire de la sexualité – Volume 1*. Paris: Gallimard.

Freud, S. 2001. Three essays on the theory of sexuality, in *The Standard Edition of the Complete Works of Sigmund Freud – Volume 7,* edited by J. Strachey. London: Vintage and Hogarth Press, 125–244.

Garfinkel, H. 1967. *Studies in Ethnomethodology*. Englewood Cliffs, NJ: Prentice Hall.

Goffman, E. 1959. *The Presentation of Self in Everyday Life*. Doubleday: New York.

Grosz, E. 1993. *Volatile Bodies: Toward a Corporeal Feminism*. Bloomington: Indiana University Press.

Gura, T. 2002. Therapeutic antibodies: magic bullets hit the target. *Nature: International Weekly Journal of Science* [Online, 6 June] Available at: http://www.nature.com/nature/journal/v417/n6889/full/417584a.html [accessed: 29 July 2009].

Heyes, C.J. 2007. *Self-Transformations: Foucault, Ethics and Normalized Bodies*. Oxford: Oxford University Press.

Klein, M. 1986. The psycho-analytic play technique: its history and significance, in *The Selected Melanie Klein,* edited by J. Mitchell. London: Penguin, 35–54.

Kristeva, J. 1982. *Powers of Horror: An Essay on Abjection*. New York: Columbia University Press.

Lacan, J. 1977. Le stade du miroir comme formateur de la fonction du *je* telle qu'elle nous est révélée dans l'expérience psychanalytique, in *Écrits.* Paris: Seuil, 93–100.

Leder, D. 1990. *The Absent Body*. Chicago: Chicago University Press.

Merleau-Ponty, M. 1945. *La phénoménologie de la perception*. Paris: Gallimard.

Mills, C.W. 1959. *The Sociological Imagination*. Oxford: Oxford University Press.

Pruzinsky, T. 2004. Body image adaptation to reconstructive surgery for acquired disfigurement, in *Body Image: A Handbook of Theory, Research and Clinical Practice,* edited by T.F. Cash and T. Pruzinsky. New York: Guilford, 223–41.

Rosenberg, N. 1990. Science, technology and the western miracle. *Scientific America*, 263(5), without pagination.

Schilder, P. 1978. *The Image and Appearance of the Human Body*. New York: International Universities Press.

Shildrick, M. 2002. *Embodying the Monster: Encounters with the Vulnerable Self*. London: Sage.

Shildrick, M. 2008a. The critical turn in feminist bioethics: the case of heart transplantation. *International Journal of Feminist Bioethics*, 1(1), 1–24.

Shildrick, M. 2008b. Corporeal cuts: surgery and the psycho-social. *Body and Society*, 14(1), 31–46.

Sullivan, N. 2007. Transmogrification: (un)becoming others, in *The Transgender Studies Reader*, edited by S. Stryker and S. Whittle. London: Routledge, 552–64.

Tait, S. 2007. Television and the domestication of cosmetic surgery. *Feminist Media Studies*, 7(2), 119–35.

Weber, M. 1978. *Economy and Society: An Outline of Interpretive Sociology*. Berkeley: University of California Press.

Chapter 10

The Abject Body in Requests for Assisted Death: Symptomatic, Dependent, Shameful and Temporal[1]

Annette Street and David Kissane

Introduction

The debates and drama around euthanasia and physician-assisted suicide death are not new (Stolberg 2007). They have raged for years in many industrialized countries confronted with an aging population, the escalation of health costs and an increase in the medicalization of the dying process. These deliberations on assisted death have been conducted on a number of fronts: issues of personal versus social rights (Bishop 2008); questions of theological, ethical or moral significance (Bishop 2008); decisions on medical authority and community values (Byk 2007, Chapple, Ziebland et al. 2006, Franklin, Ternestedt et al. 2006, Ziegler 2009); disputes on the scope of medical intervention, nursing practice and palliation (Miller, Hedlund et al. 2006) and explorations of statements of desire for death (Hudson, Kristjanson et al. 2006, Hudson, Schofield et al. 2006). The discourses that animate these debates are constructed and defended from within social, moral, religious and medical and ethical positions that situate the person requesting assistance to die, either as an autonomous site of human rights, or as someone whose personhood needs medical, nursing, psychological and spiritual care (Melin-Johansson, Odling et al. 2008, Terry, Olson et al. 2006). Missing from these perspectives is a public acknowledgment of the embodied experiences of the person requesting euthanasia and the effects that the decaying, disintegrating, dependant body-self has on the dying person.

Health professionals, particularly nurses, are very aware of the personal and social effects of the dying body but rarely discuss these embodied effects publicly. Unspoken, but potent prohibitions operate to preclude the public discussion of the smell of dying, the visceral experience of bodily disintegration (Lawton 1998, Lupton 2003) or the struggle to retain an intact sense of self (Street 1998). Yet the effects of unacceptable symptoms, fear of dependence and the shame associated

---

1   This chapter is an adaptation of a previously published paper: Street, A. and Kissane, D. 2001. Discourses of the body in euthanasia: symptomatic, dependent, shameful and temporal, *Nursing Inquiry*, 8(3), 162–172.

with a body that is disfigured, smelly and incontinent, impacts on the person as it requires them to accept decreasing control and stigma (Frank 1995). Not all people are able to accept and adjust to this loss of a predictable, controlled, clean and fragrant body (Komaromy 2000). The ongoing level of support for euthanasia (Chapple, Ziebland et al. 2006, Ganzini, Goy et al. 2008, Lindsay 2009, Ziegler 2009) suggests that our care of the dying does not deal well with the issues that concern many people.

The effects of this embodied experience on end-of-life decision-making were apparent in our study of the seven deaths associated with the Australian experience of euthanasia. These deaths have been described in detail elsewhere (Kissane, Street, and Nitschke 1998, Street and Kissane 2000), and it is not the intention of this chapter to re-examine these cases. Nor do we wish to pursue the different sides of the euthanasia debate. Rather our attention here is focused on charting four discourses of the body that shaped the decision-making of those who opted for euthanasia: the symptomatic body, the dependent body, the shameful body and the temporal body.

The texts for this study were structured around a particular moment in Australian history. On 25th May 1995 in Darwin, the Northern Territory Parliament of Australia passed the Rights of the Terminally Ill Act 1995 (ROTI Act) which was enacted on 1st July 1996 and repealed on 25th March 1997 (Northern Territory Government 1995). When the Act came into operation, most media interest was directed at the political process and the sensational stories of five of the seven people who officially sought to use the Act. These five people participated in televised interviews and also published letters and statements in the press. The first two requested euthanasia, but died before the Act became law, four died under the Act and one following its repeal died.

In this chapter the textual analysis is derived from evidence from interviews, letters written by people seeking euthanasia, medical reports, coroner's records and media reports concerning the social experiment of legalized euthanasia in Australia. We have chosen to identify the names of five people in the series of seven as they had already identified themselves publicly through appearances on national television and letters to the print media. Their cases have gained international recognition. Their relatives also contributed to the media debates. Thus there is a considerable amount of material in the public domain detailing the desires and experiences of these people. Two people maintained their privacy and they are identified in this chapter as Case 5 and 6 respectively. This public textual evidence is supported by our case study research consisting of eighteen hours of in depth audio-taped interviews conducted with Dr Philip Nitschke, the doctor who performed the legal deaths under the ROTI Act (Kissane, Street, and Nitschke 1998).

We draw upon this textual material from our research to substantiate and illustrate these discourses. In reporting this textual analysis we have made defensible, but arbitrary distinctions. The four discourses overlap, interconnect and merge in a dynamic process. Dying people move between the zippered edges of these discursive constructions with a rapidity and fluidity that is not represented in this artificial capture on paper.

The Strategies of Discourse Analysis

A 'discourse' is a useful tool for analysis as it demonstrates how particular forms of language, associated practices and social institutions combine to structure not only what it is possible for us to think or do, but also limit our potential for thinking and acting differently (Foucault 1991). Taking a discursive approach enables us to see some things, but it means we will ignore others. Seeing differently provides us with the potential to change our language, attitudes, practices, social relationships and institutional structures (Street 1998). It has been argued that the medicalized discourses of pain, symptoms, prognosis and treatment are privileged over other more marginalized discourses of nurturing/caring (Aranda and Street 1999, Benner and Wrubel 1989, Street 1992) or the body-self (Lawler 1991, 1997, Parker 1997, Rudge 1998).

One of the most helpful ways of thinking about how discourses can be analysed is captured in the words of Mills (1997: 17):

> A discursive structure can be detected because of the synchronicity of the ideas, opinions, concepts, ways of thinking and behaving which are formed within a particular context, and because of the effects of those ways of thinking and behaving.

The work of Foucault has been helpful in describing a theoretical search for such forms of discursive synchronicity. He argues for four strategies that assist in the process of deconstruction of a discursive structure (Foucault 1991). The 'master trope' and governing strategy is reversal; the other three are specific forms of reversals (Shumway 1989: 15). By this Foucault (1991) means that we must engage in a deliberate search for an alternative interpretation to that provided by tradition, to reverse the taken-for-granted assumptions underpinning social understandings. In this instance we reverse the common assumptions that advantage rationalized arguments of science or bio-ethics over the embodied experience of the person with a disintegrating body-self (Annandale 1998). Foucault also sends us on a hunt for discontinuity, the development of a suspicion of apparent historical continuity and a vigorous search for ruptures and breaks in linear and progressive movements. Specificity was also important to Foucault. He argued that periods, times, cultures and places are all different and knowledge and practices from one set of circumstances cannot be homogenized or generalized to another (Foucault 1965). Finally, Foucault was committed to an examination of exteriority, an exploration of the surface of things, the conditions of existence, always pursuing the discursive regulation and the effects on thinking and practice rather than a search for meaning in the manner of interpretive philosophers.

Textual Practices

Taking these discursive strategies into an analysis of the texts on euthanasia is an artificial endeavour. It is a task conducted in the knowledge that research interview narratives are fictions, constructions that allow messy texts to be transformed into structured coherent narratives for analysis (Lupton 2003). In this study the texts were initially subject to a qualitative content analysis to chart the patterns that surfaced concerning the content, ideas, language forms and social structures. Then use of the strategy of reversals led us to develop questions to search for what was missing or silenced in the texts. In exploring the text units it became apparent that the writers/speakers had been involved in 'narrative surrender' where they had made tacit agreements to tell their stories in 'medical terms' (Frank 1995, Charon 2006, Mattingly and Garro 2000). However, this surrender was not complete and it was in the asides and explanatory comments that the marginalized discourses of the body became apparent.

At the outset it is important to state that other discourses affected the decision-making of these seven people, but in this chapter we confine ourselves to discussing these four key discursive constructions of the body in the belief that they have been largely neglected. Given the number of people dying in Australia during the nine months of the legislation, who did not seek euthanasia, it is obvious that most people finally come to terms with the effects of the losses and disfigurement at end of life. Therefore this analysis can be seen to be limited as it only concerned with the discourses of the body-self that were present in the narratives of the seven people who requested euthanasia. This material does not deal with narratives of those who were able to come to terms with the dying body. Yet we consider this discourse analysis of the limited narrative material available on euthanasia is important because a clearer understanding of these marginalized discourses can lead to a reformulation of care.

Mapping Discourses of the Dying Body

> [T]he body serves as the medium through which the self discloses itself to others. One does not need to be an existentialist to know that a person not only *has* a body; in a sense, she is her body (May 1991: 10).

In Frank's (1991) landmark review of the sociology of the body, he argued for an understanding of the corporeal body as foundational. In his later work (Frank 1995) he contended that the body-self is a key moral problem created through reciprocal processes such that selves act in ways that constitute their bodies whilst simultaneously bodies constitute selves who act. Thus the body cannot be relegated to abstract objective concerns such as 'do I have a body?', nor can people function purely as subjects to answer the question of 'am I a body?' He contends that:

As body-selves, people interpret their bodies and make choices: the body can either seek perfected levels of predictability, at whatever cost, or can accept varying degrees of contingency. Most people do both and strategies vary as to what is sought to be controlled, where, and how (Frank 1995: 32).

Early socialization is important in the values we hold about ourselves (Slade 1994) and in the ways we inscribe our bodies in a fluctuating body image and a capacity to adorn and disguise our body surfaces (Bordo 1993). In line with this, there has been a large rise in the popularity of 'body regimes' such as diets and exercise, in which people engage to ensure the body's compliance with their own discursive sense of self, an ongoing reflexive 'project of the self' (Giddens 1991). Furthermore, it is the external appearance of the body that has most come to symbolize the self at a time when unprecedented value is placed on the youthful, sexual and trim body (Mellor and Shilling 1993: 413).

During the 1990s the body was claimed as a central concern of nursing (Benner and Wrubel 1989, Lawler 1991, Parker 1997). Nursing discursive work on the body explores the way that discourses traverse the body and the way that the body secures discourses (Hickson and Holmes 1995, Lawler 1997, May 1992, Savage 1997).

Although Holmes et al. (2006) have re-conceptualized abjection in the context of nurses' experiences of visceral care, such investigations have not been specifically linked with assisted suicide. Yet there is ample evidence to support the contention that dying people make requests of nurses for assistance to die (Hudson, Kristjanson et al. 2006, Kuhse and Singer 1994, McInerney and Seibold 1995, Scanlon 1998, van der Arend 1998, Wilkes, White, and Tolley 1993). The guidelines provided to nurses in such situations are couched in the traditional terminology of palliative care nursing or the euthanasia debates (Buckley 1998, James and Field 1996, Scanlon 1998). Missing from these analyses is any acknowledgment that nursing involves intimate bodywork (Rudge 1998) that is discursively constructed and that an understanding of the body-self is relevant to end of life decision-making.

The language framing the discourses of the body-self requesting assisted dying is a language of conventions and taboos. Medical discourses have been among the plethora of ways that the body has been systematized and discussed in relation to end of life care. In these debates the materiality and corporeality of the body is submerged under the weight of such theoretical terminology as descriptions of symptoms, prognosis, personal autonomy (Erlen 1996), palliation (Doyle, Hanks, and MacDonald 1999), personhood (Smith 1990) or burden (Bascom and Tolle 1995, Pincombe and Tooth 1996). These terms carry sets of discursive practices that shape how the body can be spoken about and acted upon.

The Symptomatic Body

The discourse of the symptomatic body derives from the dominant anatomo-clinical interests that support the medicalized dying of the person and are primarily concerned with the state of the physical body; its treatment, deterioration and prognosis (Lupton 1997). Such anatomo-clinical interests have been widely discussed and critiqued in the literature over the last forty years (Illich 1976, Lupton 1993, Willis 1983). Hence the arguments against their pervasiveness need little rehearsing here. This overarching medical discourse facilitates the exercise of medical power as it affects the way we understand, experience and regulate our bodies, providing the clinical, rational and biological basis for modern medicine's comprehension of the body as an object for cure (Foucault 1973). People are classified into categories 'dividing the healthy from the diseased, the normal from the pathological, the hygienic from the polluting, the living from the dead' (Seale 1998: 75). Disease manifestations are described and related to a generalisable pattern belonging to a recognized disease category.

When chronic illness prevails (Vamos 1993) or death is imminent, a new concept of the embodied self becomes necessary (Gordon 1990). Despite the emphasis on personhood in care for the dying, dying people know themselves and are known by others through their bodies (Turner 1992). Their bodies change, lose function and decay (Madioni, Morales, and Michel 1997). They irrevocably lose their habitual reliable body (Madjar 1998). The body is altered and suffers in myriad ways through illness, fungating wounds, skin breakdown, muscle weakness, bleeding, stomas, organ failure, and various impairments of limb. The body sets limits to experience and ultimately dictates that lives must end (Seale 1998). The authoritative medical discourse has colonized the body (Parker 1997) and it is conceptualized in a language that is monological, monoglossic, univocal and sacred to expunge the viscerality and grotesqueness of the dying body (Young 1993). Dying people learn to describe themselves objectively as body parts with changing functions or primarily as a set of symptoms (Fassett and Gallagher 1998).

The justification for the euthanasia requests of the seven people was initially couched in a litany of medical conditions, previous treatments and their effects, current physical suffering and future prognosis. Bob Dent commenced his open letter by detailing his progress to euthanasia, not in terms of his life and illness experience but as a list of ever-progressing symptoms and related treatments. He began:

> I was diagnosed with prostate cancer late in 1991. In December, I was sent to a (n) urologist in Brisbane for a bone scan and possible prostatectomy (removal of prostate gland). Before such a difficult procedure could be performed, it was necessary to check the lymph nodes in the groin area to see if the cancer had spread out of the prostate. They were all cancerous. It was now too late to remove the prostate and instead, both testicles were removed... I have lost 25 kilograms.

> My latest blood tests, taken on 2 September, indicated an acceleration of the
> cancer with the prostatic specific antigen rising to 1298 (normal is zero to four).
> The red cell picture was suggestive of infiltration of the bone marrow by the
> cancer. This was confirmed by chest x-ray. The x-ray also revealed an area of
> collapsed lung. (Dent 22 September 1996)

In this description it is apparent that the symptomatic body discourse frames
Bob Dent's capacity to describe his experience. In this narrative surrender the
'physician becomes the spokesperson for the disease and the ill person's stories
come to depend heavily on repetition of what the physician has said' (Frank
1995: 6). As a terminal prognosis usually takes time to develop, the person learns
the medical terminology over the course of their treatment through an ongoing
process of disclosure and informed consent (Hebert et al. 1997). The fluency with
which chronic patients acquire the distancing language of the symptomatic body
discourse was evident in the stories of all those who asked for euthanasia under
the ROTI Act.

Medical terminology was necessary to meet the first requirement of the Act,
that the person have a terminal illness. Under the specific requirements of the
ROTI Act two independent medical opinions were required to confirm that the
person was of sound mind, was terminally ill and had been offered the appropriate
treatments or palliation. The end result of euthanasia is a hastened death; a mistaken
prognosis would introduce an irrevocable error. Bob Dent's description of himself
illustrates the normalization process that constructs the person's experience within
the symptomatic body discourse. He depicts himself as both being subject to, and
an active participant in symptomatic surveillance: 'A plastic and reconstructive
surgeon [name supplied] agreed to do the job, and this repair is holding' (Dent 22
September 1996). In his letter he articulates the attainment of a terminal prognosis:
'Two specialists, [name supplied], who performed the 1996 TURP, and [name
supplied], oncologist, have both said nothing can be done' (Dent 22 September
1996). Similarly, after her suicide, a letter was found beside Martha Alfonsa,
which said, 'I have decided to end my life because I am terminally ill from cancer.
I have maybe a few months to live'.

Laments from Bob Dent such as: 'I have no wish for further experimentation
by the palliative care people in their efforts to control my pain' or 'If I were to
keep a pet animal in the same condition I am in, I would be prosecuted' (Dent 22
September 1996), demonstrate how the effects of his symptomatic body shaped
the construction of himself as a worthwhile person.

The Dependent Body Discourse

In our analysis three main concerns constructed the discourse of dependence: desire
for control, concern about loss of independence and fear of being a burden.

Taking Control

In Darwin, euthanasia was discussed in relation to autonomous decision making and the capacity to avoid further suffering by taking control over the their death. Nitschke explained that his decision to create a 'deliverance machine' (the computer that enabled the dying person to start the euthanasia process by pressing a key) was in response to the expressed desire of people considering euthanasia to have control in the process. Although the person was hooked up to a syringe driver by Nitschke, it took a bodily response by the person to initiate euthanasia. In her final statement Janet Mills demonstrated her desire to take control was related to her capacity to end her suffering: 'No one wants to die if they don't have to, but I know I have had no hesitation in asking for this. No one should suffer when they don't have to' (J. Mills 1997).

Losing Independence

Early socialization teaches us to be independent in our self-care; to be continent, clean, fragrant, fit and healthy. Chronic illness brings a loss of the capacity for self-care and physical independence. Our bodies are placed in the hands of others; our privacy and intimacy can be violated; and we may feel like a burden (Holstein 1997). Supporters of euthanasia usually argue that a dignified death occurs when the person has the autonomy to decide that they have had enough and wish to die.

> A competent terminally ill adult … has a strong liberty interest in choosing a dignified and humane death rather than being reduced at the end of his existence to a childlike state of helplessness, diapered, sedated, incontinent. (*Compassion in Dying v. Washington 9th Circuit*, 1996)

This self-determined death contrasts independent, rational decision-making with an embodied construction of childlike dependence. Nitschke described the frustration and sense of futility that an embodied dependence brought to Max Bell:

> … he found himself getting increasingly weak … he used to sit on the back porch…he was two steps away from the toilet, two steps away from the bucket in case he vomited, two steps away from anything. And he just sat there (Nitschke transcript – case 2).

Being a Burden

The work on burden recognizes that, for many people, there are no significant others that they can happily be dependent on (Ott 1998) and that the physical care required can be heavy, unremitting and unrewarding (Clark and Seymour 1999).

Likewise the toll extracted by the emotional burden of dealing with seemingly endless physical deterioration (Pincombe and Tooth 1996) influences how dying people come to accept their increasing dependence. In a study exploring why people request euthanasia, Seale (1995) found that those concerned with physical dependency were more likely to make such an appeal.

Concerns about dependence were borne out in our study. Bob Dent described the agony of coming to terms with dependency as: 'My own pain is made worse by watching my wife suffering as she cares for me; cleaning up after my "accidents" in the middle of the night, and watching my body fade away' (Dent 22 September 1996).

Similarly Case 6 had watched her sister die from breast cancer and she was concerned that her death would be similar. She cited her concern that she would lose continence and would be a burden to her children as the main reasons for wanting euthanasia (Kissane, Street, and Nitschke 1998).

It has been cogently argued that there is 'a valuable and necessary grace in the capacity to be dependent upon others, to be open to their solicitude, to be willing to lean upon their strength and compassion' (Callahan 1993: 144). Yet, such a contention assumes that we have available people who care for us and are willing to shoulder the burden of our care and that we are comfortable in receiving this nurturance from them. It also presupposes that these people are strong, solicitous and compassionate such that they aid us to maintain a bounded sense of self in the midst of their ministrations (Jensen and Given 1991).

The Shameful Body Discourse

The idea of a shameful body relates to the person's response to the breakdown of bodily integrity and the subsequent feelings of humiliation and embarrassment that arise from an incapacity to manage the body in a socially acceptable manner (Lombardi 2007). Shame accentuates suffering because the physical symptoms can be prolonged and exacerbated by the shame related to being social undesirable. Kalafat (2000) argued that shame plays a role in suicidal behaviour as the person, in part, wants to escape from public response to their condition. Although illness is not a moral transgression, Tangney (1996) contends that non-moral failures and shortcomings (such as incontinence) are likely to elicit shame. Shame is often the 'hidden' response and is associated with failure and loss (Gans and Weber 2000); in this case the loss of an intact self.

Broken Boundaries

The notion of an intact self is always an embodied idea; the skin is regarded as an envelope which:

[A]rmours the body against the world: it keeps the precious within and the noxious without it; it prevents fragile protoplasm from oozing into the surroundings and bars invading micro-organisms. It regulates temperature and fluid loss, and keeps in balance deeper body functions. Pimply in youth, wrinkled in age, the skin defines our extended selves, our health, and our limits (May 1991: 17).

Yet (Madioni, Morales, and Michel 1997: 161) reminds us that illness breaks the integrity of the outward bodily appearance and, in certain patients, fragments the 'psychic-envelope'. This fragmentation is evident when the body-self becomes a source of shame and anguish. Janet Mills made a televised appeal for a doctor to provide the second signature needed for euthanasia and left audiences haunted with an image of a small woman whose skin lesions covered her whole body. Her shame and disgust at her body was linked to her wish to die: 'It's bad news, because I scratch day and night. My hands and feet blister. Yes, I want to go' (patient transcript recorded in psychiatric medical record).

The effects of the radical breakdown of the body's surfaces was addressed in a study by Lawton (1998: 128) where she described those patients needing symptom control because their bodies were 'rotting inside' or 'being eaten away by their cancer' as being 'unbounded'. Unbounded bodies could be treated such that the 'boundedness of their bodies could be re-instated' (Lawton 1998: 128). It took the work of Kristeva (1982) on abjection to remind us that 'the envelope' of the body is never a safe boundary, even when we are well. She argued that the good and proper self-controlled and self-contained body, seemingly bounded by our skin, is inevitably shored up only by our idealism and ideology (Mansfield 2000). Those boundaries of this body-self are constantly broken by flows of urine, tears, shit, vomit, blood, sweat and semen (Kristeva 1982). From this perspective the body-self concept of an unbounded body being re-instated as a bounded body disregards the ongoing bodily processes to which we constantly adjust. We defend against this pollution and rupturing of subjective boundaries by shame and loathing. Thus abjection is an ambiguous state of shattered boundaries of scabs, flaking skin and leaky orifices. It typifies the dissonance between clean and unclean, the proper and the improper, order and disarray; it threatens our sense of a stable and coherent identity (Wiltshire and Parker 1996). Abjection is a source of disheartenment, a focus for shame, humiliation and disgust (Hughes 2009).

Shame

Shame is described as a global experience that is related to negative self-evaluation and depression whereas guilt is seen to be focused on a specific behaviour or situation (Alexander et al. 1999). Ferguson (2000) argues that 'unwanted identities' elicit shame and this point is pertinent here. The unwanted identity accompanying deterioration in physical functioning and appearance in terminal illness may engender feelings of shame and humiliation (Madioni, Morales, and Michel 1997), stigma, disgust, and loathing (Hughes 2009). The psycho-visceral response to the dying body-self can be disgust that it can no longer be managed as a social body; it has becomes a shameful, abject body that prefigures the post-mortem body (Hickson and Holmes 1995).

As May (1991: 15–16) clearly illustrates:

> But the deepest aversion besets the victim himself. He knows that his very existence now repels others; they recoil first, and only later talk, listen, and venture a smile. His helplessness in the midst of these shocks produces a second generation of responses less innocent than the first.

In Darwin, Marta Alfonso perceived herself as a beautiful woman whose image was important to her self esteem, typified in the use of a very youthful photo on her book of poems that she self-published when she was in her sixties. She refused curative surgery for fear it would leave her disabled. On national television she discussed the physical deterioration that illness inscribed on her body and her disgust with a body losing function (Wilkinson 1995). She took her own life when she was considered ineligible for euthanasia. Bob Dent (22 September 1996) described his shame as: 'Morphine causes constipation – laxatives work erratically, often resulting in loss of bowel control in the middle of the night. I have to have a rubber sheet on my bed, like a child who is not yet toilet-trained'.

An understanding of the body as a site of corporeality and abjection is often suppressed by health professionals (Grosz 1989). They are socialized through training, discipline and continued exposure into an acceptance of the decaying, disintegrating body, learning to 'see' the person and not the condition. Dying people and their relatives have to learn to become accustomed and accepting of the changes occasioned by the dying body. Expressions of disgust or revulsion from relatives are feared and conversations may be structured to avoid allowing such feelings to surface (Kissane 1998). Janet Mills' husband shared her anguish at the state of her body and told Nitschke that he believed that when people saw her condition they would understand and want to assist her to die (Nitschke, transcript, 4).

The Temporal Body Discourse

Humans are conscious of time in many dimensions. We waste time, lose time, take our time, get behind, get ahead, clock on and off (Street 1995). We structure aspects of our life around diurnal patterns of bed times (Street et al. 1997) and nutrition patterns of meal times (Street 1999). The healthy temporal body is well-ordered, regulated and predictable. Disease brings disruptions to the body clock: sleeping patterns are disturbed, medication times dominate, waiting for interventions, visits and treatments becomes the order of the day.

In a newspaper article Nitschke argued that 'some people calmly choose the time to die' (Nitschke 1998:1). By engaging in euthanasia, people in the study made the decision to terminate his or her life in their own time. The notion that there is a 'right time' to die and that this decision was in the hands of the ill person was repeated in many of the transcripts. Euthanasia provided control over the timing of death. In partnership with the terminally ill person the doctor becomes the agent to hasten death. Time is not constructed in a linear fashion but is related to the notion of a 'time to die'. On a televised current affairs program Max Bell expressed this desire to die, driving hundreds of kilometres from his home to Darwin, making preparations to dispose of his house and animals, to seek euthanasia. Nitschke explained his situation as:

> He couldn't eat. He couldn't enjoy his food. He was sick to death of eating yoghurt. And he found himself getting increasingly weak, and he felt that frankly, that his life was coming to an end and he didn't just want to sit there and wait for this. He said that he had had enough. He wanted to end his life (research transcript 2).

The time to die was related to the losses of a regulated, well-ordered life, a life in which meals were no longer times of enjoyment and sleep patterns were disturbed. The notion of interrupting time is inherent in the comment about not waiting to die. Similarly, Janet Mills spoke of her desire to die as: 'I know it's the right time. I can't take any more' (patient transcript recorded in psychiatric medical record). Her disgust with her decaying body was linked to her sense of temporality and preparedness to die.

Timing and control over death were also important to Esther Wild. The ROTI Act was rescinded before she was ready to use it, so she asked for an infusion to sedate her and allow her to die. She was reported saying to Nitschke (1997): 'the minute I go into unconsciousness. I don't want to wake up again. Like, I am dying at that minute'. Drifting into unconsciousness was her idea of a death with dignity. When she awoke three times over the next four days, she was angry as her desire for a controlled death had not been achieved smoothly.

Conclusions

Health professionals engaged in palliative care are shaped by their own discourses of a good death (McNamara, Waddell, and Colvin 1995). Such discourses are constructed from within professional understandings of palliation and psycho-social care without any exploration of the embodied experience of dying people and their families (Emanuel and Emanuel 1998, Turner et al. 1996). Analysis of the narrative and textual material available from the seven people who asked for euthanasia demonstrates that their concerns were not solely governed by dominant medical and psychological discourses of autonomy and personhood as regularly portrayed in the literature on euthanasia and palliative care. The discourses of the body facing death were also important to them.

Acceptance of the decaying body is a constant reflexive process – a project of the self that continues to the end (Giddens 1992). Such a project requires the dying person to constantly re-construct and re-frame a sense of self, as the body becomes more demanding, unstable, unreliable and frail. According to Lawton (1998) the consequences for those whose unbounded bodies defied symptom management were dire. Without many options, they were often sequestered away within a hospice where the taboo about commenting on the consequences of 'dirt, decay, disintegration and smell are rarely if ever, written about by hospice professionals or covered in media representations of hospice care' Lawton (1998: 139). Their condition became unspeakable. By opting for euthanasia these seven people chose not to continue to live with the unspeakable effects of forms of cancer on their bodies.

Kristeva (1982) argues that the shame we feel at our own unboundedness, or that of another who is dependent on our care, needs to be constantly repressed. Health professionals become adept at this form of repression in order to do their job (Grosz 1989). Nurses wipe up vomit and faeces, collect sputum, and deal with fungating wounds. But this repression of unconscious material concerning the unbounded body is never complete. Explaining Kristeva's (1982) position, Mansfield (2000: 80) states: 'there is a zone in which the repression of unconscious material is incomplete, where the dividing line between what the conscious mind does and does not admit is weak or blurred'.

The seven people who asked for euthanasia were unable to fully repress their horror of further disintegration and dependence. Some family members, friends, medical and nursing staff, politicians, journalists and many members of the general public supported their desires for an assisted death. These supporters often revealed the discourses of shame and dependence in their comments and commentaries (Alcorn 1998, Allen 1998, Bone 1999, Nitschke 1998).

The discourse of the temporal body is constructed around a concept of time as a pre-ordained moment or as a process of leaving. A desire to terminate the flow of life with an unruly body through medical assistance was a decision taken within a concept of the 'right time to die' (Pick 1994). With the exception of Max Bell, each person made a final decision as to the day and time of death. Marta decided not to wait for the legislation to take effect and took her own life. The others were wedded to a medical solution of an assisted death but in each instance they took time to settle affairs or assemble family members before being 'ready to die'.

A more process-oriented approach to the notion of a time to die is also a central concern of palliative care (de Raeve 1996, Gauthier 1997, Turner et al. 1996). Concerns at end of life are focused on time as a process of dying well rather than as a fixed point that is planned and executed. Brock (1997) argues that death with dignity is possible if people dying from cancer and progressive neurological conditions are able to maintain a sense of self-respect in the midst of their disease and disintegration. Understanding how people gain an embodied sense of the time for them to die is important in assisting them to face the dying process.

Although concerns around the effects of dependence and the shame of the decaying body have been expressed in a few other studies (Lawton 1998, Seale and Addington-Hall 1994, 1995), an exploration of the discourses of the body requesting euthanasia requires much more research and theorizing. If end of life care is to be designed to meet the needs of dying people, then understanding the discursive effects of the dying body can assist health professionals to work with dying people and their families to deal with their unspoken and unspeakable bodily needs.

References

Alcorn, G. 1998. Caring or killing? It's a painful question. *The Age*, 7 November, 7.

Alexander, B. and Brewin, C. et al. 1999. An investigation of shame and guilt in a depressed sample. *British Journal of Medical Psychology*, 72, 323–338.

Allen, F. 1998. Euthanasia: why torture dying people when we have sick animals put down? *Australian Psychologist*, 33(1), 12–15.

Annandale, E. 1998. *The Sociology of Health & Medicine: A Critical Introduction*. Cambridge, Polity Press.

Anzieu, D. 1989. *The Skin Ego*. London: Karnac.

Aranda, S. 1998. *A Critical Praxis Study of Nurse-Patient Friendship*. Ph.D, School of Nursing, Bundoora: La Trobe University.

Aranda, S.K. and Street, A. 1999. Being authentic and being a chameleon: nurse-patient interaction revisited. *Nursing Inquiry*, 6(2), 75–82.

Bascom, P.B. and Tolle, S.W. 1995. Care of the family when the patient is dying. *West J Med*, 163(3), 292–6.

Benner, P. and Wrubel, J. 1989. *The Primacy of Caring*. Sydney: Addison-Wesley Pub.

Bishop, J.P. 2008. Biopolitics, Terri Schiavo, and the Sovereign Subject of Death. *Journal of Medicine and Philosophy*, 33(6), 538–557.

Bone, P. 1999. Euthanasia: why I've had a rethink. *The Age*, 21 January, 13.

Bordo, S. 1993. Feminism, Foucault and the politics of the body, in *Up Against Foucault and feminism*, edited by C. Ramazanglu. London: Routledge, 179–202.

Brock, I. 1997. *Dying Well*. New York: Riverhead Books.

Buckley, M. 1998. Death rights. *Nursing Times*, 94(25), 26–32.

Byk, C. Death with dignity and euthanasia: Comparative European approaches. *International Journal of Bioethics*, 18(3), 85–102, 118.

Callahan, D. 1993. *The Troubled Dream of Life: Living with Mortality*. New York: Simon and Schuster.

Chapple, A., Ziebland, S. et al. 2006. What people close to death say about euthanasia and assisted suicide: A qualitative study. *Journal of Medical Ethics*, 32(12), 706–710.

Charon, R. 2006. *Narrative Medicine – Honouring the Stories of Illness*. New York: Oxford University Press.

Clark, D. and Seymour, J. 1999. *Reflections on Palliative Care: Sociological and Policy Perspectives*. Buckingham, UK: Open University Press.

Compassion in Dying v. Washington, 79, F.3d. 9th Circuit, 1996. Compassion in Dying v Washington, 79, F.3d. Washington.

de Raeve, L. 1996. Dignity and integrity at the end of life. *International Journal of Palliative Nursing*, 2(2),71–76.

Dent, R.B. 1996. *Open letter to parliamentarians* [letter]. *The Age* Online, 22 September [cited 25th September 1996].

Doyle, D., Hanks, G.W.C. and MacDonald, N. (eds) 1999. *Oxford Textbook of Palliative Medicine*. 2nd ed. Oxford: Oxford University Press.

Emanuel, E.J. and Emanuel, L.L. 1998. The promise of a good death. *The Lancet*, 351 (9114), Supp. 21–9.

Erlen, J.A. 1996. Issues at the end of life. *Orthopaedic Nursing*, 15(4), 37–41.

Fassett, D. and Gallagher, M.R. 1998. *Just a Head*. St Leonards, NSW: Allen & Unwin.

Ferguson, T., Eyre, H. and Ashbaker, M. 2000. Unwanted identities: a key variable in shame-anger links and gender differences, in *shame*. *Sex Roles*, 42(3/4), 133–157.

Finlay, I. 1996. Ethical decision-making in palliative care: the clinical reality, in *Facing Death: An interdisciplinary approach*, edited by P. Badham and P. Ballard. Cardiff: University of Wales Press, 64–86.

Forde, R., Aasland, O.G. and Falkum, E. 1997. The ethics of euthanasia – attitudes and practice among Norwegian physicians. *Social Science and Medicine*, 45(6), 887–892.

Foucault, M. 1965. *Madness and Civilization: A History of Insanity in the Age of Reason*. Translated by R. Howard. New York: Pantheon.

Foucault, M. 1973. *The Birth of the Clinic: An Archaelogy of Medical Perception*. New York: Pantheon Books.

Foucault, M. 1991. Orders of discourse. *Social Science Inform*, 10(2), 7–30.

Frank, A.W. 1995. *The Wounded Storyteller*. Chicago: University of Chicago Press.

Frank, A.W. 1991. For a sociology of the body: an analytical review, in *The Body: Social Process and Cultural Theory*, edited by M. Featherstone, M. Hepworth and B.S. Turner. London: Sage Publications, 36–102.

Franklin, L.L. and Ternestedt, B.M. et al. (2006). Views on dignity of elderly nursing home residents. *Nursing Ethics*, 13(2), 130–146.

Gans, J. and Weber, R. 2000. The detection of shame in group psychotherapy: uncovering the hidden emotion. *International Journal of Group Psychotherapy*, 50 (3), 381–396.

Ganzini, L., Goy, E.R. et al. 2008. Why Oregon patients request assisted death: Family members' views. *Journal of General Internal Medicine*, 23(2), 154–157.

Gauthier, P.A. 1997. Living with dignity until the end. *Canadian Nurse*, 93(3), 38–42.

Giddens, A. 1991. *Modernity and Self-identity: Self and Society in the Late Modern Age*. Cambridge: Polity Press.

Giddens, A. 1992. *The Transformation of Intimacy*. Stanford, California: Stanford University Press.

Gordon, D. 1990. Embodying illness, embodying cancer. *Culture, Medicine and Psychiatry*, 14, 275–297.

Grosz, E. 1989. *Sexual Subversions*. St Leonards: Allen & Unwin.

Hebert, P.C., Hoffmaster, B., Glass, K.C., and Singer, P.A. 1997. Bioethics for clinicians: truth telling. *Canadian Medical Association Journal*, 156(2), 225–228.

Hickson, P. and Holmes, C. 1995. Nursing the post-modern body: a touching case. *Nursing Inquiry*, 1(1), 3–14.

Holmes, D., Perron, A. and O'Byrne, P. 2006. Understanding disgust in nursing: abjection, self, and the other. *Research and Theory for Nursing Practice: An International Journal*, 20(4), 305–315.

Holstein, M. 1997. Reflections on death and dying. *Academic Medicine*, 72(10), 848–855.

Hudson, P. and Kristjanson, L.J. et al. (2006). Desire for hastened death in patients with advanced disease and the evidence base of clinical guidelines: a systematic review. *Palliative Medicine*, 20, 693–701.

Hudson, P., Schofield, P. et al. (2006). Responding to desire to die statements from patients with advanced disease: recommendations for health professionals. *Palliative Medicine*, 20, 703–710.

Hughes, B. 2009. Wounded/monstrous/abject: a critique of the disabled body in the sociological imaginary. *Disability & Society*, 24(4), 399–410.

Illich, I. 1976. *Medical Nemesis: The Expropriation of Health*. Harmondsworth: Penguin.

James, V. and Field, D. 1996. Who has the power? Some problems and issues affecting the nursing care of dying patients. *European Journal of Cancer Care*, 5(2), 73–80.

Jensen, S. and Given, B.A. 1991. Fatigue affecting family caregivers of cancer patients. *Cancer Nurse*, 14(4), 181–187.

Kalafat, J. and Lester, D. 2000. Shame and suicide: a case study. *Death Studies*, 24, 157–162.

Kissane, D. 1998. Models of psychological response to suffering. *Progress in Palliative Care*, 6(6), 197–204.

Kissane, D., Street, A. and Nitschke, P. 1998. Seven deaths in Darwin: case studies under the Rights of the Terminally Ill Act, Northern Territory, Australia. *The Lancet*, 352(9134), 1097–1102.

Komaromy, C. 2000. The sight and sound of death: the management of dead bodies in residential and nursing homes for older people. *Mortality*, 5(3), 299–315.

Kristeva, J. 1982. *Powers of Horror: An Essay on Abjection.* New York: Columbia University Press.

Kuhse, H. and Singer. P. 1994. Euthanasia – A survey of nurses' attitudes and practices. *Life and Death Matters*, 29, 10–12.

Lather, P. 1993. Fertile obsession: validity after poststructuralism. *The Sociological Quarterly*, 34(4), 673–693.

Lawler, J. 1991. *Behind the Screens: Nursing Somology and The Problem of The Body.* Melbourne: Churchill Livingstone.

Lawler, J. (ed). 1997. *The Body in Nursing: A Colleciton of Views.* Melbourne: Churchill Livingstone.

Lawton, J. 1998. Contemporary hospice care: the sequestration of the unbound body and 'dirty dying'. *Sociology of Health and Illness*, 20(2), 121–143.

Lindsay, R.A. 2009. Oregon's experience: evaluating the record. *American Journal of Bioethics*, 9(3), 19–27.

Lombardi, R. 2007. Shame in relation to the body, sex, and death: a clinical exploration of the psychotic levels of shame. *Psychoanalytic Dialogues*, 17, 3.

Lupton, D. 2003. *Medicine as Culture.* London: Sage.

Lupton, D. 1993. Is there life after Foucault? Post-structuralism and the health social sciences. *Australian Journal of Public Health*, 17(4), 298–300.

Lupton, D. 1997. Foucault and the medicalization critique, in *Foucault, Health and Medicine*, edited by A. Peterson and R. Bunton. New York: Routledge.

Madioni, F., Morales, C. and Michel, J.P. 1997. Body image and the impact of terminal disease. *European Journal of Palliative Care*, 4(5), 160–162.

Madjar, I. 1998. *Giving Comfort and Inflicting Pain.* Edmonton: Qualitative Institute Press.

Mansfield, N. 2000. *Subjectivity: Theories of the Self from Freud to Haraway.* St Leonards, NSW: Allen & Unwin.

Mattingly, C. and Garro, L.C. (eds). 2000. *Narrative and the Cultural Construction of Illness and Healing.* London: University of California Press.

May, C. 1992. Nursing work, nurses' knowledge, and the subjectification of the patient. *Sociology of Health and Illness*, 14(4), 472–487.

May, W.F. 1991. *The Patient's Ordeal.* Bloomington and Indianapolis: Indiana University Press.

McInerney, F. 2000. Requested death: a new social movement. *Social Science and Medicine*, 50, 137–154.

McInerney, F. and Seibold, C. 1995. Nurses' definitions of and attitudes towards euthanasia. *Journal of Advanced Nursing*, 22(1), 171–181.

McNamara, B., Waddell, C. and Colvin, M. 1995. Threats to the good death: the cultural context of stress and coping among hospice nurses. *Sociology of Health and Illness*, 17, 222–244.

Meier, D., Emmons, C.A. et al. 1998. A national survey of physician-assisted suicide and euthanasia in the United States. *The New England Journal of Medicine*, 338 (17), 1193–1201.

Melin-Johansson, and Odling, C.G. et al. 2008. The meaning of quality of life: narrations by patients with incurable cancer in palliative home care. *Palliative and Supportive Care*, 6(3), 231–238.

Mellor, P.A. and Shilling, C. 1993. Modernity, self-identity and the sequestration of death. *Sociology*, 27(3), 411–431.

Miller, P.J., Hedlund, S.C. et al. 2006. Conversations at the end of life: the challenge to support patients who consider death with dignity in Oregon. *Journal of Social Work in End-of-Life and Palliative Care*, 2(2), 25–43.

Mills, J. 1997. Letter written a day before death [letter]. *The Age*, 1 January, [accessed 7 January, 1997].

Mills, S. 1997. *Discourse*. London: Routledge.

Nitschke, P. 1997. Dignified death denied [online]. *The Adelaide Advertiser*, 15 May 1997 [cited May 15th 1997].

Nitschke, P. 1998. Some calmly choose the time to go. *Herald Sun*, 3 November,1.

Northern Territory Government. 1995. Rights of the Terminally Ill Act 1995. Northern Territory of Australia, Darwin: Government Publisher.

Ott, B.B. 1998. Physician-assisted suicide and older patients' perceived duty to die. *Advanced Practice Nursing Quarterly*, 4(2), 65–70.

Parker, J. 1997. The body as text and the body as living flesh: metaphors of the body and nursing in postmodernity, in *The Body in Nursing*, edited by J. Lawler. Melbourne: Churchill Livingstone, 11–29.

Pick, O. 1994. When enough is enough. *Life and Death Matters*, 29, 19.

Pincombe, J. and Tooth, B. 1996. Carers of the terminally ill: an Australian study. *American Journal of Hospice and Palliative Care*, 13(4), 44–55.

Rudge, T. 1998. Skin as cover: the discursive effects of 'covering' metaphors on wound care practices. *Nursing Inquiry*, 5(4), 228–237.

Salem, T. 1999. Physician-assisted suicide: promoting autonomy-or medicalizing suicide? *Hastings Center Report*, 29(3), 30–39.

Savage, Jan. 1997. Gestures of resistance: the nurse's body in contested space. *Nursing Inquiry*, 4(4), 237–245.

Scanlon, C. 1998. Assisted suicide: how nurses should respond. *International Nursing Review*, 45(5), 152.

Scott, P.A. 1999. Autonomy, power and control in palliative care. *Cambridge Quarterly of Healthcare Ethics*, 8(2), 139–147.

Seale, C. 1998. *Constructing death: the sociology of dying and bereavement*. Cambridge: Cambridge University Press.

Seale, C. and Addington-Hall, J. 1994. Euthanasia: why people want to die earlier. *Social Science and Medicine*, 39(5), 647–654.

Seale, C. 1995. Euthanasia: the role of good care. *Social Science and Medicine*, 40(5),581–587.

Shumway, D.R. 1989. *Michel Foucault*. Charlottesville: University Press of Virginia.

Slade, P.D. 1994. What is body image? *Behavioral Research Therapy*, 32, 497–502.

Smith, G.P. 1990. Recognizing personhood and the right to die with dignity. *Journal of Palliative Care*, 6(2), 24–32.

Stolberg, M. 2007. Active euthanasia in pre-modern society, 1500–1800: Learned debates and popular practices. *Social History of Medicine*, 20(2), 205–221.

Street, A. 1998. Competing discourses with/in palliative care, in *Palliative Care: Explorations and Challenges,* edited by J. Parker and S. Aranda. Sydney: MacLennan & Petty, 68–81.

Street, A. 1995. *Nursing Replay: Researching Nursing Culture Together*. Melbourne: Churchill Livingstone.

Street, A. 1998. Competing discourses with/in palliative care, in *Palliative Care: Explorations and Challenges*, edited by J. Parker and S. Aranda. Sydney: MacLennan & Petty, 68–81.

Street, A. and Cuddihy, L. et al. 1997. Rostering: placing the nurse in the picture. *Contemporary Nurse*, 6(3–4), 145–151.

Street, A. 1999. Bedtimes in nursing homes: exploring an action research approach for gerontic nursing, in *Nursing Older People: Issues and Innovations*, edited by R. Nay and S. Garrett. Sydney: MacLennan & Petty, 353–68.

Street, A. 1992. *Inside Nursing: A Critical Ethnography of Clinical Nursing Practice*. New York: State University of New York Press.

Street, A. and Kissane, D. 2000. Dispensing death, desiring death: An exploration of medical roles and patient motivation during the period of legalised euthanasia in Australia. *Omega: Journal of Death and Dying*, 40(1), 229–246.

Tangney, J.P. 1990. Assessing individual differences in proneness to shame and guilt: development of the self-conscious affect and attribution inventory. *Journal of Personality and Social Psychology*, 59(1), 102–111.

Tangney, J.P. 1996. Conceptual and methodological issues in the assessment of shame and guilt. *Behavioural Research Therapy*, 34(9), 741–754.

Terry, W. and Olson, L.G. et al. (2006). Experience of dying: Concerns of dying patients and of carers. *Internal Medicine Journal*, 36(6), 338–346.

Turner, B.S. 1992. *Regulating Bodies: Essays in Medical Sociology*. London: Routledge.

Turner, K. and Chye, R. et al. 1996. Dignity in dying: a preliminary study of patients in the last three days of life. *Journal of Palliative Care*, 12(2), 7–13.

Vamos, M. 1993. Body image in chronic illness – a reconceptualization. *International Journal of Psychiatry in Medicine*, 23, 163–178.

van der Arend, Arie. 1998. Euthanasia and assisted suicide in the Netherlands: Clarifying the practice and the nurse's role. *International Nursing Review*, 45 (5), 145–151.

van der Riet, Pamela. 1998. The sexual embodiment of the cancer patient. *Nursing Inquiry*, 5(4), 248–257.

Waddell, C. and Clarnette, R. et al. 1996. Treatment decision-making at the end of life: a survey of Australian doctors' attitudes towards patients wishes and euthanasia. *Medical Journal of Australia*, 165, 540–544.

Wilkes, L., White, K. and Tolley, N. 1993. Euthanasia: a comparison of the lived experience of Chinese and Australian palliative care nurses. *Journal of Advanced Nursing*, 18, 95–102.

Wilkes, L.M. and White, K. 1992. *The Phenomenon of Euthanasia: The Perspective of Palliative Care Nurses Working in Hospices in Metropolitan Sydney.* Sydney: Australian Catholic University.

Wilkinson, P. 1995. *Euthanasia* [Sixty Minutes Television Production]. Channel 9 [cited].

Willis, Evan. 1983. *Medical Dominance.* Australia: George Allen and Unwin.

Wiltshire, J. and Parker, J. 1996. Containing abjection in nursing: the end of shift handover as a site of containment. *Nursing Inquiry*, 3(1), 23–29.

Young, K. 1993. Still life with corpse: management of the grotesque body in medicine, in *Body Lore*, edited by K. Young. Knoxsville: University of Tennessee Press, 111–33.

Ziegler, S.J. 2009. Collaborated death: An exploration of the Swiss model of assisted suicide for its potential to enhance oversight and demedicalize the dying process. *Journal of Law, Medicine and Ethics*, 37(2), 318.

Chapter 11
Losing Private Kovko:
When Military Masculinity goes SNAFU[1]

Jackie Cook

Introduction

On the 21 April 2006, Australian troops serving as part of George W. Bush's 'coalition of the willing' in Iraq reported to their commanding officers the death, apparently by accident, of one of their number, inside their barracks in the Australian Embassy compound in Baghdad. Private Jake Kovko, having just completed a day's service on guard duty on the roof of the embassy building, had been laughing and joking with two fellow soldiers in the small bunk-room they shared, when his gun discharged, killing him outright.

This was to prove only the first 'accident' in the story of Private Kovko. His body, shrouded and coffined for return to his family in Australia, was misdirected in the morgue in Kuwait, and the wrong corpse dispatched to his wife and family. The Officer charged with the initial military investigation into his death left a CD ROM containing all of the files in a public computer terminal in the Qantas Lounge during her flight to Australia, and the 'inside' story leaked to the media. Subsequent Army findings of suicide were strongly refuted by Private Kovko's wife and family, whose constant media presence and online interventions fuelled a long series of debates.

What happens when a closed informational system, such as that of an army on active service, confronts an event which evokes the hyper-personalized narratives favoured by contemporary media, and the open and participatory 'personal' digital mediations of the Internet and mobile telephony? Immediately the high-masculinity of control exerted by military 'discipline' over the soldierly body begins to erode. This body, represented in that of Private Kovko, supposedly secure behind its defensive weaponry and the anonymity of its dedication to 'service', is subjected to the un-control of subtle new layers of penetration. Not only does it remain fragile, even within the 'distancing' of today's high-tech and mobile

---

1   SNAFU, a soldier's acronym for 'Situation Normal – All Fucked Up' (or 'Fouled up', in more polite formulations) has been common in military parlance since at least the Second World War. The OED which admits it into its Addenda of the 1973 3rd edition Revisions, glosses it as meaning 'chaotic', 'in confusion', and attributes it to US military slang; first known use 1942.

military engagements; it now continues to intersect and so leave traces upon all of the 'personal' social networks of communicative connection which keep serving soldiers 'in touch' with home. Operating outside military discipline, these systems register, and amplify, the vulnerability and exposure of the personal and the private, no longer expunged from the soldierly self. In analysing the various debates and layers of comment and conjecture which followed the death of Private Jake Kovko, this study suggests that this new 'personal connectedness' amounts to a major shift in the degree to which the male body is available for transgressive abjection. It is altering – permanently – the relations of sequestration and control which have traditionally marked military cultures.

'Ignored Safety System': Private Kovko's Multiple Transgressiveness

In a photograph of Jake Kovko taken during training, and released to the media after the announcement of his death (*The Age,* June 21 2006), he is shown in full camouflage, carefully posed to show alertness and the tough resolve of Australian military masculinity. The image however also provides evidence of a completely divergent narrativization: one focused upon the actual body of the soldier. This is a body we are not supposed to see or to know – except when visited by politicians for the cameras. Serving soldiers are not to be named, or rendered in any way 'real'. Numerous instances of media reporting signal the degree to which the public is not to be witness to the physicality of the modern soldier. During the Iraq campaign of 2002 there was much discussion of the near-complete disappearance of Australian forces from any media coverage. The capacity for digital feeds and satellite transmission to relay detailed reporting and live images was blocked by military demands for security and secrecy of troop movement – but at the same time, it also acted as a guarantee of the discursive purity of the idea of a 'bloodless' soldiering: a war without set-piece battles, in which citizens and non-combatants were as much in target as hostile forces, and 'peace-keeping' and 'regime stability' the primary goals. Consider too the concealment of real soldiers' identities under seemingly randomly-allocated numbers ('Soldier 17 – Soldier 19') during the Kovko Board of Inquiry hearings. Those giving testimony on the circumstances of Private Kovko's death had any hint of their identity blanked out – for to reveal the physicality of the soldier is to lift the discursive mask, and to reveal – as even the military itself does when it insists on secrecy for the maintenance of security – the intense vulnerability of militarism, as invested in the actual soldierly body, exposed to very real risk, even within this seemingly 'bloodless' conflict.

These two instances alone invite analysis of what is going on in contemporary war reporting. Whether through injury, defeat, or the interestingly-worded 'conduct unbecoming', military masculinity has always risked feminization, in Kristeva's terms: descent into the abjection of wounding, death, or indiscipline. Each of these is an erosion of masculinity, retrievable only by a literally monumental return to invulnerability, within the (concrete) form of the military memorial. Death's visceral realities: bodies irrecoverably shattered by bullets, shells, burning, bomb-blast, stab wounds, gassing or chemical exposure, are serially re-wrapped: literally carapaced in militarism itself. The dead soldier's body is 'dressed' – also a drill term, denoting much the same deliberate posture taken up towards authority. When possible, it is clad in ceremonial uniform; rests in an ornate coffin; is draped in the nation's flag; has service medals and sometimes military arms placed on top; is accorded what Australian researcher Caitlin Frye has called the 'mobile memorial' of bugler and piper and 21-gun salute; from where it moves into the absolute stasis of marble memorial and the ultimate graven formulae of name, rank, and serial number.

What I have found in the Kovko narratives – helping motivate this widespread and seemingly endless examination of the events of just one death – is growing discomfort over the degree of fit between contemporary Australian cultural values, and its core myths of military sacrifice. Eight examples of Kovko narrative, each drawn from a different text-genre and location, illustrate the depth of engagement Australians have had with these events, and the dissatisfaction that so many have expressed with the traditional means of signalling narrative closure around a military death.

Getting the Story Straight

Even the barest outline of the 'facts' of what happened to Private Kovko slips immediately into uncertainty, indicating, as any Australian serviceman or 'Digger' would recognize, an inherently SNAFU culture underlying the military experience, where disorder is as prevalent as discipline.

The response of Australian servicemen to combat conditions and to the military attempt to maintain a regulatory system of discipline inside the rapid disintegration into chaos, can be seen from the beginnings of the ANZAC tradition. In cartoons produced to portray the reality of conditions at Gallipoli in World War 1, servicemen ripped away myths of army discipline, creating instead their own image of the soldier as larrikin survivor, whose characteristics oppose military order at every level.

No surprise then that when current-affairs program *Lateline's* anchor Maxine McKew scripts her introduction for the Australian Broadcasting Corporation's TV coverage of the mishandling of the return of Private Kovko's body to his family – a procedure which ought to have been saturated in militaristic and ritual precision – she works to accentuate at every level the dis-order and error of the episode. Every discursive element of her report: its lexis, syntactic order, and modality; reproduces a charge of a culture once again revealed as SNAFU.

> Welcome to the program. We begin tonight with the *breathtaking bungle* that surrounds the *failure* to return the body of Private Jake Kovco for burial in Victoria. An *embarrassed and angry* Defence Minister Brendan Nelson *broke* the news

this morning that a casket containing, we still *don't know who,* had been flown
from Kuwait to Melbourne by *mistake.* The timing of the *discovery of this error*
is still *a mystery* and there's now to be an *investigation* as to how a much-used
private carrier *managed a mix-up* that has caused *immense distress* to the Kovco
family. Why was it, for instance, that the casket containing Private Kovco, was not
escorted at all times, by a representative of the Defence Forces? And there's an
added complication – the Defence Minister confirmed today that the *accident* that
killed Private Kovco *did not occur* while he was cleaning his weapon. On top of
that the Kovco family has gone public with its *disbelief* that the young private was
anything other than meticulous in his handling of weapons. Matt Peacock reports
on a day that's produced *more questions than answers* (Emphasis added: ratio of
30:180 words denoting disorderliness). (ABC TV *The 7.30 Report* 27/04/2006).

Here is a journalist who has taken trouble over her text. She has produced
an exceptionally high ratio of carefully thematized language: paradigmatic
choices, to simple syntagmatic connectives, at a ratio of 30:180, or 1:6. Like the
soldier-cartoonists of World War I, she is working to deflate military order,
accentuating the crises which the events reveal, and empowering journalism to
dig in even deeper, to an issue which is presenting more questions than answers.
Complications, mysteries, mix-ups, disbelief – each cuts away a layer of certainty,
containment and control – central constituents of military culture. For the media at
least, the Kovko death is an unreliable narrative – evidence of chaos where control
should lie, with fragmentary explanations, layers of obfuscation, and confusion
where there should be order. A culture which drills for meticulous control, has
delivered its exact opposite.

SNAFU 2: The Conspiracy Theories

So what do those Australians who view themselves as hard-core military make
of the 'breathtaking bungle' of the Kovko story? Out in the Internet Badlands,
wannabe warriors and veterans immersed in weapon-talk pause in their daily
round of techno-conspiracy chat (topic of the day: 'Is black clothing safe when
confronting an enemy using night-scopes'?) to conjecture whether Kovko fell
victim not to the self-avowed acts of larrikinism being suggested in the rapid
emergence of 'skylarking with guns' theories: the serving man's own assertion of
masculinity; but rather to a new form of SNAFU – one more internally erosive of
proper military conduct, and expected military outcomes. Internet Chat participant
Targan introduces a far more salient menace to today's serving soldier:

This is a sad consequence of the repeated deployments of the same units and troops
over and over again to Iraq and Afghanistan. The Coalition troops are becoming
tired, angry, para[n]oid, and dispirited. The[n] yesterday on CNN, I saw a report
that suicide among US troops in Iraq has risen 17%, and I believe it.

What *Targan* hypothesises is the presence among the Baghdad force of an invisible, internal, feminized erosion of soldierly control; a weakness and abjection stemming from the exhaustion of over-deployment.

For the blog-blokes on Dominic Knight's *Radar* blog on Fairfax Digital, which promises 'an irreverent swipe at the world of news and pop culture', such accusations need to be allied to even more personalized forms, amounting to a form of emasculation. Was Jake Kovko 'poisoned?' they ask – by which these *Radar* respondents mean specifically, psychologically weakened by the inclusion of the drug *Lariam* in his anti-Malarial prophylaxis. See this article from the *Washington Post*:

> The 1997 apparent suicide of a Special Forces soldier uncovered in the UPI-CNN investigation involved a Green Beret weapons sergeant who was in a room with two other soldiers at a base near Quito, Ecuador. He had picked up the team sergeant's weapon. He looked at the team sergeant and asked if it was loaded. Then he looked at my other friend, smiled, and pulled the trigger, said Justin Schuman, a former Army staff sergeant who retired in June. ... 'We were at a loss. We really had no idea what possessed him to do that', Schuman said. 'We knew there were some stressors in his life. He was about to get remarried, but there was nothing in particular. Nobody mentioned Lariam'.

Here the negation: 'Nobody mentioned Lariam', acts paradoxically as an assertion – for in conspiracy discourse, what is NOT mentioned immediately becomes a form of evidence. Certainly, it would suit the testosterone-gun-culture masculinity of these discussion strands on both sites to discover that it were so, reasserting not only the pragmatic survivalism of the combat-hardened Digger against the mismanagement of command, but re-cementing it into a new generation of betrayal: an internal (feminizing) erosiveness, acting unseen.

'Inside a Young Man's Mind': The Psychological Instability Narratives

As a next step in this feminization through interiority, pop.-psychological explanatory narratives have been marshalled – and deployed very strategically, most often by the military themselves. Four different attempts at indicating a pre-disposition within Private Kovko towards suicide have been made in media reports, each claiming to be based either on military witness statements, or on tabled documents presented by the Defence Forces. And all of them focus on markedly un-military behaviours.

In the first, an extract from Kovko's diary outlines a dream, which is then said to be about suicide. Here the extract is used in an emotionally-charged media piece – all the more expressive for the seeming facticity of the descriptions used to capture the reality of Kovko's experiences on post in Baghdad, and for their contrast with the terse realist prose; in the best Hemingway tradition, a marker of masculine 'action' writing.

You live close in the army. Armpit close. The three men were crammed into a room the size of a small child's. But you can never get close enough to see inside a young man's mind. Jake Kovco wrote his thoughts down with unflinching honesty in his journal. A month before he died, he recorded an unnerving dream in which he shot himself in the head with his pistol while in his room, to see what it felt like. He described the blood gushing from his wounds, eyes, ears and mouth as he felt the bullet's exit hole on the top of his head. He wrote: 'I know it wasn't about killing myself … I'm very happy with my life', but admitted he had experienced similar feelings four years earlier when he was going through 'a rough patch'.

In a second such attempt at 'seeing inside a young man's mind', it is revealed that Kovko has himself been drafting works of fiction; action-thrillers, with scenarios which appear to be revolving obsessively around hidden chambers and live burial – or at least so it might seem, when the two brief extracts cited do precisely that. In one, we are told, Kovko considers a plot in which 'a librarian uncovers a hidden chamber deep below the library he works at'. The other, granted a brief dramatization on TV, is more fully realized:

CONOR DUFFY: In the first story the main character is called Sergeant Kurt Lowe. The beginning of the story was found in his [Private Kovko's] room by military police after his death.

STORY EXTRACT [read by actor]: Sgt Kurt Lowe hunkered down even further into his hastily dug pit. 'Any lower,' he thought. 'and I'll become the dirt I'm lying in'. He secretly wished it could happen. Above his head, bright red and green tracer rounds flew over the battle hardened soldiers with an ear splitting crack followed by a deep thud.

In the third example, the music and lyrics of The Cranberries, playing in Kovko's shared bunk-room at the time of the gun's discharge, are represented as significant to events. Yesterday the inquiry heard that The Cranberries song the men were singing along with was titled *Dreams*. The song's lyrics include the lines: 'Oh my life is changing every day, every possible way' (*theage.com.au,* June 21, 2006).

The words were eerily prophetic: 'oh my life is changing every day in every possible way. Though my dreams, never quite as it seems'. Did Private Kovco's thoughts turn erratically to his own dream? 'And they'll come true, impossible not to do'. (*theage.com.au,* June 24, 2006).

And in the fourth explanatory scenario, 'the larking-about-which-went-wrong' strand, barrack-room sex stunts and sing-along falsetto vocality introduce the idea of a joke beyond tolerability: a joke about yet another form of emasculation. Pte Kovco added to the frivolity by pulling his shorts up high above his waist so his testicles spilled out the sides.

'He used to do it all the time, it was pretty funny', Soldier 17 said *(theage.com. au,* 20 June 2006).

Soldier 17 said the gunshot happened as the three men laughed, joked and sang along to a song from pop group The Cranberries, mimicking the high-pitched wailing of singer Dolores O'Riordan.

'I thought he might have done it in a joking fashion, because the song we were singing was in a female, homosexual way', he said of the sudden shot. 'Almost as if to say, "this is so gay I'd rather be dead"'.

Here the resistive masculinities of larrikinism, in breaking open the genres and styles of military control, also appear to admit a great deal of play across sexualized identity – all of it enacted as forms of 'body work', playing over what are jokes precisely because they are forms expressive of vulnerability.

'The Slippage Between Description and Creation': Why Kovko Carries 'Performative Power'

As Private Kovko slips from the disciplined controls of military masculinity; first into the established larrikin modes of Digger resistance, and then into the pop-cult expressivism of musical lyrics, pulp-fiction action-hero projections, and bar-room banter, he is becoming no longer either the solider the army trained, or the man his family knew. Instead, he is now constantly in motion: shifting between the many text-generic streams of personalized public communication, in ways that rapidly escalate his availability for deployment in almost any narrative formation. Ian Kortlang, media consultant, commenting on the case for ABCTV's *7.30 Report,* puts it this way, in reply to a question from Reporter Matt Peacock, on the Government's attempts to keep control over this story:

Matt Peacock: You couldn't imagine a worse scenario for this Government here, could you? That it's the first death and this happened?
Ian Kortlang: Well, he's become iconic. I mean, a young family, a very strong courageous widow, a young kid. We all watched that two days ago and then for this to be screwed up – and that's a very polite way of putting it – screwed up, is almost unbelievable.

Kortlang, like Maxine McKew in the extract cited earlier, feels licensed here to accentuate the gaps opened everywhere in this story – or stories, as Kovko's death has already become. It is, as he says, 'unbelievable' – a phrase used again and again, in relation to any number of possible details of the Kovko death, in public discussion on the Internet sites. The evaluation itself however juxtaposes interestingly with the term 'iconic' – normally reserved for those cultural symbols of long provenance, massive proportion, and core social value: Ulleroo. The Sydney Opera House. Cricket. To what degree then, and in what ways, is Kovko now 'iconic'? In Kortlang's formulation at least, precisely because of the *impurity* of his status: the ever-increasing incapacity to attach any stable or reliable meaning at all to the Kovko case. Kortlang's incredulity, standing in for so many thousands of others, for whatever reasons, attaches in particular to the military discipline and orderliness which ought to have been evident in the return of Kovko's body to Australia: because they would have rehearsed what was going to happen. They would have rehearsed as they have the minister arriving, the coffin being draped in the Australian flag. All that was done. Unfortunately, they had the wrong person.

At every narrative level, Kovko has become 'the wrong person'; an anti-icon of sorts, representing chaos where order is promised; slippage instead of certainty; abjection rather than secure control. But with this fall into incertitude, Kovco himself has also lost agency. The body which cannot express control, also cannot command it. Within narratives of military masculinity, once your own systematic, disciplined order breaks down, your capacity to command disappears with it. Kovko is no longer the 'meticulous' soldier – and every element of the military's attempted re-assertion of order must now position him outside of itself. Everywhere, forces are scrambled to effect just such a distancing action.

'The further... from the front line, the worse the situation': Mismanagement Spreads Across Defence

The website of the *Australia Defence Association,* 30 November 2006, was headed with a far broader accusation than either the media or the general public had produced. In 'What is Wrong with the Department of Defence'? This pro-defence lobby outlines three explanations for what it terms 'bungles, scandals and damaging allegations', ultimately of course sheeting them home to politically-motivated cuts in defence force budgets. Specifically however, these errors are still carefully distanced from 'our... operational professionalism ...' It is bureaucrats, not soldiers, eroding 'our' capacity for control – those individuals that Private Kovko's wife, Shelley, is reported to have labelled in an email to her husband: 'those dickheads'.

> Our defence force, while small, is highly respected internationally. ADF operational professionalism is acknowledged as being at the forefront of Western countries. The further back you move from the front line, however, the worse the situation gets.
>
> A succession of recent bungles, scandals and damaging allegations in the Department of Defence and the Australian Defence Force increasingly risks public confidence in the ADF. First, for an organization disproportionally comprised of [sic] 18–25 year olds, demographic and multicultural trends increasingly make recruiting harder. This is not helped by a healthy economy; defence force salaries and conditions are just not sufficiently competitive. Then there is the problem that the military justice system still results in far too much injustice. The ADF

will certainly not overcome its recruiting problems in particular while Australian mums and dads are increasingly reluctant to trust their children to a defence force with a public reputation of being seemingly incapable of stamping out workplace bullying. Second, the defence force is working at its highest operational tempo, and across the broadest range of tasking and greatest diversity of operational theatres, since at least the mid to late 1960s. Yet the defence force is only two thirds the size it then was; third, this high operational tempo comes after generally static or declining defence budgets throughout the 1972–2000 period.

It is only the strongly sustained push towards a single solution: more funding; which prevents this text breaking open under the pressure of its own inconsistencies. Here an international reputation for operational excellence – a very soldierly assertion of *esprit de corps* – is immediately undermined by the detailing of low-quality recruiting, bad public image, outmoded and ineffective equipment, and overwhelming deployment demand – each of them explanatory strands to which elements of the Kovko story have already been elsewhere connected. With this contribution Defence Australia may have intended to defend serving personnel such as Jake Kovko from the highly personalized narratives streaming across public and online media – but have instead managed only to broaden the chaos. Uncontrol, previously located in the acts – however explained – of Private Jake Kovko and a few anonymous Kuwaiti morgue workers, is now represented, and by a self-avowed expert and insider group, as both rampant, and systemic, within defence culture.

At which stage it is necessary to re-focus, and to consider those final strands of the Kovko discussion which overtly attempt forms of narrative closure: which seek, through whatever means, to reassert discourses of control. In the first of these, media professionals review the performance of their peers – but yet again, in the very act of attempting resolution, exacerbate the breaches.

Mismanagement in Media – Public Relations and Media Ethics

In a web commentary on his blog 'A good yarn', entitled 'Lessons from the Private Kovco bungle', public relations manager Chris Newlan explains that:

> I had an interesting conversation last night with a former Defence PR rep about the Government's appalling mismanagement of the aftermath of Private Jake Kovco's tragic death in Iraq.

He then offers 'some important observations for crisis communication specialists', relating to ways of 'managing' information flows at moments of such crisis:

> multiple spokespeople – four official spokespeople: Prime Minister John Howard, Defence Minister Nelson, the Chief of Army and the Chief of the Defence Force – made comment regarding the Private Kovco's death, the

subsequent bungling of the repatriation of his body and backflip regarding the
circumstances surrounding the incident.

For Newlan, this produces a confusing 'plethora of messages reaching the
public, which only added to the confusion'. He suggests that 'a single spokesperson
would have been far easier to manage in this situation'.

This drive to manage is of course specifically the role of a PR professional
– yet there are also disturbing elements within this mission. Here, the definition of
'messages' for the public appears actually to mean 'message' – a single, integrated,
controlled release through a sole source. So it is too that the second charge of
uncontrol relates to 'impatience – it would appear the rush to bring the news of
Private Kovco's death to our attention led to the wrong information reaching the
Defence Minister about the circumstances surrounding the incident'. Worse: 'The
conflicting information has led to claims of a cover-up'. For Newlan there must
still be – somewhere – a single, manageable 'truth' in the Kovko story; released
only when it reaches a sole information source: the Defence Minister. Why?
Because news of military casualties is always a political risk.

> Does the Prime Minister or ambitious Defence Minister want to be front and
> centre every time a soldier dies in the Middle East, particularly in an environment
> where public support for the Iraq War is limited?

Having located the optimal sourcing for 'the' flow of information, Newlan's
PR instincts are telling him to close it down again – for as long as possible.

De Mortuis Nil Nisi Bonum: Closure Through a Return to Privacy

Such drives to close down on all discussion, in whatever areas of public debate, are
common on almost every website sampled for this analysis. Typical is a response
on a yahoo talk site:

> It is less than a week *to mother's day.* This *young man's mother, and his wife
> and mother of his children,* are enduring *personal grief* over their loss, and don't
> need to see this crap here. Talk about it in your *loungerooms* if you must – we
> are all curious I know, and some have their opinions well formed. I just *sincerely*
> doubt the validity of exchanging your ideas and opinions here, so soon after the
> event, when the *family is so raw. Lock* the thread yahoo.

The image of Kovko is once again starkly clear: the private man; the family
member. It is expressed even more forcefully by Kovko's in-laws, who attempt the
same sort of shut-down in a post to another active Kovko discussion list:

Come on don't you read, suicide has been ruled out as we the family ruled it out on the 21st April this year. We are very proud of both our son-in-law Jake and our daughter Shelley and believe as Shelley does that this was a horrible accident. We sincerely hope you all watched Shelley at the media conference on 20th September when she spoke from her heart about how it has been for her for the last 5 months. She and her children has [sic] certainly been subjected to a lot of speculation and now we hope she can try and get on with the rest of her life. (Posted by: Lorraine at September 21, 2006 08:36 PM)

This is of course cultural work of another kind: preservation of self and of family, conducted more in the public or semi-public (new media) spotlight than is usually the case, but still a core part of the drawing together of close social networks at a moment of rupture. What it intersects however, painfully for those directly involved, is a parallel set of 'wound healing' strategies and performative acts, used to re-assert military order as prime sign of well-ordered national power. That this may endorse those more patriarchal aspects of a family's image of an ideal son, husband brother or father, is incidental to its motivation – which is, as ever, about erasure of the abject realities to which the soldierly body is subject.

Cementing Over the Cracks: The Body in the Monument

Since the dead body cannot be healed, the nation must – and the first act in sealing the nation's wound is the draping of the coffin in its flag. *Badbrhu* on the RPG (Role Playing Games Forum) is among a surprisingly large number of online posters who reacted negatively to this:

Two things pissed me off about Kovko's case. A news bulletin I saw showed Aussie troops carrying a metal transport coffin – just like the Yanks use – onto a plane and it was draped in a Aussie flag – just like the Yanks do – (different flag obviously). What are we now the Friggin' 51st state or what! Inter operability is one thing but come on.

How even more discomforting it then becomes, to view the most typical of the Australian press coverage of the flag-draped Kovko funeral, and to detect precisely these 'closure' strategies in play. Headlined 'Bloody good soldier' farewelled, John Donegan's photograph in *The Age* shows Kovko's coffin carried, shoulder height, through Sale cemetery, by fellow soldiers. All are shown from behind; the foreground occupied by a semi-focused mid-torso shot of a soldier, stiffly to attention. Jordan Chong's report:

The first Australian soldier killed in Iraq has been buried with full military honours in Sale this afternoon. His casket arrived on a gun carriage at Sale cemetery for the 1pm burial ceremony, greeted by a guard of honour of about 50 soldiers from his unit, the 3rd Battalion of the Royal Australia Regiment (3RAR).

Military honours   Three Roulettes flew over the cemetery during the burial ceremony and shots were fired in salute before a military band then played the *Last Post*. A soldier carrying a folded Australian flag, as well as Private Kovco's medals and regimental beret, followed behind on foot.

Every element of military ritual now in place, the 'family of nation' is able to express the final grief which returns Private Kovko, soldier, to Jake Kovko, family man.

PM pays respects   After the funeral, dignitaries at the service – including Prime Minister John Howard and Defence Minister Brendan Nelson – hugged members of Private Kovco's family and offered messages of support and sympathy. Mr Nelson appeared quite emotional.

But in the final gesture, the military itself sets an end to the Kovko story, explicitly re-connecting the soldierly body with the regimental tradition and ritual which will ensure the ongoing position of both.

Soldier 'stood proud'   Corporal Cameron Wagstaff, one of the soldiers who dressed Private Kovco for his funeral, said: 'The thing I remember about Jake is that he wanted to stand proud with his mates, with the medals on his chest'. Colonel Mumford said Private Kovco's name would be inscribed in stone memorial tablet at the Sydney's Holsworthy army barracks.

It seems appropriate to give the last citation in this multi-text analysis, to an historian of military death. Associate Professor Bruce Scates, author of *Return to Gallipoli: Walking the Battlefields of the Great War*, is a member of the Army History Unit. As part of the Kovko response, he wrote on the *Sydney Morning Herald's* website of the degree to which the return of the military dead has been an ongoing problem for Australia. Currently working on the taskforce assessing the lost World War One bodies from Fromelles, in France, he comments on the same sorts of drives towards closure signalled in orderly gravesites and monuments, which I have outlined here:

The agony of the Kovko family reminds us of a grief that has shadowed generations of Australians. The vast majority of our war dead was never returned. They lie in foreign fields, their bodies blending with the soil of any of the dozens of countries Australians have been sent to fight and die in. In the case of the Great War, more than 20,000 of about 60,000 dead are still listed as "missing". Families were told their remains had "vanished without trace", but that simple phrase conceals a much more sordid reality: bodies that sank in the mud, withered in the sun or were simply blown to pieces.

The physicality of the abjection that Scates records: the 'sordid reality' of the body at war, contrasts with both the military drive to re-order such realities; and the popular community view that 'closure' comes only with a return to the certitude of a known and secure identity: a confirmed place within the circle of nation/family. For Scates, unflinching in his commitment to historical accuracy, no such certainty or orderliness or comfort is, or should be, possible.

> Each war dead must be individually recovered, identified if possible, buried as an 'unknown' if not. Exhuming the missing of Fromelles, disentangling long-commingled bodies, will be a grim, lengthy and inconclusive enterprise. But long, grim and inconclusive is an apt description of the Great War. There should be no easy answers for the dead of Fromelles, no simple solution that literally buries the problem. Ninety years after the battle of the Somme, its pain and pointlessness still echo.

Conclusion: Lest *We* Forget

In sum, what is consistent across all of these Kovko stories has been trouble over text construction: no one source ever quite able to satisfy or convince its readers/viewers/listeners/participants. Again and again boldly asserted statements slip, revealing inside their own constitution intolerable degrees of tension, which will not settle into certainty or persuasiveness.

One thing however has become evident. Such slippages occur not only on the surface of the Kovko stories, constituted after the event, in the various acts of representation. Instead, they go right to the heart of the matter. Everywhere we look, someone crucial in the events we are attempting to interpret has themselves been immersed in acts of 'textualizing'. Kovko, dreamer, diarist and would-be writer, at the time of the fatal gunshot, was emailing his wife – and singing along to lyrics by The Cranberries. His name on a coffin was transcribed phonetically into Arabic and back into Roman notation by Kuwaiti morgue workers, morphing between Australian-Croatian KOVKO and Bosnian JUSO. It is a slip that should remind all of us not to point the finger of blame. That same name slides just as persistently in almost all sectors of Australian commentary, where it is variously spelled *Kovko* and *Kovco*.

Despite all attempts to attach him to a coherent narrative, Private Jake Kovko remains elusive; his story a matter of fragmentary possibilities, rather than the single straightforward line now allocated to him, on the nation's military memorials. Somewhere inside the complexity of the many stories offered about him, he encompasses the dilemmas of embodying today's military masculinity, where the once-hard and invulnerable male body, toughened and disciplined by its training and regimentation, is more than ever penetrated – not merely by the enemy's high-tech weaponry and e-scoped targeting, but by a new form of corrosive 'feminization': a softening from within. In a form of abjection Kristeva did not consider, the socio-psychological 'connection' of the soldierly-self into the private and the domestic: the feminized interiority of emotional connection, is reasserted – by those new and still only half-understood communications media and mobile technologies which 'bring you home', 24/7.

This chapter suggests that in an irony which is receiving far less critical attention than it deserves, it is this second Western incursion into the Middle East: the Iran and Afghanistan engagements, which have seen the potential of the new electronic connectedness fold back upon the high-tech nations. Where the first Gulf War: the campaign won for the US media by CNN and Fox, with their 'embedded journalists' and the release of military imaging direct to a fascinated public, carried the new technological invulnerability of Western military might to unprecedented heights, this second era has reversed the flows. Not only do we now receive on our TV screens and web news, counter-images of warfare 'on the ground': endless civilian casualties and chaos, reported from the local coverage produced by Al Jazeera and its new cohort of rival Gulf-State news channels, but we are increasingly able to access the 'home life' feeds of the family members, veterans, and even serving personnel, directly impacted by the 'human' events which war produces. It is a new vision of abjection: one in which our dangerous and ill-disciplined humanity once again spills forth. If military culture is to reassert control over these new incursions, it will need to reassess what it all means. They are going to need to re-read the lessons of Kristeva, from inside the re-technologization of the body within its digital communications networks: to learn to see Web 2.0 and 3G communications as themselves a form of psycho-social feminization of the military citadel. How they might come to react, is the next stage in an ongoing story.

References

Australia Defence Association. 2006. http://www.ada.asn.au/.

'Badbrhu', posting to http://forums.rpghost.com/showthread.php?t=43049.

Chong, J. 2006. Bloody good soldier farewelled, http://www.theage.com.au/articles/2006/05/02/1146335701778.html.

Cranberries lyrics: http://www.zombieguide.com/news/category/cranberries/.

Duffy, C. 2006. Kurt Lowe story, ABC Radio *PM,* July 18.

Knight, D. 2006. *Radar* blog on Fairfax Digital, Kovko Radar Blog, November.

McKew, M. 2006. The *7.30 Report,* http://www.abc.net.au/7.30/content/2006/s1625518.htm.

Newlan, C. 2006. Lessons from the Private Kovco bungle, http://chrisnewlan.typepad.com/a_good_yarn/2006/04/index.html.

Peacock, M. and Kortland, I. 2006. *The 7.30 Report,* 27 April http://www.abc.net.au/7.30/content/2006/s/625518.htm.

Scates, B. 2006. *Return to Gallipoli: Walking the Battlefields of the Great War.* Cambridge, Cambridge University Press.

Scates, B. 2006. *smh.com.au,* 17 July, http://www.smh.com.au/news/opinion/unknown-then-and-even-more-so now/2006/07/16/1152988409020.html?page=fullpage#contentSwap1.

Silkstone, D. 2006. Music and mystery: the last hours of Jake Kovco, 24 June, theage.com.au.

PART III
Containment of Bodies

Chapter 12

Strange yet Compelling:
Anxiety and Abjection in Hospital Nursing

Alicia Evans

Introduction

Fifty years ago, Menzies (1959) published her paper on nurses' anxiety[1]; a paper that was to become a classic study of hospital nursing (Rafferty and Traynor 2002, Wiltshire and Parker 1996), being extensively cited in the nursing literature on the organization and practice of nursing (Rafferty and Traynor 2002). Menzies (1959) took a psychoanalytic perspective, arguing that the constant and close proximity of the sick patient was anxiety-provoking for nurses; the closer the relationship and the more concentrated it was, the more likelihood the experience of anxiety for the nurse.

However, Menzies wrote at a time when, according to Lazarus and Folkman (1984), the concept of 'anxiety' was starting to decline. Having been influential in the first half of the 20th century, it was starting to be replaced by the idea of 'stress'. While psychoanalytic theory tends to continue to refer to 'anxiety', from the 1960s, psychoanalysis also fell from favour (Lazarus and Folkman 1984). It is important to note the distinction between the terms and concepts of 'anxiety' and 'stress' as the latter is steeped in a more behaviourist tradition. The concept of stress involves the idea of a stressor that is located externally and acts like a stimuli, causing the person either to feel 'stressed' or to cope with the stress, for example (Wiltshire and Parker 1996). Although Menzies does use the term 'stress' at times (see Menzies Lyth 1988), the concept she is working is that of anxiety, and is given through her work at the Tavistock Institute of Human Relations as a psychoanalyst (Menzies Lyth 1988) where psychoanalytic methods were applied to consultancies (Rafferty and Traynor 2002).

A contemporary of Menzies, the influential French psychoanalyst Jacques Lacan, criticized the shift to what he considered a more experimental approach to anxiety and one that gave rise to the notion of stress as an empirical object that acts on the subject (Lacan 1962/2002), often referred to as a 'stressor'. He highlighted

---

[1]   This was a report from a study of a nursing service of a London general hospital. The senior nurses had engaged Menzies to assist them with the problem of nursing student allocations as they had become highly problematic. Menzies regarded this as a presenting problem though and focused instead on the heightened anxiety of the nurses.

the experiments conducted with Pavlov's dog, arguing that the presence of the dog's master had both been overlooked and discounted (Lacan 1962/2002), a point he would make more of in arguing his psychoanalytic theory of anxiety.

In this chapter I refer to Lacan's (1962/2002) theory of anxiety to consider both anxiety and abjection in nursing practice, a practice that Menzies (Menzies 1959: 98) described as 'distasteful, disgusting and frightening' by ordinary standards. I argue that a psychoanalytic reading renders anxiety and abjection in nursing both particular to each nurse and devoid of an empirical object, although in abjection there is in addition, a certain jouissance[2].

In the context of hospital practice, with its associated anxieties, I argue that the nurse is in a position to respond from her anxiety to designate something of what she witnesses in practice. If she is able to do so, then her anxiety functions to marshal other hospital staff to the emergency treatment of a patient[3]. In addition, the nurse addresses herself to the patient who is horrified at their own physical condition. Her capacity to stand and face the patient, without turning away in disgust, can function to assist the patient to also face that which is evoked from the changes in their bodies. While this nursing practice may be considered distasteful work, there is something compelling about it that keeps many nurses at the bedside. I will argue that a jouissance of the abject is implicated in this.

A Psychoanalytic Theory of Anxiety

As has been mentioned, Lacan (1962/2002) argued that what had been overlooked and discounted in the accounts of the experiments conducted with Pavlov's dog was the presence of the dog's master, and the dog's response to the desire of his master. Whereas Pavlov's dog experienced the approach of his master who desired something of him, so too the human subject experiences the approach of an Other that desires (Lacan 1962/2002).

This Other of the human subject is both the structure of language that the subject is subordinated to and their unconscious; the subject's unconscious being produced by their 'entry' into language.

> It is because there is language that there is unconscious, insofar as language is constituted by a set of discrete elements, and it therefore suffers the laws of the logic of sets: that is to say, what Bertrand Russell and others discovered at the beginning of the century, that there is no universal set, that there is at least one element missing … (Vegh 1990: 193).

---

2   The term 'jouissance' is defined later in this chapter.

3   The nurse is designated as female in this chapter for both ease of style and because of the female gendered nature of nursing.

In the way that something is always missing in language, the Other is not complete; a certain lack exists in the Other. For the subject to experience this lack in the Other is to experience anxiety; an anxiety that has been referred to as 'castration anxiety' as this lack signals to the subject that something is profoundly missing or absent. To defend against the devastation of this experience of lack, the subject perceives that the Other desires something of them, a something that if given, will make the Other seem whole (Lacan 1962/2002). Clearly this is not a conscious or deliberate process in any way.

Anxiety arises when the subject experiences the approach of this desiring, lacking Other. The question arises: 'what does he want of me?' (Lacan 1962/2002). Yet what is desired is not known, for the Other's desire is of the unconscious. In addition, there is also the characteristic of an absence of doubt that comes with anxiety. Indeed there 'is the dimension of appalling certainty that is in anxiety' (Lacan 1962/2002: lesson 6).

Although Lacan (1962/2002) argues that anxiety is not without its object, this is not an empirical object. There is no empirical or tangible event, experience or person that is the object of anxiety, rather the subject's anxiety is produced by the immediacy of their experience of lack in the Other (Lacan 1962/ 2002).

However, the immediacy of this experience may be provoked by an actual event or interaction for example, although this does not make of the event or interaction an object of anxiety. Merely the event or interaction gives rise to the subject's anxiety by provoking in them something that makes present the lack in the Other. In this way, an event or interaction can provoke anxiety in one subject and not in another.

The 'Real' in Lacan's Theory

Freud's second topography (the id, ego and super-ego) was not reworked by Lacan, unlike much of Freud's other theory. Rather Lacan developed his own topography: the registers of the 'symbolic', 'imaginary' and 'real'. These registers are joined but heterogeneous (Lacan 1977). It is necessary to articulate something of this in order to consider further Lacan's psychoanalytic theory of anxiety.

Put rather simply, the symbolic register (or 'order', as it is also called) can be considered to be all that is symbolic, that is, it is all that is of language and symbols. The imaginary register is all that is of images and fantasy. It is out of this register that identifications are made and a sense of consistency and wholeness are generated. The register of the real is that which is lacking in the symbolic register (Lacan 1977). The register of the real can neither be symbolized in any way in language, nor imagined in any way (Lacan 1962/2002).

The relationship of the register of the real to anxiety is such that while the approach of a desiring and thus lacking Other produces anxiety, this experience of lack is also a 'signal of the real' (Lacan 1962/2002: lesson 13), not dissimilar in some ways to how Freud (1926/1979) theorized anxiety as being a signal of danger, that is, in relation to a loss. This real though is not synonymous with reality (Lacan 1977). The real is that which the subject experiences beyond both signification and image (Lacan 1962/ 2002). The real is where ' … all words cease and all categories fail … ' (Lacan 1955/1988: 164).

Responding in the Context of Anxiety

This is not to say that one cannot respond in a moment of anxiety, when faced with something of the real. When experiencing anxiety, the subject can either introduce doubt and become inhibited, or they can act in the immediacy of the moment. This act will be non-reflective and conducted with the certainty that comes with anxiety (Lacan 1962/2002). Indeed, it is from this certainty that one is able to act in this moment. For '[t]o act is to operate a transfer of anxiety' (Lacan 1962/2002: lesson 6). However, this is not, of course, a deliberate choice; it bears more on one's capacity to respond in this moment of anxiety.

One of the ways to respond to an encounter with the real, and thus to anxiety, is by way of designation; that is, to name something of this encounter. This naming is not of the order of description but rather ' … a designative naming is to name in its pure, demonstrative, deictic function, it is only to point out' (Etkin 1995: 73). This pointing out, this naming, is non-reflective, conducted as it is in the moment of the encounter. What this 'designation as act' in the real allows is for a hole to be made (Lacan 1971/2002: lesson 2), a hole, or cut that will not be without its effects.

Abjection

It was Kristeva, a psychoanalyst and academic (Skelton 2006) who made the concept of 'abjection' famous. However, Kristeva's (1997) concept of abjection reverberates with Lacan's (1962/2002) theory of anxiety, which is perhaps not so surprising as she attended Lacan's seminars until 1974 (Kristeva as cited in Roudinesco 1990). It was Lacan, in an interview on French television in 1973, who said his theory of anxiety is founded on the 'object' as it relates to the abject, and what he later called *objet petit a* (Lacan 1990). This 'object' is clearly not an empirical object though.

Abjection is related to a threat beyond what is tolerable, even thinkable; something close by that 'does not have, properly speaking, a definable *object'* (Kristeva 1997: 229). Indeed the only quality of object that it has is that it opposes the subject, and yet it is endured because it is imagined that is what is desired of the subject (Kristeva 1997).

In that abjection is caused by a disturbance of identity, system and order (Kristeva 1997) it can in some ways be mapped against Lacan's (1955/1988) concept of the real in that it cannot be either symbolized (in a language system and order) or imagined (as is required for identification). Kristeva's abject 'object' is jettisoned 'into an abominable real, inaccessible except through jouissance' (Kristeva 1997: 236).

Yet there is something else with abjection, as Kristeva defines it, as it also has a quality that both summons and repulses, a fascination that draws one to it (Kristeva 1997). This non-object of abjection sits on the border, something marginalized that is neither incorporated nor expelled; a non – object that both beckons and repels (Kristeva 1997) and in doing so, is compelling.

Secondary repression is related to abjection in that abjection can appear in the symptom; the tumour as symptom can be an example of the abject (Kristeva 1997). '[R]epugnance, disgust, abjection … they tumble over into non-sense or the impossible real, but they appear even so in spite of "myself" (which is not) as abjection' (Kristeva 1997: 238).

The Symptom and Jouissance

In Kristeva's theory of the abject can be heard the psychoanalytic theory of the symptom. Freud (1926/1979) theorized that symptoms are formations of the unconscious and represent a compromise between two opposing forces. Lacan concurred with Freud, only theorizing the symptom in linguistic terms (Evans 1996).

The French term 'jouissance', a complex term, is not easily translated into the English language, however, Allouch (a French psychoanalyst who attended Lacan's seminar) contends that the way Lacan works the term 'jouissance' corresponds with Foucault's working of the term 'pleasure' (Allouch 2007). In other places, 'jouissance' is translated as 'enjoyment' (see Lacan 1975). However the term 'jouissance' was also employed by Lacan in a number of different ways, one of which was to express the satisfaction that the symptom can bring, as paradoxical as that might seem given that there is also suffering associated with the symptom (Evans 1996).

In the symptom the drive impulse has some fulfilment and thus some satisfaction, some jouissance, yet this can be outside the subject's awareness. Jouissance is also associated with the abject, as while the abject is neither wanted or known, it can only be accessed via jouissance (Kristeva 1997), thus explaining how the abject both repels and attracts. That is, just as the symptom represents a compromise between two opposing forces, so there is this play of opposite forces with abjection.

Hospital Nursing and Anxiety

In order to consider something of nursing practice in relation to this theory, a number of vignettes from practice will be presented and theorized. Consider, then, these field-notes from a research study undertaken on a medical ward of an

Australian metropolitan hospital; notes in this instance that were taken during a change-of-shift handover report.

> The handover report moves on. A male patient has 'chopped his own finger off in an argument with his wife'.
>
> RN Patterson says, 'The fingertip is in the ward fridge'.
>
> One of the nurses says, 'Our fridge? Here? Gross!'
>
> RN Patterson says, 'Yeah. He chopped his finger off and it's in the fridge'.
>
> The man has, until now, refused to have his finger 're-implanted'. The nurses are not so sure the fingertip will be any good now.
>
> RN Patterson says, 'I'm happy to throw the finger out'. She had made enquiries of the theatre staff. They'd said if it wasn't reattached, to throw it out into a 'yellow bin'. RN Patterson says throwing it into a yellow bin 'brings back memories'.
>
> RN Gale says to the nurse who sounded horrified, 'I'm going to get it out and wave it at you … '.
>
> Another handover: The graduate nurse says, 'It was pretty yucky'. The partially blind man in bed ten has a hernia. Around one third of his bowel has collapsed into, and is now in, his scrotum. The graduate nurse describes, partly by gesture, how she needed to help the man urinate by putting the urinary bottle in place. 'It pulsates' she says (Evans 2005: 8–9).

Within the walls of the hospital the nurse can be exposed to sounds, sights, smells and experiences quite extraordinary by usual community standards: a finger can be designated as rubbish and disposed of into a yellow bin. The response to these events is particular to each nurse; in some anxiety may be provoked, in others not so. These events, which could by ordinary standards be described as frightening, distasteful and disgusting (Menzies 1959), can be spoken about, at least in this instance, in spite of any associated anxiety or horror.

Herewith another example of something provocative of anxiety, perhaps even horror, which was experienced by one nurse and not the other. Dartington (1998), in a paper where she puts forward an argument about inhibition of thought in hospital nursing, offers the following recollection from her first visit to a surgical ward as a nursing student.

> I stood at the end of the bed of someone with tubes coming out of every orifice. He was gripping so tightly to the bedframe that his knuckles were white. I felt

giddy and faint. In my imagination the man was being tortured, a thought so terrible I could not even voice it to my friend, who was asking sensible questions about the temperature chart. Later, as I sat recovering in the cool corridor, I felt foolish. It occurred to me that the new patients arriving on the ward might have similar waking nightmares, and like me feel ashamed of themselves (Dartington 1998: 103).

While the object of anxiety is unknown (Lacan 1962/2002), the experience of anxiety is not. It can be heard when at the handover: the horror of the finger disposed of as garbage; the return of memories; the 'yucky' bowel that pulsates in the scrotum. It can be heard when at the bedside, perhaps the first time a disturbing image is witnessed: the tubes, the thoughts of torture, the need to recover in the cool corridor.

However, it is not the tubes, the white gripping knuckles, the pulsating scrotum or the finger-come-garbage that is the object of anxiety. One nurse feels faint and giddy while the other asks sensible questions; one nurse is horrified about the unattached finger and the other threatens to wave it at her. While the object of anxiety is unknown (Lacan 1962/2002), something of some encounters, at some moments, provoke anxiety for the nurse.

However, while what provokes the nurse's anxiety is particular to each one, perhaps there is something about the practice of nursing that is more provocative of anxiety than other practices. Menzies (1959) argued that it was the proximity of the patient that was so provocative; a patient who was ill or injured, and often seriously so. 'Nurses are confronted with the threat and the reality of suffering and death as few lay people are' (Menzies 1959: 98).

Operating a Transfer of Anxiety

While at times something of the experience of anxiety can be spoken of, at other times there are experiences that leave the subject speechless. Take this example, also witnessed on a medical ward in an Australian public hospital.

> Nurses are running in and out of a patient bedroom ... RN Patterson is doing cardiac compression on a patient in the room. ... Someone yells out 'Call a code blue.' A nurse picks up the phone. She has a blank expression on her face and she doesn't say or do anything. She is frozen like this for no more than a few seconds when another nurse yells out to her 'It's okay. I'll do it' as she picks up another phone, dials and calls the code (Evans 2005: 206–7).

One nurse freezes, while the other nurse is able to take action. The nurse, who is momentarily unable to speak, faces something that she is unable to respond to – it renders her speechless. In this moment she cannot assimilate her experience; something has her in its grip.

While we will never know what this nurse's experience actually was, nonetheless there is a situation, a lack of speech in a given moment, which can be theorized, albeit in somewhat tentative terms perhaps. The nurse is speechless; something of her experience cannot be brought into words. She picks up the phone to call the code but is unable to find the words to speak. This is suggestive of an encounter with the real; something encountered that is beyond signification and image. In the moment when the subject brushes up against the real, in the moment when the nurse is frozen, without words or image, this intense brush with the Other's lack (of what is missing, of lack of symbol or image) is productive of anxiety (Lacan 1962/2002).

The nurse experiences events as they unfold on the ward, the sudden changes in the patient's condition for example, and encounters something that might at first be experienced in the register of the real. While one nurse is immobilized by anxiety though, the other is able to act. Thus the nurse who is able to respond in the context of anxiety (that is, to act and thus 'to operate a transfer of anxiety' (Lacan 1962/2002: lesson 6)) is able to function for the patient who requires the code to be called. Rather than perceiving the situation as a stressor for the nurse, the nurse's anxiety here can be considered to be functional. This that the nurse encounters, something as yet undesignated, she must be able to name and quickly. The nurse's act is both non-reflective and one of designation in this moment of anxiety; she names that which she encounters and in this way she produces an effect: 'This is an emergency' or 'This is a cardiac arrest – call a code' or 'This is nothing to worry about' for example.

In this way, if the nurse is able to operate a transfer of anxiety, then her anxiety has an extraordinary function within the organization of the hospital – her anxiety functions within the organization as a beacon of approaching danger. Her anxiety-producing action mobilizes other people to address that danger and thus she initiates the emergency treatment of the patient. The nurse calls the code.

The Real of the Body

While this encounter with the register of the real might be experienced in an emergency (this brush with something that profoundly lacks) it might also be provoked by nurses' work with some patients' bodies in some disturbing moments. That is, if a patient's body in some moment cannot be either symbolized or imagined, if there is an experience of the patient's body that is beyond signification and image for the nurse, then there may be an experience of the real of the body for the nurse.

Consider, for example, this extract from a nursing student who was working in the Emergency Department when a male patient was admitted and resuscitated after having a cardiac arrest (van der Riet 1997).

> He looked vulnerable and alone. In this sea of technology a human body looked
> out of place. I tried to imagine that this body had a life with his family … I didn't
> feel like I could touch him, he was cold and bluish like a cadaver. It was still
> difficult to think of him as human … (van der Riet 1997: 100).

The nursing student is grappling with something horrific. If, as this extracts
suggests, there was something of the patient's body that was beyond signification
and image in this moment for the nurse, then this would be an encounter with the
real of the man's body and thus an experience of anxiety; something perhaps not
at all surprising.

Abjection and Horror in Nursing Practice

While an encounter with the real of the body may have occurred for the nursing
student in practising in the Emergency Department, the palliative care hospice
is another site that one might reasonably expect to encounter this. For example,
something of the disturbance to one's identity, system and order that characterizes
abjection (Kristeva 1997) might be heard in the following field-note from Lawton's
(1998) study at a hospice.

> A similar comment was proffered by the husband of another patient in the
> hospice, Clare, who had advanced breast cancer and gross lymphoedema in her
> arms and legs. He frequently pointed to the 'brutal' way in which Clare's cancer
> was eating her body away. In one particular emotional outpouring he told me that
> he'd been in the armed forces for seventeen-and-a-half years and had witnessed
> many deaths. Yet he had never seen anything quite so 'cruel and disgusting' as
> what was happening to his wife. The husband of another patient suggested that it
> would have been much easier if his wife had been run over by a bus than to see
> her 'deteriorate and rot away so slowly' (Lawton 1998:140).

In this account there is portrayed an experience of the body that is suggestive of
an encounter with the real of the body. While a patient's cancer may represent
something of the abject for the patient themselves (as it is their symptom), it is not
the patient's cancer *per se* that is the abject 'object' for the nurse. An encounter
with the real of the body and of abjection is something beyond this because the
thought and image of the body being eaten away, for example, is clearly of the
symbolic and imaginary registers.

Nonetheless there may be something of the horror of the experience of
witnessing the decaying body in this way that produces abjection for the nurse,
and as can be heard in this account, for the patient's loved ones. Something of the
experience that provokes horror; brushing up against an unnameable, unimaginable
object of the real can produce anxiety.

While this account of the effect of disease and dying on a patient's body occurs in a hospice, it would be surprising indeed if the majority of nurses could not describe at least one patient whom they had nursed whose life had become a living hell due to their ill-health. The horror story is not an unfamiliar one in the nurse's repertoire. This is not to trivialize the horror but rather to substantiate its place within the world of the nurse's practice. What the nurse does in the face of the patient's abjection and maybe her own, provoked by something of this, is what is of importance. Just as the nurse operates a transfer of anxiety in her act of designation in the emergency situation, perhaps also there is something of this with the patient (and also the relative) who is horrified.

Perhaps there is an act of designation in the way the nurse addresses and dresses the patient's failing body. In that the nurse addresses the patient, stays with them, stares into that patient's horror without pulling away in disgust, could be considered an act that assists the patient. In this way the nurse might designate by her presence that something can be faced, something of the real for the patient.

Abjection and Jouissance in Nursing Practice

While it might be considered offensive to associate rotting, decaying bodies and nurse's jouissance, nonetheless the nurse's work keeps her close to this that others might prefer not to see. Better to be run over by a bus than to be this body that the nurses, nurse. Rather another death than this cruel and disgusting one that the nurse is witness to; not once but many times (though clearly not in the same capacity as the patient's loved ones).

The hospital nurse is surrounded by sights and smells, and she has experiences that can provoke anxiety, even horror at times. However, it could be argued that these are just things the nurse must withstand in order to undertake the technical work that interests her. Perhaps for many this is so. However the nurse often does much more than withstand.

The disturbance that abjection produces is caused by a non-object on the border that both repels and beckons (Kristeva 1997). If abjection is experienced by the nurse it is one that can only be accessed via jouissance, suggesting that for the nurse there is a jouissance experienced in some way in this work that horrifies.

For the nurse, something of a jouissance, perhaps even one that is not known, draws her back to her work, a work that brings with it experiences that may give rise to considerable anxiety for her and an experience of something of the abject. However, in this work that brings with it this abjection, there is a jouissance. Perhaps even it is this jouissance, this enjoyment, which allows her to work with something unnameable, something that is at times frightening, horrific and disgusting to her too. For as repelling and disgusting as diseased and dying bodies can become, or as shocking the sight of the body traumatized in ways not before seen, many nurses remain at the bedside. There remains something compelling about this practice of nursing.

Anxiety and Abjection in Nursing Practice

It is five decades since it was famously argued that nursing work was both anxiety-provoking and included practices that others might easily find distasteful, frightening and disgusting (Menzies 1959). The nurse's practice can situate her within the strangely compelling site of the hospital; a place where a finger becomes a piece of garbage and scrotums pulsate, swelling beyond all imaginable proportions.

Yet what actually produces anxiety for the nurse in these encounters cannot be defined, for anxiety, in a psychoanalytic reading, does not have a tangible object and is particular to each subject (Lacan 1962/2002). It can be witnessed though, in the moment when the nurse brushes up against this 'object' with neither form nor substance, this object of the real. She may even fail to speak; stunned as she is whilst in its grip.

Yet while one nurse fails to speak, another nurse, in a moment that precedes any reflection, transfers her anxiety into action. In doing so, her action summons the necessary people to the medical emergency. She has acted on the certainty of her anxiety and in the immediacy of the moment of that anxiety. In this can be witnessed a conceptualization far removed from a notion of 'stressors in nursing', a notion that considers stress to be outside and bearing down on all nurses in the environment. Rather anxiety is experienced in all its particularity and for each one.

However, this is not to dismiss some of the difficult working conditions that may face the nurse, but rather to appreciate how a concept of anxiety can bring a richness to a consideration of the nurse's practice. In addition, the transfer of anxiety into action can illustrate how anxiety can be functional and necessary to the nurse's practice, rather than be considered something to eliminate.

As well as this, with the experience of anxiety comes another non-object – one that both repels and attracts, a marginal object that sits on the border refusing to leave when repelled: the abject (Kristeva 1997). It also cannot be known but can be experienced, sometimes perhaps when confronted with the decaying body, yet clearly particular to each one. An 'object' that the nurse faces as she looks into its eyes: it remains on the border, threatening, as she tries not to let it touch her.

Yet still the nurse works in this environment where perhaps much abjection is experienced. Nurses' work involves a practice that can be described as 'distasteful, disgusting and frightening' (Menzies 1959: 98), but this disgust the nurse does not shun. Rather the nurse is able to somehow tolerate this disgust, perhaps even finds it compelling, and in being able to tolerate it may illustrate to the patient, by her actions, that it can be tolerated, that indeed the disgust that is experienced can be withstood.

Conclusion

The nurse's anxiety, in the conceptualization presented in this chapter, is understood in terms that go beyond the idea that there are stressors in the environment that bear down upon the nurse. In this conceptualization, the nurse's anxiety is functional. For without both the experience of anxiety and the certainty that comes with it, the quick designation of what is required for the patient would not work so well. The nurse calls the code.

In addition to anxiety, the nurse is exposed to experiences that suggest an encounter with abjection, both as witness to it when the patient experiences it and when it is experienced firsthand. In this too, perhaps the nurse has a function of designation. When the patient experiences abjection by what is evoked by their physical condition, she faces their horror, not turning away in disgust at what it is she witnesses. This standing and facing, dressing and addressing the patient, perhaps allows the patient to withstand something of this experience; to face their own horror.

This is her practice and one not without its jouissance. No matter how horrific the story might be some days, no matter how distasteful the experience, the nurse remains at the bedside. In all this there remains something compelling for the nurse in her practice – perhaps thankfully so.

References

Allouch, J. 2007. Jacques Lacan and Michel Foucault: misunderstandings and convergences, in *Lacan Love: Melbourne Seminars and Other Works*, edited by M.-I. R. d. Zentner et al. Melbourne: Lituraterre, 27–57.

Dartington, A. 1998. Where angels fear to tread: idealism, despondency and inhibition of thought in hospital nursing, in *The Unconscious at Work: Individual and Organisational Stress in the Human Services,* edited by A. Obholzer, et al. London: Routledge, 102–109.

Etkin, G. 1995. Nothing returns from the real: The structure of psychosis, in *Papers of the Freudian School of Melbourne: Psychosis: Who Speaks?,* edited by D. Pereira. Melbourne: The Freudian School of Melbourne, 61–76.

Evans, A.M. 2005. *Discourses of Anxiety in Nursing Practice: A Psychoanalytic Case Study.* Unpublished PhD thesis. Melbourne: The University of Melbourne.

Evans, D. 1996. *An Introductory Dictionary of Lacanian Psychoanalysis.* London: Routledge.

Freud, S. 1926/1979. Inhibitions, symptoms and anxiety, in *On Psychopathology,* edited by A. Richards and translated by J. Strachey. Ringwood, Melbourne: The Pelican Freud Library, volume 10, 229–333.

Kristeva, J. 1997. Approaching abjection (abridged), in *The Portable Kristeva,* edited by K. Oliver. New York: Columbia University Press, 229–47.

Lacan, J. 1955/1988. *The Seminar of Jacques Lacan, Book 2, The Ego in Freud's Theory and in the Technique of Psychoanalysis 1954–1955,* translated by S. Tomaselli. Melbourne: Cambridge University Press.

Lacan, J. 1962/2002. *The Seminar of Jacques Lacan, Anxiety, Book 10,* translated by C. Gallagher. London: Karnac Books.

Lacan, J. 1971/2002. *The Seminar of Jacques Lacan, On a Discourse That Might Not Be a Semblance, Book 18,* translated by C. Gallagher. London: Karnac Books.

Lacan, J. 1975. *On Feminine Sexuality: The Limits of Love and Knowledge, Book 20, Encore 1972–1973,* translated by B. Fink. New York: Norton.

Lacan, J. 1977. *The Four Fundamental Concepts of Psychoanalysis*: Translator's note, translated by A. Sheridan. Ringwood: Penguin Books.

Lacan, J. 1990. *Television. A Challenge to the Psychoanalytic Establishment,* translated by D. Hollier et al. London: WW Norton and Company.

Lawton, J. 1998. Contemporary hospice care: the sequestration of the unbounded body and dirty dying. *Sociology of Health and Illness,* 20(2), 121–143.

Lazarus, R.S., and Folkman, S. 1984. *Stress, Appraisal, and Coping.* New York: Springer Publishing Company.

Menzies, I.E.P. 1959. A case-study in the functioning of social systems as a defence against anxiety: a report on a study of the nursing service of a general hospital. *Human Relations,* 13, 95–121.

Menzies Lyth, I. 1988. *Containing Anxiety in Institutions.* London: Free Association Books.

Rafferty, A.M. and Traynor, M. (eds). 2002. *Exemplary Research for Nursing and Midwifery.* London: Routledge.

Roudinesco, E. 1990. *Jacques Lacan & Co: A History of Psychoanalysis in France, 1925–1985,* translated by J. Mehlman. Chicago: The University of Chicago Press.

Skelton, R.M. (ed.). 2006. *The Edinburgh International Encyclopaedia of Psychoanalysis.* Edinburgh: Edinburgh University Press.

van der Riet, P. 1997. The body, the person, technologies and nursing, in *The Body in Nursing: A Collection of Views,* edited by J. Lawler. Melbourne: Churchill Livingstone, 95–108.

Vegh, I. 1990. The Real, the Symbolic, the Imaginary and the structure of neurosis, perversion and psychosis, in *Papers of the Freudian School of Melbourne: Crucial Questions for Psychoanalysis,* edited by O. Zentner. Melbourne: The Freudian School of Melbourne, 187–97.

Wiltshire, J. and Parker, J. 1996. Containing abjection in nursing: the end of shift handover as a site of containment. *Nursing Inquiry,* (3), 23–29.

Chapter 13

Subjectivity and Embodiment:
Acknowledging Abjection in Nursing

Janet McCabe

Introduction

On a regular basis nurses encounter situations during which the body or bodily functions shape the nursing care that is provided. From the public health nurse working with the homeless and drug addicted to the medical surgical nurse dressing wounds on an in-patient unit – embodiment becomes a mediating factor in how care is structured. However, despite the centrality of the body and embodiment to nursing work, nursing theorists have tended to either approach the body from a strict biomedical perspective or have simply avoided discussing the role of embodiment in nursing. For example, nurses regularly interact with bodies that do not fit within established norms; bodies that leak, bodies that are disfigured and deformed, bodies that have committed heinous acts, bodies that reveal disabilities. Sometimes bodies and/or the actions of nurses threaten an individual's assumptions about what both the patient and nursing practice should be. For example, historically individuals with developmental disabilities have been considered either asexual or sexually deviant, as such, nurses working with this population may have these assumptions challenged when their work involves providing sexual health care. Others may see the sexual activity and sexuality of this population as something transgressive, something that challenges the defined boundaries of a specific embodiment and subjectivity. This contradiction presents a threat to the perceived self and thus may trigger abjection, as it has been described by Julia Kristeva (1982). Clearly then, the concepts of both embodiment and abjection are essential to nursing practice, and are vital mediators in nursing work, as such they should be represented within theoretical nursing literature.

Despite the importance of embodiment current theoretical nursing literature not only disregards nursing experiences regarding the breakdown of bodies, and alterations to accepted bodies, but these theories also neglect how these situations may effect the subjectivities of those involved and instigate abjection within the nurse. The concept of patient presented in the existing nursing literature is often one of an autonomous, self-created human being, who is an active participant in nursing care; often, the body is considered of secondary importance. This perspective overlooks the idea of person as subject, and ignores the role nurses play in the construction of subjectivity. It also overlooks situations that carry the potential to invoke the elements of abjection that are inherently present in nursing work. The lack of attention to these aspects of nursing work presents a risk to the profession, and speaks to a lack of professional awareness regarding the contribution of nurses to the control of patients in order to maintain social norms. This control could be interpreted as a means of containing what is considered abject and abject embodiment; containment in this sense affects and reinforces social norms and the subjectivity of the nurse and patient. The interplay between embodiment and abjection may lead to the fortification of norms as they relate to the asexuality and/or sexual deviancy that have historically been linked to the sexual activity of individuals with developmental disabilities.

This chapter will explore the concept of person as presented within theoretical nursing literature to demonstrate this inattention to subjectivity and embodiment. The works of Kristeva (1982) and Foucault (1980a, 1980b) and Fawcett (2005) will be used to frame this discussion. In describing the causes of abjection, Kristeva (1982) states that it is the challenges to the fixed identity of the subject and the transgression of established boundaries (either physical or metaphorical) that result in the perception of a threat to the self. To clearly illustrate the relationships between subjectivity, abjection, and embodiment, the 1980 film, *The Elephant Man*, will be used because the film demonstrates transgression, abjection, and subjectivity on many levels. While the film addresses abjection from a medical standpoint, it also illuminates abjection in relation to sexuality – juxtaposing scenes of tenderness with those of horror at the sight or thought of a simple kiss. Also, the film exposes how various contexts influence the subjectivity of the eponymous central character, Merrick, and often causes others to question their sense of self, and may be effectively applied to nursing work; specifically, nursing work that addresses the perceived problematic nature of individuals with developmental disabilities who are sexually active. However, before these concepts can be discussed in the context of the *The Elephant Man*, and applied to nursing work, subjectivity and abjection both merit further explanation and exploration.

Exploring Subjectivity and Abjection

Subjectivity, or the sense of self, is not only an abstract principle; it is how we come to see ourselves as distinct from those around us (Mansfield 2000). Abjection, literally, the act of throwing away becomes by extension the act of distancing oneself from something that is perceived as a threat or source of contagion, as an act of defending one's own subjectivity. The concept of person in nursing literature is dominated by the perspective that the individual is a free and autonomous human being. This notion was prevalent during the Enlightenment, and is central to the works of individuals such as Rousseau and Kant. The self envisioned during the Enlightenment is autonomous, and is subjected to forces exerted on it by external sources, such as society (Mansfield 2000). Both Foucault and Kristeva reject this idea, and suggest that the self is constructed and experiences constant change.

For Foucault the self is linked to the concept of power/knowledge. Foucault suggests that power exists before the subject becomes aware of its very existence and it is this pre-existing power that shapes what we consider our individuality. Thus, the self is created not by us, but rather for us through its mechanisms (Foucault 1980b). Systems of power, which exist in all social relations, require a body of knowledge on which all claims of truth are based (Foucault 1980a). The combination of power and knowledge, results in the creation of subjects (Mansfield 2000). Subjects which then govern their own bodies and the bodies of others in relation to specific subjectivities and rules based on socially constructed categories. Foucault stated that 'the individual which power has constituted is at the same time its vehicle' (Foucault 1980b: 98). In embracing our subjectivity, we actually confirm and reaffirm the powers which have created it.

While Foucault identifies the constitution of the subject in relation to power/ knowledge and interprets the subject as its product, Kristeva approaches the subject from a different angle. Following in the footsteps of Sigmund Freud, Jacques Lacan, and Melanie Klein, she provides a psychoanalytic explanation of the body. To fully comprehend her interpretation of abjection, we must first attend to her understanding of the subject or self. For Kristeva the self (the 'I', the ego) is never stable; rather, it is *le sujet en processus* (McAfee 2004). As suggested by Mansfield (2000), the self is never a complete and separate entity and as a result, our sense of self, our subjectivity always involves other people. The sense of self is what is contained within an imaginary boundary drawn around the body. And as with any borders, those of the self must be defended against threats by means of a reactive defence system. Abjection is the defence system which functions to maintain and uphold the borders of the self.

The abject always threatens the identity of either the subject and/or society and questions the fundamental ideas on which they are based. The danger posed to society and the self by the abject is a threat because it disturbs the symbolic order on which society is built; it disrupts the categories, and classes into which subjects are sorted (Oliver 1993). Douglas (1966) points out that the disturbance caused by polluting forces (the disgusting or abject) is due to a blurring of categories and classifications. Foucault suggests that categories of subjects are the result of power/knowledge generated by the dominant discourses, and enforced through disciplines. For example, nursing creates categories of the good patient, the difficult patient, the non-compliant; medical discourse creates the categories of the disabled and the mentally ill, and justice systems have defined the criminal. These categories outline and define the norms by which subjects are expected to act and present themselves. It is when these categories are violated, or the boundaries are blurred, when one is presented with the disgusting, polluting, or the abject, that the seeming unity of an individual's subjectivity is challenged. As previously mentioned, inattention to the importance of subjectivity and embodiment within nursing literature may result in nursing actions that function to purify or contain the abject, or abject work.

The Nursing Concept of Person

Although the person (patient, human being) is a central concept within nursing knowledge, the dominant conceptualizations of this idea are problematic on two levels: first, the concept of person as presented at the level of the *metaparadigm* of nursing, secondly how dominating worldviews influence this concept within nursing philosophy and impact on conceptual models and nursing theories. In examining nursing literature, it becomes evident that the person is represented as self-creating and that embodiment is always secondary to this belief. This concept inevitability poses a challenge to nurses because they work with bodies and subjects that fall not only outside of societal norms, but also physical embodiments and nursing actions that are considered abject (e.g. seeping wounds, foul smells).

In her proposed organization of nursing knowledge, Fawcett (2005) outlined a structural holarchy[1]. Each component of this apparatus is recognized as a whole unto itself and also as a contributing part of the larger whole, the whole in this case being the body of nursing knowledge. The components of this holarchy include: the *metaparadigm*, philosophies, conceptual models, theories and empirical indicators. Fawcett organizes these components into a hierarchy based on their level of abstraction, the *metaparadigm* being the most abstract, and the empirical indicators the most concrete.

Fawcett's (2005) nursing *metaparadigm* identifies the concepts most central to the discipline in order to communicate what the discipline is and is not. She presents the concepts of human being, environment, health, and nursing as most central to the discipline. Human beings are viewed as active participants in nursing care and include both individuals (if recognized in a specific culture) and collectives that interact with nursing, for example: families, communities and special interest groups. According to Fawcett, nursing is defined as the actions that are carried out by nurses in conjunction with, or on behalf of, the person, for example assessment, planning and evaluation. There is no acknowledgment at the level of the *metaparadigm* that nursing actions, or the environment, contribute to the patient as a subject, or how the individual is seen by others, and thereby by her/himself. However, the activities that Fawcett (2005) outlines are those that can lead directly to the creation of specific subjects – of patients as compliant or non-compliant, troublesome, or difficult. And these subjectivities typically lead to actions on the part of the health care team that function to mitigate these negative subjectivities.

In *Sailing Beyond: Nursing Theory and the Person*, Drevdahl points out that 'individuals are the *result* of social workings' (1999: 5) and that it is within discourses, such as nursing, that identities are created and differences established. In contrast, Fawcett provides no propositional statements to connect the concept of person to the concepts of environment, health, or nursing in a way that establishes

---

1   Holarchy, a term first used by Hungarian writer Arthur Koestler, refers to a hierarchy of holons – a holon being both a specific part, but also a part of the larger whole.

how the latter affects the way in which individuals see themselves or are perceived by others. While she does acknowledge that human beings are in 'continuous relationship with their environments' (Drevdahl 1999: 6), the power of this environment in shaping the person is not addressed. Consequently, her concept of person ignores the subjective nature of the human being, especially as this concept relates to health and illness, and affects the subsequent levels of the holarchy.

Philosophy, the second level of the holarchy, outlines three world views that are valued and believed by the discipline, and thus have contributed to the discipline of nursing (Fawcett 2005). Fawcett re-labels these worldviews as the reaction worldview (bio-medical perspective), the reciprocal interaction worldview (holistic perspective), and the simultaneous action worldview (unitary perspective), and maintains that they have shaped and guided both the profession and the discipline, and have interpreted the concepts set forth in the *metaparadigm* in different ways. It is at the philosophical level that nursing literature neglects embodiment as an important aspect of the conception of the person in favour of one that envisions a self-creating human being whose body is of secondary importance.

Over time, nursing has engaged with, and been influenced by, a number of different worldviews, which in turn have uniquely affected the ontological and epistemological priorities of both the profession and the discipline, and thus affected the concept of person. In the 1970s, nursing theorists attempted to shift nursing away from the biomedical perspective that had played a dominant role up to that point (Thorne et al. 1998). Fawcett refers to this biomedical perspective as the reaction worldview, which saw the person as the sum of their parts, each of which could be looked at objectively and individually. Thorne et al. (1998) contend that it was at this point that a polarization, as represented by the holistic and unitary perspectives, occurred in the understanding of the embodied person within nursing.

The unitary perspective (simultaneous action) interprets human beings as continuously changing, self-organized energy fields, recognisable only through behaviour patterns (Fawcett 2005). This perspective emphasized knowledge development based on inner experiences, choices and values (Fawcett 2005). This worldview influenced Rogers' (1980 and 1992) conceptual model 'the science of unitary human beings', which in turn contributed to the theory of 'health as expanding consciousnesses' as presented by Newman (1997). Rogers defined unitary human beings as 'irreducible wholes' (Rogers 1992: 29), identifiable through energy field patterns, Newman in her theory of health as expanding consciousness saw each client situation as a pattern, both unique and whole. Both Rogers' conceptual model and Newman's nursing theory present the person as self-organizing; both disregard the person's physical embodiment, seeing it as reductive because humans exist through their behaviour patterns. Such a conceptualization is ironic, considering the fact that behaviour occurs with and through bodies.

On the other hand, the holistic perspective (reciprocal interaction) interprets the body as part of the person; a part which can have meaning only in relation to the whole human being (Fawcett 2005, Thorne et al. 1998). The relationship between the environment and the person is seen as reciprocal, with a person's behaviours changing in response to factors within the environment. Many nursing theories, such as those of Orem (1997) and Roy (2000) are situated within the holistic perspective. Holism suggests that persons can only be understood when all of the discrete parts are considered in unison; this would suggest that while the physical body is a part, it still can only be understood in relation to the whole.

All three worldviews minimize the importance of embodiment, either by perceiving the body as an objective entity (bio-medical perspective), or completely ignoring it as a critical aspect of the person (holistic and unitary). Some scholars, however, see these views as problematic because it is through the body that we present ourselves to the world, and on which first impressions and judgments are made. In addition, not one of these dominant worldviews addresses the subjectivity of persons; rather, they view the person as logical and self-organizing. This conceptualization of person makes it impossible for nurses to acknowledge the creation of the subject, and their role in the perpetuation of these ideas about specific subjects. The failure to provide attention to situations in which the embodiment of the person is of primary concern or those situation that provide defining moments to the subjectivity of nurse or patient, may reflect the fact that philosophically nursing has sublimated the abject aspects of the profession, and in doing so contributed to a purified view of the profession and its patients.

An interesting example to bring these aspects of nursing care to the forefront is that of the nursing care of burn patients. These patients violate social norms which dictate the requirement of a perfect body, and the actions taken by nurses of dressing and covering the wounds (and the subsequent pain that is inflicted) violate norms of nursing in terms of care and protection. Nurses perceive themselves as individuals who protect others from harm, not as inflictors of pain and suffering. As such, nurses take actions to purify these experiences as made evident through the language used in their discussions about wound healing (Rudge 1998). The use of language in relation to assessing burn wounds is full of words and phrases that sanitize leaky bodies:

> While doctors and nurses can talk about a graft 'looking good', patients still talk about their skin with a degree of uncertainty … One patient talked about (and laughed rather darkly) about leaving bits of himself behind on chairs, and how he was horrified how the grafts could get blood blisters and pustules, and how the grafts seemed to leak all the time (Rudge 1998: 234).

This is an example of how nurses interpret the status of patients in purely clinical terms, simply as a part of a larger whole. This may be done completely unconsciously, in order to contain or purify the abject, to make others conform to the norms and boundaries of prescribed subjectivities. Although these wounds violate the clean and proper body, the use of sanitizing phrases helps the nurses to normalize the abject. In addition the focus placed on the healing process of the wound as opposed to its current physical status, regardless of how the patient sees the situation purifies the space in which the profession engages in such abject acts. This behaviour demonstrates how failure to acknowledge subjectivity and the priority placed on embodiment within nursing work may result in ignoring how nursing actions, contain, control and purify what is considered abject.

Although nursing literature does not deny the existence of the body, it also does not clearly recognize/acknowledge its importance. Not only is the body an important dimension of the person, it is often (in the case of health and illness) the aspect of the subject that is the most visible; the problems or issues with the body are usually the reason for the patient seeking health care and, therefore, interacting with nurses. Consequently, the person must be acknowledged as having a physical embodiment. However, the literature tends to disembody the person, by presenting it as separate to the person, or as an aspect that is not overly important. Building on the work of Foucault (1977) on increasing visibility through disciplinary mechanisms, Thorne (2001) writes that during health and illness 'the subjective reality of an individual renders one part of that person more visible, more prominent, and more relevant than any other' (Thorne 2001: 261). This is extremely evident in nursing: it is the body that nurses see first and it is the body at which much of nursing work is directed. Drevdahl (1999) has argued that, unfortunately, nursing has taken a simplistic approach to conceptualizing the person and that this view of the person facilitates nursing's avoidance of issues that surround subjectivity. Regrettably, it is often the case that social injustices are aimed at those who fall outside the norm or violate boundaries of what is considered appropriate for their subjectivity.

Subjectivity, Embodiment and Abjection in *The Elephant Man*

The character of John Merrick in David Lynch's *The Elephant Man* is based on the experiences of Joseph Merrick, whose life was divided between a back alley freak show and The London Hospital during the late 1800s (Victorian Era). Since his death, suggested causes of his deformity have included neurofibromatosis and Proteus Syndrome, Merrick's physical embodiment was far from normal as defined by those around him, because he was afflicted with numerous deformities and skin lesions. The film demonstrates how, in various contexts, this condition and its violation of what is considered normal or appropriate for a specific person is challenged. In this way, the film is a visual representation of the intersection of subjectivity, embodiment, and abjection, and, as such, is an excellent vehicle for exploring the concepts of abjection and the abject.

In this film John Merrick is the object; the abject is what he represents to others. His physical embodiment disturbs, it represents 'what does not respect borders, positions, rules; the in-between, the ambiguous' (Kristeva 1982: 4). And in this sense what is abject becomes both seductive and repulsive. Merrick's internal conflict arises from the contradiction between how others perceive him and how he perceives himself. In the Victorian Era, physical deformities resulting from accidents were readily accepted because they were the result of commonly occurring, easily classifiable causes of deformation, and therefore did not threaten the collective sense of self. Because the reason for his deformity was obscure, Merrick represents confusion – in the freak show both his owner and the patrons view him a cross between a man and an animal. Later, in the hospital, the nursing staff vacillates between perceiving him as a medical condition and a human being. In this way, Merrick's physical presence blurs/encroaches on boundaries, and incites fear in others. This blurring of boundaries, the ambiguous nature of Merrick's physical embodiment, stimulates an unconscious process of abjection in those around him, and in these instances the notion of the abject as both repulsive and seductive/familiar becomes clear.

This process of abjection is seen in several forms. First, there is the abjection of self – Merrick's physician Dr Treves is challenged at this level when he is confronted by the charge nurse, and accused of repeating history with Merrick. She points out that rather than helping him, Treves has put Merrick on display and exposed him to the harsh judgment of the masses. This forces Treves to consider how he has profited from Merrick. The abject in this instance is what Treves 'sees' as uncannily familiar between himself and Bytes (Merrick's former manager); his own sense of self as a physician, one who cares and protects, is challenged when he is able to identify similarities between himself and Bytes. Both Treves and the former manager profited from putting Merrick on display for society. The manager profited financially and Treves gained the respect of his medical colleagues in identifying Merrick as a medical anomaly; the doctor was now widely sought out by patients.

The second form of abjection is evidenced by Merrick's physical body – it represents a transgression of the existing norms, and thus may be considered as an example of the abject. Merrick's body (as object) challenges others, and confuses established social norms about the acceptable appearance of a man, thereby threatening other people's sense of self. Because he is interpreted by others as a violator of boundaries, Merrick is the object of abjection. As the self develops over time, so are areas of the body and orifices mapped out as pure or impure, clean or dirty, Kristeva refers to this as the 'clean and proper self'. In this context, abjection defends the self against real or perceived threats to the established boundaries which define the 'clean and proper self' – what one is and what one is not. This process of differentiation (abjection solidifying the difference between self and it, self and the other) is obvious in the scenes involving other people's reactions to, or treatment of, Merrick; it becomes apparent through the language used to describe him. For example, a constable attempting to shut down Merrick's act in the freak show, states that the 'exhibit degrades everyone who sees it as well as the poor creature himself'. Then, when he is admitted to The London Hospital, Merrick is treated as the abject; the priority given to his anomalous embodiment becomes apparent because his selfhood is completely medicalized into a condition.

After Merrick enters the hospital, a new interpretation or truth is offered for his appearance – a medical explanation. The discourse of medicine forces Merrick to become a new subject. He is no longer the subject of the freak show (and, as such, the freak); he now becomes subject to medical discourse – the patient. He is no longer treated as an animal (as established by his former manager) but rather as a man, and thus begins to occupy this new subjectivity. At this point, attempts are made to purify and control Merrick in accordance with prevailing social standards. He is given new clothes and a room of his own; he is also taught the traditions of the encompassing culture. However, even while occupying this new subjectivity, Merrick remains an anomaly because his body remains deformed and, therefore, an object of abjection.

In the context of the film, the efforts to cleanse and purify that which disgusts, could be considered a form of physical control, an attempt to fit Merrick into the subject of a man through dress and the imparting of socially appropriate manners and gestures. Unfortunately, no matter how hard Treves and others try, they never succeed in making him completely fit this imposed subjectivity. Thorne (2001: 261) writes:

> In the context of human health and illness experiences, it seems worth remembering that there may be countless occasions in which the subjective reality of an individual renders one part of that person more visible, more prominent, and more relevant than any other.

Treves never succeeds in purifying and cleansing that which others find repulsive in Merrick because he cannot eradicate what has been rendered the shockingly visible. In the end, acceptance of Merrick might return those around him to a time when they had no borders, to a time when there was no sense of self. As a result of this, they may fear that the borders of self will collapse and therefore feel constrained to remain vigilant in maintaining them (McAfee 2004). The physician cannot cure Merrick's deformities and it is the reaction of others to his body that contributes to the instability of Merrick's subjectivity. Consequently, Merrick is continually caught between two disparate subjectivities.

Subjectivity, Embodiment, Abjection and Nursing Work

While *The Elephant Man* presents shocking visual examples of abjection, embodiment and subjectivity, these processes are also evident in nursing work. However, the concept of the person, as it is defined in the nursing literature does not acknowledge those situations when a person's body (object) violates norms (abject), and instigates the unconscious process of abjection within the nurse. In addition, the concept of person, as it is presented in the nursing literature, tends to overlook the person as subject, and disregards the fact that the borders, which result from abjection, not only create and solidify the 'I' but also create the

'Other'. Kristeva (1982) states that, in response to the abject, the subject situates or separates her/himself. Within nursing, abjection, subjectivity, and embodiment are all important aspects of care. These aspects can be explored through an examination of the provision of nursing care to individuals with developmental disabilities. Specifically, as it relates to the sexual health of this population and by linking asexuality to the purification of nursing space and the containment of the abject.

Abjection, embodiment, and subjectivity can be drawn from attitudes towards the sexual conduct of individuals with developmental disabilities. Typically, this population is required and/or considered to be asexual and childlike. The lack of inclusion of embodiment in nursing theory speaks to how, in part, health care professions may inadvertently perpetuate these stereotypes. Failure to attend to embodiment may lead to professional failure to address the issues that are a consequence of a given embodiment. Nurses are not immune to broader social assumptions regarding the subjectivity of a given embodiment. Assumptions about the sexuality of individuals with developmental disabilities are rooted in social movements throughout history. In part, the developmentally disabled subject has emerged as asexual because of the eugenics movement and the forced sterilizations that ensued. In the early to mid-1900s, the developmentally disabled or 'feebleminded' were seen as contributing to a rise in criminal behaviours. Crime and the decay of social morality were linked to the unfit and defective and measures were sought to control these segments of the population (Carey 1998). Both segregation, in the form of institutionalization, and sterilization were seen as viable options. Those individuals who threatened the moral fabric of society were literally contained, enforcing asexuality, through physical containment. When Park and Radford (1998) reviewed the documentation of the Alberta Eugenics Board, they found that cases of sterilization of the 'feebleminded' were justified by descriptions of their sexual behaviour as abnormal. The mass sterilization of the developmentally disabled led to the opinion that the control of their sexuality was not only an option, but a necessary one. This in turn contributed to the perception that these individuals were either asexual or predatory. Forced sterilization and the development of a dangerous label are examples of how society has historically reacted to the developmentally disabled individual as a target of abjection.

Typically, individuals with developmental disabilities have been classified into two separate categories: those who pose a threat and those who are vulnerable and in need of protection (Anderson and Kitchin 2000, Block 2000). The perception of the person as either vulnerable, or a source of social threat, thus results in the perception that people with developmental disabilities are either incapable of sexual activity (asexual) or sexual 'monsters' who cannot control their sexual urges (Anderson and Kitchin 2000). The media reinforces the idea of the asexual developmentally disabled individual through another means of containment, exclusion; sexuality remains 'a privilege of the white, heterosexual, young, single and non-disabled' (Tepper 2000: 285).

The perception that individuals with developmental disabilities may not have an interest in, or the capacity to understand, sexual relationships is also perpetuated by nursing literature aimed at student nurses. In one nursing fundamentals textbook the following passage appears – 'those with very low cognitive functioning are unable to seek out or understand sexual relationships' (Wilkinson and Van Leuven 2007: 783). As a result of these socially enforced subjectivities, the sexual expression or interest of a patient with a developmental disability may cause abjection in nurses.

In this context, the abject is not the individual, but rather is a perceived transgression from the established norm of asexuality; that is, the perception of a sexual individual with developmental disabilities challenges the sense of self in others who have self-defined as non-disabled. To the nurse providing sexual health education, the question may surface: could I be attracted to that? Also, there may be a perceived risk of contamination in the sense of the nurse transgressing the boundary of 'proper nursing' if s/he assists an individual with developmental disabilities to obtain or maintain sexual relationships. Nurses may feel that they are contributing to the transgression of an established boundary (person as asexual), and in doing so compromise their own subjectivity as nurse. In this case, the source of abjection becomes not only the abject body (the patient), but also the mental images that may be evoked by this interaction. The internal 'I' that Kristeva speaks of is thus threatened by visions of developmentally disabled individuals engaging in sexual experiences. This may cause even further abjection if the individual is displaying interest in sexual experiences that fall outside the heterosexual, monogamous relationship because such sexual conduct may be seen as transgressive and dangerous. The myth of asexuality functions as a means to of containing what is considered abject.

Holmes, Perron, and O'Byrne (2006) note that the work of nurses exposes and engages them in health practices that challenge the clean and proper body and that this may lead to fear and anxiety on a personal level. They also suggest that situations or persons that cause abjection within the nurse may lead to attempts to control or purify. The nurse's experience of abjection as it relates to the sexuality of the individual with a developmental disability may result in the unconscious oppression of this sexuality and the enslavement of the individual to the imposed subjectivity that they are expected to occupy – that of asexuality or promiscuity. Just as the example of the burn unit nurses demonstrated how nurses become entrapped in a new subjectivity as a result of self-abjection, this is also evident in some nurses' reactions to the sexual subject with developmental disabilities.

Conclusion

The goal of examining the concept of person, as presented in theoretical nursing literature is not meant to completely abolish the work of scholars that have come before us, but rather to gaze on these ideas with a critical eye. We must question why concepts have emerged, and what these concepts communicate about the perceived values of both the nursing profession and the nursing discipline, the implications this has on the development of knowledge, and as a result, the future direction of the nursing. In examining subjectivity, embodiment, and abjection both in *The Elephant Man* and in the work of nurses, it is clear that there is a need to reconceptualize the concept of the person as it is currently defined in the nursing literature. We need to acknowledge abjection and how nurses are directly involved in the construction of the person because abjection directly affects our perception of health practices and bodies. In addition, this new understanding may facilitate a discussion of how situations and persons that evoke fear (and abjection) lead to nursing behaviours which unconsciously aim to control the patient. How the discipline 'constructs' the person will not only affect the development of future conceptual models and theories, but will also affect how we come to understand both the profession and the discipline and our contribution to health care in general. Nursing needs to accept that 'the body of the patient and perhaps, to a lesser degree, the body of the nurse, is lived in ways that are untidy, messy, and unpredictable' (McDonald and McIntyre 2001: 238); in doing so embrace both the embodiment and subjectivity of the person as an important aspect of care.

This chapter has examined how nurses deal with embodiment on a daily basis. If nurses continue to objectify patients, and distance themselves from the embodied experience, their activities involving physical bodies will become devalued (Benner 1990). At times our physical bodies are linked to, and represent, the subjectivities that have been created through power/knowledge and discourses. Lack of attention to the body, or a failure to include the physical body, in the concept of person disregards the reactions and experiences of nurses as they relate to the breakdown or alterations of bodies and subjectivities and risks controlling patients in attempts to maintain the clean and proper body.

The ultimate example of the power of abjection, and subsequently, the need for others to contain and purify the abject is disturbingly evident in the closing of *The Elephant Man* when Merrick takes his own life. Throughout the entire film Merrick has struggled between self-identifying as an animal and a man. In a sense, it is Merrick's attempt to protect himself, to defend his boundaries against perceived threats, to affirm his true identity as a man and as a human being, which motivate his death. In his final moments, Merrick, knowing that this action will kill him, removes the pillows from his bed, and lies down to sleep, like a 'normal' human being, thus affirming his sense of self as a man, and also sure in the knowledge that his actions will at the same time result in his death.

References

Anderson, P. and Kitchin, R. 2000. Disability, space and sexuality: access to family planning services. *Social Science & Medicine*, 51(8), 1163–1173.

Baruch, E.H. and Serrano, L.J. 1988. Julia Kristeva, Summer 1980, in *Women Analyze Women: In France, England, and the United States*, edited by E.H. Baruch and L.J. Serrano. New York: New York University Press, 129–148.

Benner, P. 1990. The moral dimensions of caring, in *Knowledge about Care and Caring: State of the Art and Future Developments,* edited by J.S. Stevenson and T. Tripp-Reimer. Kansas City, MO: American Academy of Nursing, 5–17.

Block, P. 2000. Sexuality, fertility, and danger: twentieth-century images of women with cognitive disabilities. *Sexuality and Disability*, 18(4), 239–254.

Carey, A.C. 1998. Gender and compulsory sterilization programs in America: 1907–1950. *Journal of Historical Sociology*, 17(4), 74–105.

Douglas, M. 1966. *Purity and Danger: An Analysis of Concepts of Pollution and Taboo.* New York: Routledge.

Drevdhal, D. 1999. Sailing beyond: nursing theory and the person. *Advances in Nursing Science*, 21(4), 1–13.

Fawcett, J. 2005. *Contemporary Nursing Knowledge: Analysis and Evaluation of Nursing Models and Theories*. Philadelphia, PA: F. A. Davis Company.

Foucault, M. 1977. *Discipline & Punish: The Birth of the Prison, translated by* A. Sheridan. New York: Vintage Books.

Foucault, M. 1980a. Truth and power, in *Power/Knowledge and Selected Interviews and Other Writings 1972–1977 by Michel Foucault*, edited by C. Gordon. New York: Pantheon Books, 109–133.

Foucault, M. 1980b. Two Lectures, in *Power/Knowledge and Selected Interviews and Other Writings 1972–1977 by Michel Foucault*, edited by C. Gordon. New York: Pantheon Books, 78–108.

Holmes, D., Perron, A. and O'Byrne, P. 2006. Understanding disgust in nursing: abjection, self, and the other. *Research and Theory for Nursing Practice: An International Journal*, 20(4), 305– 315.

Kristeva, J. 1982. *Powers of Horror: An Essay on Abjection*. New York: Columbia University Press.

The Elephant Man (dir. David Lynch, 1980).

Mansfield, N. 2000. *Subjectivity: Theories of the Self from Freud to Haraway.* New York: New York University Press.

McAfee, N. 2004. *Julia Kristeva.* New York: Routledge.

McDonald, C. and McIntyre, M. 2001. Reinstating the marginalized body in nursing science: epistemological privilege and the lived life. *Nursing Philosophy*, 2(3), 234–239.

Miller, W.I. 1997. *The Anatomy of Disgust*. Cambridge, MA: Harvard University Press.

Newman, M.A. 1997. Experiencing the whole. *Advances in Nursing Science*, 20(1), 34–39.

Oliver, K. 1993. *Reading Kristeva: Unraveling the Double-Bind.* Bloomington, IN: Indiana University Press.

Orem, D.E. 1997. Views of human beings specific to nursing. *Nursing Science Quarterly*, 10(1), 26–31.

Park, D.C. and Radford, J.P. 1998. From the case files: reconstructing a history of involuntary sterilization. *Disability & Society*, 13(3), 317–342.

Rogers, M.E. 1980. Nursing: A science of unitary man, in *Conceptual Models for Nursing Practice*. 2nd Edition, edited by J.P. Riehl and C. Roy. New York: Appleton – Century – Crofts, 329–337.

Rogers, M.E. 1992. Nursing and the space age. *Nursing Science Quarterly*, 5(1), 27–34.

Roy, C. 2000. The visible and invisible fields that shape the future of nursing care system. *Nursing Administration Quarterly*, 25(1), 119–131.

Rudge, T. 1998. Skin as cover: the discursive effects of 'covering' metaphors on wound care practices. *Nursing Inquiry*, 5(4), 228–237.

Tepper, M.S. 2000. Sexuality and disability: the missing discourse of pleasure. *Sexuality and Disability*, 18(4), 283–290.

Thorne, S., Canam, C., Dahinten, S., Hall, W., Henderson, A. and Kirkham, S.R. 1998. Nursing's metaparadigm concepts: disimpacting the debates. *Journal of Advanced Nursing*, 27(6), 1257–1268.

Thorne, S.E. 2001. People and their parts: deconstructing the debates in theorizing nursing's clients. *Nursing Philosophy*, 2(3), 259–262.

Wilkinson, J. and Van Leuven, K. 2007. *Fundamentals of Nursing: Theory, Concepts & Application.* Philadelphia, PA: F.A. Davis Company.

Chapter 14

Encountering the *Other*:
Nursing, Dementia Care and the Self

Dave Holmes, Sylvie Lauzon, and Marilou Gagnon

Introduction

For centuries nurses have cared for the most vulnerable of us. Through this professional practice, they encounter patients who embody corporal and individual differences – patients who embody otherness. The nature of nursing itself implies that those who care must do so in situations where the images of sickness are as difficult as they are often violent. To oversee this aspect of practice would suggest that nurses are capable of distancing themselves from the images of mutilation, amputation, necrosis, and contamination rising out of bodies that excrete, expire, transpire and putrefy.

The mind, much like the body, can manifest itself in different ways in the presence of disease. For example, mental illnesses and degenerative diseases (such as dementia) disrupt the mind and evoke feelings of empathy, sadness, disgust and abjection on the part of those who provide care. Nurses are exposed to and confronted by many forms of disruptive health issues and practices that challenge the order of the clean and proper and engage them on the personal level of anxiety, and perhaps fear.

We believe that the process of abjection has been historically ignored by the nursing discipline and consequently, under-theorized. The objective of this chapter is to partially address the existing gap on abjection and the way it is experienced within nursing practice, particularly regarding dementia care. Our challenge will be to explore the concept of abjection, as defined by Julia Kristeva, in order to shed a new light on the care provided to people living with dementia. We will also discuss the mechanisms involved in the social exclusion of the demented (the abject) towards more sophisticated apparatuses of exclusion (read captivity) such as health care institutions and nursing homes. Many of these apparatuses of exclusion used to rely on strict regulations where disciplinary technologies were coupled with care. Nowadays, these apparatuses are softening disciplinary regimes that characterized them. These regimes are slowly replaced by architectural practices and spatial arrangements; yet still such apparatuses exclude some populations from the social sphere.

Frail and Vulnerable: The Elderly Living with Dementia

Dementia is no longer considered a disease in itself but a syndrome accompanying a variety of neurological (e.g. Alzheimer's disease), vascular (e.g. multi-infarct), inherited (e.g. Huntingdon's disease) or infectious (e.g. AIDS) diseases. Characterized by a loss of intellectual and affective functions, which are severe enough to interfere with a person's daily functioning and quality of life, dementia is a brain disorder that can be classified into two broad categories based on its anatomical structure: cortical and subcortical dementias (Cleveland Clinic Health Information Center 2007).

Cortical dementias are caused by disorders affecting the cerebral cortex, which plays a critical role in cognitive processes such as memory and instrumental functions (language, gestures, perceptions). Patients suffering from cortical dementias like Alzheimer's and Creutzfeldt-Jakob disease show severe memory impairment and important limitations in all instrumental functions. On the other hand, subcortical dementias like Huntington's disease, Parkinson's disease and AIDS Dementia Complex arise from lesions affecting areas of the brain beneath the cortex. Such dementias will mostly affect the patients' executive functions and bring intellectual inertia (Masson and Morin 1997).

Dementia is found all over the world but is now more prominent in developed countries. Using the Delphi consensus method, Ferri et al. (2005) estimate that 24.3 million people are currently suffering from dementia and that 4.6 million new cases are diagnosed every year. These authors also project that, given the same morbidity rate and no effective prevention or curative strategies, the number of people with dementia will double every 20 years to reach 81.1 million in 2040. Yet, the rates of increase will not be uniform: 100 per cent in developed countries, but more than 300 per cent in India, China, South Asia and Western Pacific regions.

Although possible in all age-groups, dementia is usually found amongst the elderly and prevalence rates of dementia increase considerably with age (Ferri et al. 2005). Using 5 year bands from 60–64 years up to 85 years and older in each of the 14 World Health Organization regions, Ferri et al. (2005), reported that prevalence rates almost doubled from one age band to the other, in all regions. For example, in North America, the rates are the following for each 5 year band: 0.8 (60–64), 1.7 (65–69) – 3.3 (70–74) – 6.5 (75–79) – 12.8 (80–84) – 30.1 (85 and over).

A secondary analysis of the Canadian Study of Health and Aging (N=10,263) (Hill et al. 1996) also showed that dementia was age-related but suggested it was linked to sex as well. Using a randomly selected representative sample of people aged 65 and over, living in the community (n=9,008), the authors reported that in the 65–74 age-group, there were 28 cases per 1,000 for women and 19 for men whereas, for the 85 years and over, the cases were more than ten-fold, 371 and 287, respectively. Of the various forms of dementia, Alzheimer's disease was more common in women than men (69 per cent vs 53 per cent), but the proportion of vascular dementia was greater for men (30 per cent vs 14 per cent).

Prevalence of dementia in long-term care institutions has not yet been clearly established. However, several anecdotal observations and few recent studies now suggest that the majority of residents of institutional care suffer from dementia. In the United Kingdom, Matthews and Dening (2002) found that dementia prevalence was 62 per cent, ranging from 52 to 71 per cent among institutions. In Taiwan, a stratified randomized sampling of elder residents from over 60 institutions indicated that the prevalence rate was 61.8 per cent in assisted living facilities and 64.5 per cent in the nursing homes (Chen et al. 2007). Needless to say, dementia definitely shortens life. When comparing life expectancy at age 65, the Canadian Study of Health and Aging workgroup (1996) has found that people without dementia can expect to live 14.6 years at age 65 but only 1.2 year when they are afflicted by the syndrome.

As indicated earlier, dementia arises from several disorders. In fact there are over 50 known causes of dementia, some of which being treatable, but Alzheimer's disease remains by far the most frequent etiological factor, causing between 50 to 70 per cent of all dementias. In Canada, (Canadian Study of Health and Aging Working Group 1996), it was found that 64 per cent of dementias were caused by Alzheimer's disease.

Dementia of the Alzheimer's type is a progressive and irreversible disease characterized by a gradual onset. According to the DSM-IV-TR (2000), it is portrayed by the development of multiple cognitive deficits manifested by both memory impairment (impaired ability to learn new information or to recall previously learned information) and one or more of the following cognitive disturbances: aphasia (language impairment), apraxia (impaired ability to carry out motor activities despite intact motor function), agnosia (failure to recognize or identify objects despite intact sensory function) and disturbance in executive functions. Executive functions refer to a set of cognitive abilities that control and regulate other abilities and behaviours, examples include planning, organizing, sequencing, abstracting.

Due to significant advances in the biological understanding of Alzheimer's disease, its diagnostic reliability has considerably improved over the years. The definite causes of the disease still remain unknown, but many scientists believe it is probably linked to a combination of genetic, environmental and life-style factors. Several risk factors such as age, the gene APOE4, sex, head trauma, education, and diabetes have indeed been identified, but data remain inconclusive and the underlying mechanisms, far from being elucidated (Gendron 2008). To date, there is no curative treatment for Alzheimer's disease, but its evolution can be delayed with the use of medication such as cholinesterase inhibitors (donepezil, galantamine, rivastigmine) and NMDA receptor antagonist (memantine).

In sum, living with dementia is probably one of the most perplexing experiences there is. Because of this ravaging cognitive deterioration, people suffering from dementia gradually lose the meaning of the reference marks by which they led their entire life. Memory lapses produce severance in all aspects of ones life, cognitive disturbances cause limitations in daily activities and usual means of communication slowly become unproductive. Gradually cognitively cut from themselves and others, people become increasingly dependant on their environment (human, physical, social) and respond to stimuli with behaviours that are often incomprehensible to others: agitation, apathy, clinging, delusions and hallucinations, disinhibition, hoarding, sleep disturbances, repetitive questions, resistiveness to care, wandering are examples of such behaviours. In the late stages of dementia, people become more and more frail and need assistance for all activities of daily living. Eventually, they are confined to bed and almost completely unable to communicate. They usually die from complications associated with dementia such as fall-related injuries caused by reduced mobility or lung infections secondary to bed confinement.

The caregivers' experience is also quite bewildering. Because of the current limited understanding of dementia's underlying mechanisms, there are very few treatment options. Moreover, since there are only partial explanations of the behaviours expressed by people suffering from dementia (Algase et al. 1996, Smith et al. 2004), caregivers are often left with a rather small repertoire of effective practices. They then turn to strategies with which they are most familiar even though they know these strategies will not bring the intended outcomes. Left with feelings of powerlessness and incompetence, caregivers tend to progressively distance themselves from people with dementia.

Embodying the *Other*

Humans are social beings who materialize their existence in a process of becoming, one that transforms the body and the mind into perceptible entities. Cregan (2006: 3) states that 'embodiment – the physical and mental experience of existence – is the condition of possibility for our relating to other people and to the world'. In fact, our physicality is the very means by which we define our existence as social beings because the body is a symbolic vehicle that delineates how meaning is shaped, presented and represented in society (Cregan 2006). Within the social sphere, 'we relate to each other through our embodied being and the fact of our social interrelationships shapes the way we constitute our embodied being' (Cregan 2006: 5). Consequently, the body should be conceived as an object of communication and a technical means that transits the mind into the social sphere.

For people living with dementia, the manifestations of disease threaten the locus of control over the body and the mind by revealing the uncertainty of the clean and proper. Through a slow process of degeneration, those whose integrity is breached not only become the object of personal abjection, but the object of social abjection – the recipient of disgust. Based on Kristeva's work (1982), we can understand how the physical manifestations of dementia irrupt into and disrupt the symbolic order (Cregan 2006) by translating the decay of the mind and its inability to control bodily functions. As such, the body becomes an object to be read and deciphered during the progression of an insidious disease that distorts the human mind. For individuals living with dementia, the body is a medium through which the disease manifests itself slowly by coercing the mind into a defective state. Mostly associated with Alzheimer's disease, dementia is a disease of the mind and its main symptoms include 'loss of memory, disorientation, impaired abstract thinking and impulse control, and changes in personality and affect' (Mattson Porth 1998: 916). Individuals who bear the progressive degenerative changes of dementia embody a broad range of social, moral and cultural meanings around corporeality, selfhood, suffering and mortality (Persson 2005). However, it is not until the defective mind is manifested through impaired bodily functions and disruptive behaviours that the demented person becomes abject.

Based on the work of Kristeva (1982), the concept of abjection allows us to explore the experience of illness and the way it is socially and culturally enacted through the human body and its bodily functions. For people living with advanced dementia who fail to control basic bodily functions such as elimination, disgust is associated with failure to contain bodily products – or failure to reject what is not of the body. According to Kristeva (1982) 'one must abject (expel) the waste and enter the clean and ordered symbolic state to function effectively as social being' (Cregan 2006: 96). Yet, the late stage of dementia is characterized by urinary and faecal incontinence. Based on the work of Miller (1998), we can understand that those who come in contact with the demented are frequently exposed to an orifice that possesses the power to pollute and contaminate: the anus (Holmes et al. 2006). Disgust is a defensive mechanism that is enacted in order to strengthen one's own subjectivity and to preserve a self *propre* (clean, proper, self-controlled). Such a response can be explained by the fact that the sight of incontinence reveals doubts about personal integrity and autonomy (Holmes et al. 2006). Through the ritual of cleaning the anal zone and the genitals (containing another dangerous orifice), the demented is provided with temporary relief from social disgust.

The mouth is an orifice that is recognized by Miller (1998) as dangerous 'by virtue of its physiological functions and their consequent connection with disgust and danger' (Holmes et al. 2006: 306). For people living with advanced dementia, the mouth is an important orifice because it is the entrance to the digestive tract and the vehicle through which verbal communication is made possible. The mouth is also a facial feature that bears the signs of advanced aging, dehydration, thermoregulation and lack of autonomy in performing oral hygiene. At every stage of dementia, disturbing behaviour related to this orifice have been described in demented individuals such as verbally aggressive behaviour, vocally disruptive behaviour, biting, aphasia, water intoxication, cophrophagia (consumption of faeces), urodipsia (consumption of urine), anorexia, voracious appetite and indifference to food (Helizen et al. 2004). For the onlooker, the mouth signifies degenerative changes resulting in a clear lack of autonomy in regulating its physiological functions and its clean and proper use in communication, ingestion and socialization. As such, it enters the symbolic realm in which 'the abject evokes filth and is associated with pollution of the body and mind' (Holmes et al. 2006: 307).

Based on Kristeva's work, we can understand that 'abjection goes beyond the perception of the body' (Holmes et al. 2006: 308). In fact, 'the abject challenges established systems of order, meaning, truth and law' that produce the manageable subject (Holmes et al. 2006: 308). By presenting a defective mind, individuals living with advanced dementia confront the onlooker by embodying the disruption of a clear system of order (abjection) through which human beings learn to maintain and secure their integrity and autonomy. Furthermore, they resist ideological truth by demonstrating the power of dementia over life and by reaffirming the 'law of nature', one that we learn to resist through the abjection of what is both manifest (concrete) and imaginary (symbolic) about a progressive, painful and debilitating death. By living in a degenerative state, the demented becomes the abject by embodying the unbreakable interrelationship between life and death, its sight evoking the pollution of the body and the mind. Eventually, the demented becomes unmanageable and is sentenced to behaviours that are judged to be repulsive such as wandering, agitation, assault, auto-mutilation, hypersexual behaviour, psychotic behaviour, sundowning[1], inappropriate social behaviours and repetitive behaviours. Confronted by the defective mind of the *Other*, contamination becomes a permanent threat for integrity of those who come in contact with people living with dementia, proving that 'the abject cannot be fully expelled; it leaves a trace embedded within the unconscious to provoke unease' (Holmes et al. 2006: 313).

People suffering from dementia come regularly in contact with health care providers, namely nurses. As stated earlier, these individuals often induce fear and anxiety by the very nature of their condition. Commonly described as an unpredictable person, the demented cannot successfully communicate according to the norms established by society. In contemporary Western societies, bodies that are seen to transgress or blur culturally important boundaries and codes are often sources of apprehension. For instance, encounters with actively psychotic individuals confront the 'normal' and induce fear on the part of the latter. These 'others' are commonly seen as threats to social order and hence the need for exclusion in closed spaces (Sibley 1999) such as nursing homes, asylums or prisons. According to Bauman (1995), two strategies are deployed by the dominants (normals) to undermine effects strangers have. These strategies are *anthropophagic* or *anthropoemic*. *Anthropophagic* strategies involve the annihilation of strangers by devouring them and transforming them into something that remains indistinguishable from one's own while *anthropoemic* strategies

---

1   'The term *sundowning* is interchangeable with *sundowning syndrome* and *nocturnal delirium*. Sundowning syndrome is a common set of behaviours for the patient with a memory-impairing illness. The patient may experience increased anxiety, increased confusion, delusions or paranoia that may appear or increase, restlessness, and wondering. Symptoms typically surface when the sun goes down' (Sharer 2008: 27).

involve the 'vomiting' of strangers, banishing them from the limits of the orderly world and having them excluded from all communication with the dominant group.

These two strategies are applicable to mentally ill or demented individuals. As such, they are deployed in order to return to a sense of order and control where the established boundaries are respected by all. The 'others' are responsible for creating chaos within a highly regulated society. Their liminal state (something between human and something else) creates uncertainty which can result in intense fear and disgust. When addressing the disabled individuals' cases, Lupton (1999: 136) suggests that like dirt, people categorized as disabled have been dealt with 'though policies of policing, regulation, exclusion and avoidance in the effort to re-established' social order.

Nursing the *Other*

Protecting the Self from the unclean and polluted *Other* is a reaction that nurses may experience when caring for people living with dementia. But the social (as well as the professional) constructions of nurses, in a way, forbid the verbalization of emotions such as disgust and repulsion. The caring nurse is supposed to be able to sublimate these negative feelings in order to maintain ethical standards, but behind the appearance of tolerance and calm, nurses may experience dramatic personal responses when they come in contact with the demented – the abject. Parker (2004) suggests that the nature of nursing work unveils the abject and by doing so commands ways to manage the feelings surrounding abjective situations. By suggesting that nurses draw upon a range of unconscious defenses to manage the tensions evoked by the disturbances and threats to their own integrity, Parker (2004) reveals an unchartered territory of nursing practice. In effect, the impact of abjection on the care of abject individuals has traditionally been silenced in nursing (Holmes et al. 2006). Yet, the very nature of abjection is to distance oneself from the abject even in the face of extensive social to do otherwise (Holmes et al. 2006).

As part of the degenerative progression of dementia, individuals exhibit extremely disturbing features that testify to the pollution of the mind, the body and the bodily functions which allow us to secure our integrity as human beings. In this sense then, the meaning of caring for the abject 'seems to touch on moral aspects of human existence, the question of our willingness or unwillingness to be violated in a relationship' (Hellzen et al. 2004: 3). When coming in contact with the demented, the nurse might be disturbed by the transgression of boundaries that typically maintain the clear distinction between us (the clean and proper) and them.

Securing one's inviolable, distinct and autonomous mind and body is a defensive mechanism that is deployed in the face of the abject. In effect, the concept of abjection describes the recognition of and retreat from the knowledge of our own ambivalence as well as the detachment from the Other – a being who embodies what must remain outside the boundaries of the clean and proper zone. For those working with demented patients, such an imperative is translated in the way care is perceived and provided on a daily basis. Through different practices, nurses secure their boundaries while providing each other support to contain negative feelings, to minimize contamination and to regain control over the chaotic experiences of abjection.

Securing Boundaries

As health care professionals, nurses are thought to systematically reject their own response to abjective situations (Holmes et al. 2006). In order to secure boundaries of the clean and proper self, the professional persona is deployed during patient-nurse interactions to create a safe zone to provide care. Moreover, nurses learn to present themselves in ways that hide their own negative feelings evoked by their work (Parker 2004) – a process defined as 'emotional labour' by Walsh (2009). Yet, those working with disruptive individuals, such as people with dementia, tend to focus their nursing care on personal protection (Hellzen et al. 2004). This defensive mechanism attests to the failure of the professional persona in securing the boundaries of nurses who care for the abject. As such, those who are exposed to disruptive behaviours (violence, verbal abuse, sexual behaviours, etc.), bodily fluids, bodily orifices and physical signs of degeneration will feel (unconsciously) the urgency to protect their body and their mind from being violated by the Other. On the other hand, focusing on personal protection may become detrimental for the care of abject individuals who are perceived to be dangerous, polluted, contagious and repulsive (Hellzen et al. 1999, 2004). Therefore, we could argue that the professional persona, as an important strategy to secure one's own boundaries, may lead to an intensification of the perceived threat in nurses working with demented individuals. Incidentally, such a phenomenon, we would assert, results in an impoverishment and distancing of care in the name of personal security. This is Kristeva's idea of disavowal that attempts to control for abjection but like all defence mechanisms is only partially successful as the abject always is already present in the use of the defence.

Containing Negative Feelings

Being in a therapeutic relationship with abject individuals implies an array of negative feelings such fear, disgust, nausea, impatience, anger, grief, insecurity, helplessness, humiliation, powerlessness and meaninglessness (Hellzen et al. 1999, 2004, Parker 2004). While these emotions bear the potential to have a profound impact on the psychological and physical health of nurses, they are silenced by professional and ethical discourses (Holmes et al. 2006). Furthermore, their impact on the way nurses provide care requires further exploration and even more so in the context of long-term care for individuals living with dementia. Hellzen and colleagues (2004: 9) suggest that 'ordinary professional ways of being repellent (control, power, etc.) or being hatefully repellent' are behaviours that may emerge as an indirect consequence of feeling violated by the abject individual. While trying to contain negative feelings and secure their own boundaries, nurses describe being caught in the evilness and disturbance of the 'Other' (Hellzen et al. 1999, 2004). Confronted with the difficulty of maintaining the professional persona, those who care for abject individuals report feelings of helplessness and despair in the face of abjective situations. For some, it is difficult to find meaning in the care provided to defective individuals – the care being perceived to be equally defective (Hellzen et al. 1999, 2004). As exemplified by Hellzen and colleagues (1999: 660),

> It is difficult for carers to see any meaning in their work when most of the care activities they performed could be seen as failures, e.g. having the patient spit in your face or being hit in the face with his fists when helping him to dress, being chased with a spade when being together outside or getting the tray thrown at your back when serving dinner.

For nurses, powerlessness becomes an important issue since they feel inevitably 'soiled' and 'infected' by the abject individuals whose power to contaminate is greater than those deployed to remain clean and proper (Hellzen et al. 1999, 2004). They may also report being victimized by this power dynamic, especially when they are not able to intervene effectively in abjective situations (Hellzen et al. 1999). In effect, the unpredictability of demented individuals results in a lack of control over the outcomes of the patient-provider relationship: 'I think he's the biggest problem here … It's hard because he has good periods, when he is nice and gentle and we can sit down and talk and suddenly he is like a monster (an expression used by the nurses interviewed)' (Hellzen et al. 2004: 6). By perceiving themselves as good, nurses attempt to re-establish a sense of cleanness, thus washing away the dirt – personified as the abject individual they see in their 'therapeutic encounters' (Hellzen et al. 2004). Incidentally, such a phenomenon may result in a perpetual repression of nurses' negative feelings in favour of their clean, proper and professional selves.

Minimizing Contamination

In order to be productive as health care professionals, nurses working with demented individuals develop strategies to minimize their own contamination. Described by Parker (2004: 213) as the *nursing look*, this strategy 'refers to a form of concrete and practice-orientated knowledge in a receptive persona, which is a metaphor standing for the range of senses through which nurses pick up cues about the patient'. Although Parker's work is based on medical nursing practice, we believe that it could be applied to all forms of nursing practice where abjection occurs. For instance, by using the nursing look, those who care for people living with dementia are certainly able to identify and minimize the potential for their own contamination. Whether it is the smell, the sight, the sounds, the speech or the touch of the abject, nurses will immediately recognize the threat and attempt to secure their boundaries. For example, a nurse will pick cues about a demented patient whose aggressive behaviours are escalating and as a result, avoid contact and/or pre-medicate in order to not be exposed to disturbing visual, physical and verbal exchanges with that specific patient. The *nursing scan*, is another strategy proposed by Parker (2004: 213) to explain how nurses constantly scan their terrain of responsibility in order 'to locate patients spatially, identify spatial related problems, ascertain location of technologies that may be required and make the terrain safe for patients'.

When caring for demented individuals, nurses certainly deploy this protective surveillance to minimize their own risk of being contaminated. For example, nurses from a specific unit will confine patients to their room or when outside, to a designated area that is inherently populated by the same patients. Furthermore, nurses will permanently localize themselves at the nursing station, always going back to this safe zone between every intervention. This reaction has been observed by Holmes (2001, 2003, 2005, 2006, 2007) following his many research endeavours in both psychiatric settings and forensic psychiatric settings. It is at the nursing station that those who care for demented individuals perform a cleansing ritual – the nursing 'handhover'. At the end of a shift, each nurse passes on her assessments and interventions to a colleague who will, through her comments, minimize the contamination brought on by the abjective situations of the day. For example, the colleague will turn a distressing incident and a confession into a comic routine, which serves to wash away the pollution from the care episodes of the day. This very ritual validates one's professional stance when interacting with abject individuals while minimizing the 'perceived' impact of abjection on the way care is provided on the unit.

Regaining Control Over the Chaotic Experiences of Abjection

It seems logical to assume that nurses working with demented individuals experience chaos in the face of abjective situations. According to Hellzen (2004), one way to create order is to provide pathological explanations for the 'evilness' of patients by explaining, for example, how brain damage is probably worse than it appears or how the sudden manifestation of violent behaviours is related to the progression of Alzheimer's disease. By making abjection part of the ordinary, nurses focus on a rational interpretation of chaotic events, leaving no room for their own feelings when confronted with a disruptive human being (not a pathology). The feeling of losing control of the patient-provider interactions is rarely discussed in a climate of objectification. As a result, this lack of openness gives rise to feelings of guilt and despair for nurses who consider that their actions are not always 'right' (Hellzen 1999). Incidentally, the most favourable way to regain control of the abject individual (and his behaviours) and of our own actions as nurses is to medicate. This is a current practice in nursing homes and psychiatric settings

(Voyer et al. 2005). Yet, the administration of medications is rarely described as a power strategy to manage the chaos brought on by abjective situations. Not only is medicating presented as the best intervention to be implemented for those suffering from their defective mind and body, it is a mechanism that protects nurses from contamination, while testifying to the efficacy of their care.

Final Remarks

Encountering the demented person is a challenging nursing experience which requires not only empathy, solicitude and knowledge but also the courage to acknowledge feelings of fear, repulsion and unease. Although official nursing discourses discourage the expressions of these 'negative' feelings, we assert that it is only when dealing openly with these disturbing feelings and emotions that genuine patient-centred nursing care can take place.

References

Algase, D.L. et al. 1996. Need-driven dementia-compromised behavior: an alternative view of disruptive behavior. *American Journal of Alzheimer's Disease and Other Dementias*, 11(6), 10–19.

American Psychiatric Association. 2000. *Diagnostic and Statistical Manual of Mental Disorders*. 4th Edition. Washington, D.C: APA.

Bauman, Z. 1995. *Life in Fragments: Essays in Postmodern Morality*. Cambridge: Polity Press.

Canadian Study of Health and Aging Working Group. 1994. Canadian study of health and aging: Study methods and prevalence of dementia. *Canadian Medical Association Journal*, 150, 899–913.

Chen T.F. et al. 2007. Institution type-dependent prevalence of dementia in long-term care units. *Clinics in Geriatric Medicine*, 21, 83–92.

Cregan, K. 2006. *The Sociology of the Body*. London: Sage Publications.

Ferri, C.P. et al. 2005. Global prevalence of dementia: a Delphi consensus study. *The Lancet*, 366, 2112–2117.

Gendron M. 2008. *Le mystère Alzheimer*. Montréal: Éditions de l'homme.

Hellzen, O. et al. 1999. Unwillingness to be violated: carers' experiences of caring for a person acting in a disturbing manner: an interview study. *Journal of Clinical Nursing*, 8, 653–662.

Hellzen, O. et al. 2004. The meaning of caring as described by nurses caring for a person who acts provokingly: an interview study. *Scandinavian Journal of Caring Sciences*, 18, 3–11.

Hill, G. et al. 1996. Dementia among seniors. *Health Reports*, 8(2), 7–10.

Holmes, D., Perron, A. and O'Byrne, P. 2006. Understanding disgust in nursing: abjection, self and the 'other'. *Research and Theory for Nursing Practice: An International Journal*, 20(4), 305–315.

Masson, H. and Morin, M. 1997. Démences vasculaires et autres démences, in *Précis pratique de gériatrie*. 2nd Edition, edited by M. Arcand and R. Hébert. Saint-Hyacinthe: ÉDISEM, 185–199.

Matthews, F.E. and Dening, T. 2002. Prevalence dementia in institutional care. *The Lancet*, 360, 225–26.

Mattson Porth, C. 1998. *Pathophysiology : Concepts of Altered Health States*. 5th Edition. Philadelphia : Lippincott.

McAfee, N. 2004. *Julia Kristeva*. Routledge : New York.

Miller, W. 1998. *The Anatomy of Disgust*. Cambridge, MA: Harvard University Press.

Parker, J. 2004. Nursing on the medical ward. *Nursing Inquiry*, 11(4), 210–217.

Persson, A. 2005. Facing HIV: body shape change and the (in)visibility of illness. *Medical Anthropology*, 24, 237–264.

Sharer, J. 2008. Tackling sundowning in a patient with Alzheimer's disease. *Medsurg Nursing*, 17(1), 27–29.

Sibley, D. 1999. *Geographies of Exclusion*. New York: Routledge.

Smith, M. et al. 2004. History, development, and future of the progressively lowered stress treshold: a conceptual model for dementia care. *Journal of the American Geriatrics Society*, 52, 1755–1760.

The Cleveland Clinic Foundation Health Information Center. 2007. Types of dementia. Available at: http://www.clevelandclinic.org/health-info. [accessed on July 20 2009].

Voyer, P. et al. 2005. Symptoms of psychological distress among older adults in Canadian long-term care centres. *Aging and Mental Health*, 9(6), 542–554.

Walsh, E. 2009. Prison nursing: The knowledge/power connection. *APORIA*, 1(2), 7–14.

Chapter 15

Dirty Nursing: Containing Defilement and Infection Control Practices

Allison Roderick

Introduction

'Infection control is in your hands'. This statement and many others like it remind people, particularly in the health care environment, that infection control is a personal matter, a matter to be personally and individually controlled. Having worked in many hospitals on two continents I always find it surprising that people think that hospitals are bastions of *asepsis* – that is, *without infection*. The reality is that hospitals are absolute cesspools of disease and illness. This is not to say that hospitals are unclean or unhygienic, but rather people seem surprised that there are infections, germs and bacteria there within. If you follow the lines of logic, that a hospital contains a collection of the 'sick and infirm' altogether in one place, then to continue this logic, do you then expose the weak and infirmed to even more disease and illness?

In the organization of the clinic and the movement of health care away from the municipality of family, wife and mother, was the emergence of institutions to house the sick and the infirm. In this present age in the developed world we see a falling away of traditional diseases and illnesses – such as measles, dysentery, consumption and the emergence of 'super bugs' such as Methicillin resistant *staphylococcus aureus* (MRSA) and the ever fearful and worrying risk of mutating viruses such as H1N5 (Bird Flu) or H1N1 (Human Swine Flu). This chapter is an attempt to understand infection control practices as experienced by the nurses in an intensive care unit (ICU).

During a pilot study of infection control practices in ICU, the experience of nurses who cared for a patient requiring 'additional precautions' for the super bug MRSA were explored. In this study, the nurses represent the boundaries, the borders of the less certain and invisible world of infection control and microbiology. It is not the patient that causes the abjection in this case, rather the lack of clear boundaries and as Kristeva (1982: 4) suggests where borders have become object.

Setting the Scene of Additional Precautions: Isolation

Infection control in the health care setting is a highly regulated apparatus. It provides guidelines to the safe management of every kind of situation that employees and organizations will encounter. Infection control practices can mean the difference between a health care organization's gaining accreditation or not; it can shut centres down, cause public outcry as well as media hysteria.

All health care professionals, by the very nature of their work, engage in infection control and prevention. The 'infectious patient' is managed through the use of both standard and additional precautions. Standard precautions as its name suggests, is the minimum standard that is used with everyone through the use of protective attire mainly gloves and goggles for blood and bodily fluid contact, along with personal hygiene – especially the washing of hands between patients and procedures. Additional precautions, the focus of the pilot study, are used in addition to these standard precautions for patients with infections that are highly transmissible or of great concern.

These additional precautions include standard precautions but may emphasize different aspects such as the wearing of protective attire for *all* contact with the patient and their surroundings, rather than *just* when there is risk of blood or bodily fluid exposure and may include placing the patient(s) in isolation rooms. Standard precaution, to a greater or lesser extent is part of the everyday fabric of care: but infection control becomes visible when precautions are used in addition to these.

This means of understanding the infectious patient and therefore infection control practices, has been dominated by the medico-scientific paradigm. Douglas stated 'the bacterial transmission of disease was a great 19th century discovery. It produced the most radical revolution in the history of medicine. So much has it transformed our lives that it is difficult to think of dirt except in the context of pathogenicity' (2002: 36). Douglas's claim that our understanding of pathogenicity[1] was *the most radical* revolution did not only dominate the 19th century but continues to this day. There is no doubt that medical breakthrough, with resultant consequences in morbidity and mortality[2] have been widely affected by this greater understanding of pathogens and appropriate treatment with antibiotics and antiviral medications. What this study shows, however in terms of practice, is that this revolution has its limitations.

The Intensive care unit (ICU) in which the pilot study took place was a level 3 ICU. This ICU cared for a wide spectrum of patients and it was responsible for retrieval/air-evacuation, the management of complex medical and surgical conditions from various forms of organ failure, heart attacks and even organ

---

1   Pathogenicity refers to something i.e. bacteria that cause disease. Not all bacteria however would be referred to as a pathogen; it is only when they cause disease.

2   Morbidity (rate of disease/illness) and mortality (death rate) are commonly used terms in ICU. This data together with other clinical information systems aid in understanding the effectiveness of patient management.

transplantation. The ICU was located in a busy tertiary government hospital. The ICU consisted of 15 patient care spaces or 'bays' around the perimeter of the unit with a central workstation that housed emergency resuscitation equipment, medication, stationery and monitors where every patient in the entire unit could be viewed – that is, viewed through the 'lens' of heart rhythms and internal pressure monitoring. Each bay was the image of the next, containing typical objects such as bed, workbench and cupboards filled with a plethora of syringes, medication, bottles and dressings, and typical equipment such as the patient monitor, cables and the ventilator[3] and a range of electrical pumps that could deliver intravenous fluid and medication to the patient. Each bay was separated by 'walls', with the bottom half solid thereby creating privacy for the unconscious or infirm, whereas the upper portion was glass to allow maximum surveillance for staff to what was happening around them. Privacy was created with the use of long drapes at the perimeter of the bay that simply prevented the patient or procedure from being viewed. They did not however prevent smell, light or sounds – and although creating a sense of privacy, they really only *symbolized* a private space to work, and in many cases, mourn.

In this ICU there were two designated isolation rooms. They appeared identical to all the other bays with the exception they had *complete* walls and two heavy doors instead of the long drapes. Unseen was the *lamina flow air-conditioning unit* – which could adjust the pressure of air flow to ensure a negative pressure which prevented air from escaping the room. This is particularly important in the case of patients with highly transmissible respiratory infections.

Patients were placed in the isolation rooms for a range of infections, the most common being the super bug, MRSA[4]. It was common during the pilot study for there to be more than two patients who required isolation concurrently. Those patients who had a respiratory infection were always contained in the 'isolation bay'; however it was common practice for patients to be grouped together or cohorted around these isolation rooms. For example, a case that comes to mind is one wherein three or four patients requiring *additional precautions* were located next to each other. At other times, when scanning the ICU you may simply see a red 'STOP' sign attached to the drapes of the bay, alerting staff that this patient requires additional precautions.

Patient care by nursing staff within the isolation room, or with a patient requiring additional precautions was essentially no different to the 'normal' patient. All patients, irrespective of their condition, still require monitoring, intravenous infusions and medications to be managed, and procedures to be

---

3   The ventilator is more commonly referred to in the media as life support or the respirator.

4   MRSA is commonly referred to in the media as a 'super bug'. The name comes from the fact that MRSA is resistant to many common and typical antibiotics used to treat these infections. As a result MRSA is very difficult to treat and causes 'great' concern if it is transferred to other patients in hospital.

done. Here, the following excerpt from field notes provides a simple example of additional precautions for a patient. This account shows a space that is bound by the symbolism created by the 'infectious patient' and yet the simple activity of fitting an oxygen mask was managed no different to a patient who was not infectious.

> I watched Kate apply a plastic apron over her uniform and gloves to assist Ted with his oxygen mask. There was a problem with part of the tubing and this required a new piece of tubing from the cupboard which was three meters away from where Kate was. I watched as Kate removed all her protective attire, wash her hands, leave the bay and collect the tubing from the cupboard three meters away. She returned with the tubing, reapplied the plastic apron and gloves and connected the new tubing. A task that only took five seconds and yet was prolonged by the extra steps of gowning and gloving. A little later a similar thing happened again when Kate required the Electrocardiogram (ECG) machine. She retrieved the ECG machine applied the plastic apron and gloves, attached the ECG to the patient. On completion she again removed her protective attire and this time washed down the ECG machine with soapy water and then washed her hands, she then returned the machine. Returning to the bay she reapplied the protective attire … .

When rendering down the procedures observed in the above field notes they all can be considered as simple, not very technical or challenging nursing activities. Fitting an oxygen mask or performing an ECG is considered normal, everyday activities of a nurse in the ICU. Also the simple 'donning and doffing' of personal protective equipment such as plastic aprons, masks, goggles and gloves is also not technically difficult. Washing one's hands or '*hand hygiene*' is often the simplest of techniques and is even something of which people outside of the health profession are aware and commonly practice for hygiene, social and/or religious reasons. However, it is *not* the above-mentioned procedures that cause tension in the management of the patient who requires additional precautions.

The Invisible World of Infection Control and Microbiology

When Leeuwenhoek[5] first noted the tiny eels under the microscope the cook, so the story goes, did not eat for a week. As Douglas stated earlier the discovery of pathogens as the cause of disease and illness produced an incredible revolution in medicine and science. However, my question for this study was how does this revolution equate to practice? Pathogens are now made visible through the use

---

5   Anton van Leeuwenhoek (1632–1723) often acknowledged as one of the fathers of microbiology because of his work with lenses and the discovery of microscopic 'animals' on a slide.

of the microscope. How does the nurse know where a super bug is if it remains invisible away from the Petri dish or the microscope? The following participants had much to say about the invisible nature of pathogens.

> There is no visual evidence, no sign other than [pause] you'd be looking after your patient normally one morning, doing what you normally do and they *(the laboratory)* ring up with a result of MRSA positive and then it dramatically changes.

This example from Anna describes how there was no definitive physical evidence for Anna to identify the patient having MRSA. Nurses could argue that there is no new evidence that this is a resistant pathogen. It is quite normal for patients to be in ICU for multiple infections, for bodies to leak, for wounds to ooze foul smelling discharge and to hear the noise of patients coughing and spluttering through copious amounts of spit and phlegm. These signs did not signify that this was a super bug; these signs signified the patient's ill health which was why they are in ICU. Anna went on to say: 'it's big and invisible. It is just a result on a screen. It probably scares people more because you don't know where it is, where you've taken it. You don't know if it's on you'?

This account also resonated with other participants even when they were wearing the protective attire. Elle during interview describes how:

> You assume that you are 'clean' and that your practice is good but you then touch something that you assume is clean and then scratch your nose and walk into another bay – are you then still clean? What can we really assume in this business as far as infection control is concerned? Must we assume that everything is contaminated and nothing is clean?

The cleanliness and contamination of objects in and around the room becomes questionable. Jen goes further to say:

> We presume our hands could have MRSA on them, that is why we wash them. If we wash our hands first and then remove our plastic apron we could possible re-contaminate ourselves when removing the plastic apron, do we wash our hands again? However, if we remove the plastic apron first (and) if our hands are contaminated with MRSA, we could be contaminating our clothes unknowingly with MRSA and putting others at risk.

Anna demonstrates that to her this diagnosis of a super bug is not something that can be observed, '*it is just a result on a screen*'. Elle and Jen express how that even with the wearing of protective attire and the isolation of the patient they felt that they needed to guess or assume where the pathogen might be and whether it was on them. Also prior to the diagnosis of MRSA the patient was bound, intact and contained within the boundaries of human flesh. Prior to the diagnosis of MRSA the nurse moved freely around the patient and their surroundings, carrying out routine activities without any thought of the patient's boundaries. However, once diagnosed with MRSA, as well as the movement of the patient to the isolation bay, the donning and doffing of protective attire, the continuous questioning by the participants 'is it on me?': this is not only a recognition of the physical boundaries put in place by medicine and science to contain the spread but also a recognition of the blurred borders of the patient with the nurse.

Pathogens are considered as an unseen, invisible and incognisant element of human existence which through the labelling as 'a super bug' becomes visible. This visibility, however, is not confirmed by physical evidence – like blood or pus – and is not definite in the space where practice takes place. Anna suggests that 'it is big but invisible', and Elle questions that fact if she accidentally gets the pathogen on her would she then transmit it somewhere else, therefore putting others at risk. Jen believes that everything to do with the patient should consequently be considered unclean and contaminated. Foucault declares that 'there is disease only in the element of the visible and therefore *statable*' (2003: 116). From the perspective of the microbiologist there is disease because of the presence of pathogens, which is known and readily visible in the laboratory. But in everyday practice, how is this revelation of a pathogen or disease made visible when there is no real evidence to signify its presence — other than on a computer screen from the laboratory results.

From the examples given by the participants, they struggle to understand the divisions between clean and dirty. The binary nature of science; *sepsis* and *asepsis* (with infection or without infection) is much less clear in practice. This super bug does not possess the usual signs and symbols that signify *filth, defilement or dirtiness*. Human excrement is unremarkably dirty. As a nurse, first one notes the offensive odour, then on raising the sheets to survey if this is merely odour or is there other 'offensive' evidence. Once the object is viewed, gloves are donned, new linen obtained, toilet tissue, rubbish bags and explanations to the patient (yes, even the unconscious one) 'just going to clean you up now – better out than in'. Excrement is evidence of human filth, and is visible. The problem is that the infectious patient forces us to imagine and visualize that which is not visible. It causes us to question the 'boundedness' or the lack of boundaries of the human body.

In trying to understand the visible/invisible nature of infection control Kristeva suggests that 'it is thus not lack of cleanliness or health that causes abjection but what disturbs identity, system, order' (1982: 4). Here we see from the examples from the participants that that the scientific classification system of organizing disease and in particular pathogens requiring isolation is an ambiguous system. The orderly lines of the binary nature of science do not assist nurses to practice; they cannot visualize what is invisible. The identification of what would be considered clean and what is considered dirty or contaminated is indistinct, in-between and does not respect the borders that have been created by the use of additional precautions: the plastic aprons, the gloves, or the hand washing. Douglas goes on to say 'in short, our pollution behaviour is the reaction which condemns any object or idea likely to confuse or contradict cherished classifications' (Douglas 2002: 37). The participants condemned all objects as dirty rather than confuse the 'cherished classification' of clean and dirty. In attempting to manage the risk of the infectious patient the concept of additional precautions condemned all objects whether infectious or not from a microbiological perspective. Nurses are now socialized to think that the infectious patient can be contained through the use of additional precautions such as isolation and protective attire. But the very object of isolation with its correlate protective attire creates a confusing reclassification of clean and dirty.

As mentioned earlier excrement is obviously dirty. The signs and symbols of additional precautions, brand one patient and their environment dirty versus the next patient and their environment as clean. The nature of the super bug MRSA is that it typically can be found on skin, and therefore wherever skin can be, it is assumed that MRSA can be as well. The imagery of a single skin cell being lost or a finger print reminding you of where someone has been conjures up images of risk and terror.

But understanding this risk creates the reclassification of clean and dirty. Bodies however, have always leaked, shed skin cells or left its fingerprint. It is only when the body falls apart or are not contained that we recognize that we are all unbound. Lawton's (2000) study of hospice patient describes how patient's bodies become 'unbound' and eroded away by cancer. Lawton describes how bodies began to 'fall apart' and how we as adults had come accustom to the notion of intact and contained bodies and that this lack of control represented an 'unbound' body (2000: 128). Sjöholm goes on to say that this erosion, these uncontained bodies is… 'contamination the breaking down between inside and outside, an aesthetic of contamination is a phenomenon through which I am moved or touched, by my fellow being. The touch appears with intensity and feverishness where the separating limit between inside and outside runs most thinly' (2005: 96). These unbound bodies lacked clear borders or boundaries, the patient's skin which you once considered intact, a clear defining limit is now blurred.

Creating Order: The Line

One means of creating order is through the use of additional precautions. Science and medicine through the use of guidelines would have us believe that by wearing the protective attire while in contact with the patient and their surroundings and then removing the protective attire when no longer in contact with the patient or their surroundings is that simple. To remember how puzzling this is, I return to the participant Jen and her dilemma working out where MRSA was!

> We presume our hands could have MRSA on them, that is why we wash them.
> If we wash our hands first and then remove our plastic apron we could possible

re-contaminate ourselves when removing the plastic apron, do we wash our
hands again? However, if we remove the plastic apron first (and) if our hands are
contaminated with MRSA, we could be contaminating our clothes unknowingly
with MRSA and putting others at risk.

Jen's dilemma was how to approach the risk and potential of contamination of
her hands and whether she needed to wash them first or not before removing her
plastic protective apron. She feared she could become re-contaminated whatever
order she went through the process. So using the binary approach of science by
removing the contaminated object first (the plastic apron) and then washing her
hands, she questioned if her hands would contaminate her clothing that the plastic
apron had protected. Douglas approached this by saying 'if uncleanness is matter
out of place, we must approach it through order' (2002: 41). When we view the
body as an intact, bound body then infection, pathogens and more importantly
super bugs must be viewed from the stance of the unbound leaking body. In such
a situation, the nurse's protective attire becomes the boundary of the less than
certain world of clean and dirty when pathogens are known to be present.

Practice, and in particular nursing practice in the ICU, does not occur in a
vacuum. Even the least ill patient in the ICU needs 'tasks' such as monitoring:
poking and probing to understand the inner workings of disease and illness and
matching these findings to treatment orders, medication, and disease trajectory.
The following field note is an account of a routine central venous catheter '*line*'
insertion[6].

> The procedure went slowly and as is the case with the majority of line insertions
> a check X-ray is performed (to check for the correct location of the line and to
> see if there have been any complications as a result such as a pneumothorax)
> with a mobile X-ray machine. The nurse wore the typical garb of plastic apron
> and gloves. I watched as the radiographer also dressed in the protective attire
> (they also placed the X-ray board in a plastic bag to protect it as well). According
> to Jenny what is contaminated should remain in the bay or quickly disposed
> of. It's like there is an unwritten rule that you are not to leave the bay wearing
> protective attire.

Why is this so? Do you drop bits?

> But a dilemma arises when doing the X-ray. To perform the X-ray in the
> ICU bay, staff (in this case Jenny) is required to stand six feet away from the

---

6   A central venous catheter (CVC) is very similar to an intravenous cannula and is used
for the administration of fluid and medication. It is a technical procedure that requires a
medical officer under sterile/surgical conditions inserting a long catheter usually into the
subclavian vein so that the tip of the catheter sits just outside the heart in the vena cava or
just within the 'first' chamber of the heart (the right atria).

X-ray machine. This means leaving the isolation bay. Question: do you remove or leave on the protective attire for a three second procedure such as the X-ray. Some people say that you shouldn't be seen walking around with the stuff (the protective attire) on. *Why?*

Moments later I watched as the nurse walked to the edge of the bay, leaning her body out into the main unit she called out for assistance with endotracheal suction and turning the patient. She did not step beyond the line made between the two isolation doors. It was if there was a line – an imaginary line between the two doors. How come only minutes ago she walked freely outside her bay and now she gets to the imaginary line and stops?'

The observation of Jenny in the first part of this field note is not necessarily an unwritten rule rather in simplistic terms she is describing infection control policy, that is, the isolated patient and their surroundings are infectious. Outside of the isolation room the protective attire and precautions is not required because it is not infectious. However when doing a chest X-ray there is a risk of radiation exposure and so all staff (or those not having an X-ray) move about 6 feet away from the X-ray machine. The question is raised. Do you remove the protective attire to do a three second procedure when you are not touching anything else? But what happens when you move outside of what was and will become again that 'set' boundary of what is clean and what is not.

This account also demonstrates that weighing up of different rules – the X-ray is an exceptional circumstance – risk of radiation[7]. But the requesting for assistance for endotracheal suction or turning the patient is routine and not a high risk procedure and so warrants a change back to routine practice – the stopping at the imaginary line. The imaginary line was made between the two doors of the isolation bay, in the normal bay it was created by the perimeter made by the heavy privacy drapes.

There were other accounts of the imaginary line. Anna when asked about the imaginary line said:

It's really REAL. It is definitely there. You know its not there. But it's definitely an image of it there. Even if you come out to look at your charts[8] you feel you shouldn't be and that you'll infect your chair. And by washing you hands inside are you being contaminated by everything

---

7   There is risk of exposure to radiation during the X-ray procedure albeit a minimal risk.

8   The observation charts, notes, medication charts (the paper work for the patient) in this unit was always located outside of the isolation bay or on the perimeter. These charts were also always oriented so that they faced the central workstation. For a nurse to check a treatment order or to record observations required them to step outside of the isolation room and into the clean space.

inside and if you wash you hands outside are your contaminating everything outside.

This line represents the real (in the psychoanalytical sense) of what is clean and what is dirty. Everything outside of the isolation room is clean, contained and not infectious. Everything in the isolation bay was deemed infectious – again there is no evidence that the chair, the notes, the syringe on the bench is dirty or contaminated. The patient is infectious, so due to this everything in the room is infectious – everything is deemed dirty. The imaginary line between the doors and drapes divided one space as clean and one space as dirty. In this space everything could be deemed clean or dirty.

However, the imaginary line was not *just* imaginary. Gary describes being reprimanded by a member of the infection control team for wearing the protective attire outside of the isolation bay – even when he had not yet been inside the isolation room so as to become 'dirty'. These accounts echo Douglas, in that what is unclean is that which is out of place and the need to approach uncleanness with order, the use of boundaries and the invisible line, and the symbols of protective attire create that order: objects have become border – what is unclean is an apron.

Borders have Become Object

The normal, typical non-infectious[9] ICU patient is bound. Previously the body has been described as bound by skin and embodied in flesh however infection control challenges the notion of this boundedness. There is much discussion, most notably on this topic from Douglas (2002), Kristeva (1982) and Reineke (1997) who all focus their attention on the physical: blood, phlegm and excrement or the socially defiling elements of taboo and sin. However, Sjöholm (2005: 96) suggests that contamination is that which runs most thinly. This thin line between clean and dirty is better understood when considering Foucault.

> But this order of the solid, visible body is only one way – in all likelihood neither the first, nor the most fundamental – in which one spatializes disease. There have been, and will be, other distributions of illness … Has anyone ever drawn up the specific geometry of a virus diffusion in the thin layer of a segment of tissue (Foucault 2003: 1).

The presence of a resistant bacterium such as MRSA is the thin line, the specific geometry of a *virus*[10] or bacteria in a thin segment of tissue. Until now the means

---

9   The reference to the patient being non-infectious is a contradiction. The body is inhabited by many harmless bacteria. Humans and bacteria live in mutual harmony. Therefore the idea that a patient is not infectious is not entirely correct.

10   MRSA is bacterial not viral.

of understanding infection control and its practices has been through the lens of science and medicine. But from the accounts of the participants there is a new way of looking at these practices. On the one side we have the normal everyday running of the ICU with 'normal' patients who do not require additional precautions – clean. On the other side we have an isolation bay (either by design or because it has been designated as such). Within these walls and/or drapes we contain the patient who is deemed infectious – dirty. As Cinderella's slipper is an emblem of hope, so too is personal protective attire and the imaginary line this generation of health care workers' slipper. The presence of the abjected boundary challenges this reality of an unproblematic border of clean versus unclean. Moreover, unlike in the rhetoric of infection control, it is not the patient that is abject in this case, but rather the anxiety caused by the lack of clear boundaries where, as Kristeva suggests, borders have become object.

The nurse represents the *boundaries*, the borders of the less certain and invisible world of infection control and microbiology. The patient *is the reason for the isolation* and additional precautions. They have a pathogen that requires them to have these precautions. It is *assumed* that everything in contact and all that is within the isolation room is infectious. The nurses cannot see the pathogens they assume that they are contaminated with them: hence they take the precautions. From the accounts given in this chapter the nurse is the *uncertain boundary* because they move constantly between *clean* and *dirty*. The nurses constantly collect equipment such as ECG machines, an oxygen mask, or check the patient's chart. To perform their everyday and routine duties they move between the *uncertain* and invisible world of the infectious patient in isolation into what is *considered* as the certain world of clean, *normal* world of the ICU.

However, boundaries are less clear than science would have us believe. The signs and symbols of additional precautions, the isolation room or the imaginary line only make the outside world less certain. It is assumed and accepted that the isolation room is *infectious*. But the nurse, as the one that moves between these two spaces cannot visualize what trails behind them as they move between these two spaces. It is sacred on both sides. On one side is that which represents sin and filth – infectious objects and borders. On the other side – represents a world that is considered as clean, *un-infectious – sacred.* Douglas (2002: 7) reminds us that pure and impure are at 'opposite poles' and it is this binary code which *troubles* the nurse. But where does the nurse fits in this polar world. The nurse is in-between, the nurse in these examples does not belong to either world. Science and medicine would have us understand that the patient is or is not infectious – they are one or the other. The nurse travels between these two worlds, yet they do not belong to either world. On the one side the nurse represents the sinner's reverence for all that is clean in the world – the recognition of the clean and revered world that could easily be contaminated. On the other side the nurse exists and symbolizes an unstable world of dirty unbound bodies – an uncertain space. The nurse must move between the two sides – clean and dirty. On the dirty side the nurse must enlist the *additional precautions* to protect themselves from the defilement of the isolation room through the donning of protective attire and the profuse washing of hands. Moving from the isolation room is known for what it is guilt and reverence – though the patient is not blamed for the pathogen that has inflicted them, that course through their veins or leaks like a miasma from wounds, spit and excrement. There is hope of atonement for the nurses through the sacred washing of hands and the removing of defilement, taboo and contamination, so as to reinstate themselves in their ceremonial clothing (normal uniforms) and then finally by passing the veil of the imaginary line from the isolation room and into the clean.

In such a scenario, the nurse represents a less certain world, and therefore would atonement be enough? Are their hands clean, have their sins left their mark and could they infect another with their sin? This is the non-presentable and less certain space of understandings of infection control. This unstable identity Kristeva (1982) would suggest is the non separation of object and subject. And like Kristeva the constant challenge of ascribing beings and borders, the difference between dung and it enabling me to live and then the corpse, signifying the other side, the place where I am not. Yet in the unclear borders of infection control as nurse, *'I'* am abject. The participants in this study, each nurse, is an *'I'* that is abject because, 'I' must cross the uncertain boundaries and borders between filth and clean. Sjöholm says '"*I*" reject myself and come to be in and through this very rejection … . The problem however, is that the self is expelled in the same process' (2005: 97). The precautions and crossing the line enable me to be in the place where I am not; *infectious* yet I am not infectious. I am *defiled* as everything in the isolation room is defiled.

Conclusion

Under the microscope, on the Petri dish is the certain world of disease causing pathogens. We are reminded of the revolution that science and medicine has pressed upon humanity through the recognition of microscopic *animals* – bacteria, viruses, fungi and parasites – pathogens. The rhetoric of infection control and microbiology is clearly defined: *sepsis or asepsis* – with or without infection. Away from the microscopic lens is the less certain world of clean and dirty. The ICU represents the clean and certain world of everyday practice. Behind the heavy double doors or beyond the 'STOP' sign is the less certain world of the isolation bay. Science would have us understand that the patient is infectious but through the practices of additional precautions the boundaries become less clear and certain. Borders have become object. But the borders are not clearly defined like a Petri dish. The nurse moves between the certain and less certain worlds of clean and dirty. The nurse is in-between clean and dirty – purity and filth. Yet in the unclear borders of infection control as nurse, I am abject. *'I'* must reject myself. In this rejection, the nurse does not deny or reject their contamination. The nurse through the symbol of additional precautions recognizes that they *are* always contaminated, that they *are* always at risk of passing filth, sin and life on to others. In rejecting myself, *I* deny the certain world of *sepsis and asepsis* and understanding the more certain world of life – that cannot be contained.

References

Douglas, M. 2002. *Purity and Danger: An Analysis of Concepts of Pollution and Taboo.* London: Routledge.

Foucault, M. 2003. *The Birth of the Clinic.* London: Routledge.

Kristeva, J. 1982. *Powers of Horror: An Essay on Abjection.* New York: Columbia University Press.

Lawton, J. 2000. *The Dying Process: Patients' Experience of Palliative Care.* London: Routledge.

Reineke, M.J. 1997. *Sacrificed Lives: Kristeva on Women and Violence.* Bloomington: Indiana University Press.

Sjöholm, C. 2005. *Kristeva and the Political.* London: Routledge.

Chapter 16

Regaining Skin: Wounds, Dressings and the Containment of Abjection

Trudy Rudge

Introduction

The study on which this paper is based is an ethnography of wound care procedures in a burn trauma unit (Rudge 1997, 1998). In such a unit, wound care procedures could mean providing a shower where the patient's dressings[1] are removed and their entire body is washed or bathed. When the person requires graft care when grafts[2] are newly applied, then the patient is washed in bed, with their burnt areas attended to in this way while trying to keep the graft and surgical sites as still as possible. Each patient who agreed to participate in this study was admitted to the unit after sustaining a major burn trauma[3]. The patients formed the central focus of the study and were observed while different nurses undertook their wound dressings on three to four occasions each week of their admission. Each patient participant was interviewed about the experience of burn trauma, dressing processes and on discharge, their overall impressions of the experience. Nurses were interviewed about learning to be a burns nurse, the process of wound care and beliefs about burns nursing. Medical records and nursing documentation were another source of data, as were meetings where wounds and wound management were a focus of discussion.

When a person suffers a major burn trauma, they have a long and arduous treatment regimen to recover from the initial trauma with daily assaults on their burns and skin because of dressings, surgical interventions and other forms of treatment (Wiechman and Patterson 2004). The dressings, meant to act as covers (one of skin's functions), are poor substitutes that fail to contain bodily fluids, adding to a patient's insecurities. This is made worse by the fact that contemporary

---

1 Dressings are materials that provide a sterile cover and can be impregnated with treating substances such as antibiotics or other substances that work on clearing or healing the wound.

2 Grafts are skin removed surgically to cover areas that have been cleaned during surgery. Grafting uses different techniques, but the main idea is to put a biological cover on the surgically cleaned area that was previously burnt.

3 Major burn trauma is a person with 20–50 per cent of the total body surface burnt to varying degrees.

treatment regimes assert that for better healing, a moist healing environment is required, which promotes ooze, adding to the failure of the traumatized skin to contain bodily fluids – from at least the patient's perspective (Bland 1996, Gardner 1996, Rudge 1997). Moreover, a major burn is a life-threatening event, and the men in this study all experienced the loss of masculine invulnerability through their brush with death (Yu and Dimsdale 1999). Their interviews, interactions with nurses and feelings about their bodies reveal how they are rendered abject, and that this sense of abjection is set to continue long past their supposed 'cure' by surgical and nursing treatments.

Kristeva (1982) highlights how transgressions and leaking boundaries destabilize and result in the use of the defence mechanism of abjection. Nurses who are witnesses to the trauma, and cause trauma in the treatments required to recover skin, and are caught in cycles of management of pollution as they seek to replace/become the containers for the patients through replacement of dressings, universal precautions, infection control practices and the nurses' emotional labour. This never-ending cycle of cleaning, containment, disciplining and civilizing of the burnt body leads to their positioning as abject, as self-sacrificing maternal functions in the practices of burns nursing. Such a positioning is seldom acknowledged with a variety of outcomes for the players in the drama of burns care, the wound and wounding (psychical and physical) leaking out from the dressings and practices designed to contain the uncontainable. Recognition of such a situation can lead to terror and abandonment; or to compassion and forbearance in the in-between spaces of care.

Why the Psychoanalytic?

To conceptualize the process of healing of burnt bodies and burnt out nurses, a psychoanalytic approach to emotions, bodies and identities was identified as providing a more nuanced analysis. Such analysis explores these traumas, without passing judgement on their experience, as well as recognizing the seriousness with which we should attend to such matters in the work nurses do with their clients. These matters are integral to the work of the unit being studied, and in many others where the work that nurses undertake is witness to or attests to disruptions to identity and social order (see Evans, Pereira and Parker 2008, Madjar 1997, Parker 2004, Wynn 2002). Kristeva's work on the *The Power of Horror*, a work which identifies a key emotional and psychic structure around horror and disgust is central to our understanding of what it is that nurses do in such locations. In this work, Kristeva uses metaphor, textual and structural analysis and a refiguring of Freud's work on the structure of the human psyche to identify abjection's source. She asserts that abjection is the emotion on which all other emotions are founded – it is our emotional life's primer. Abjection's presence signals how our lives are fundamentally uncertain, problematic and disordered even though the forms of systematized control, rules or societal values we put around us for protection from life's braided horrors, fail.

While many theorists (Frosh 1987, Lechte 1990, Oliver 1993)[4] have asserted that Kristeva's work does not lend itself easily to a gendered analysis, because many believe that her approach is essentialist and does not explore the masterful power of the psychoanalyst. However, counter to this, I consider that the concept of abjection is of particular salience when exploring the nature of abjection in wounds and their intersection in particular with gendered and sexed bodies of nurses and patients. Moreover, the effects of abjection are readily identified as present for nurses and patients of whatever gender in the situation of burn trauma and treatment. Embodiment is a key element of the process of abjection and its correlate body, the abject body. I have outlined elsewhere (Rudge 1997, 1998, 2009) the particular issues about skin that encourage a psychoanalytic analysis. Using Anzieu's (1989) work on *skinego* and Lacan's (1977) figuring of the mirror stage in psychoanalytical development, I have shown that skin, as an embodying fabric, has a strongly determinate effect in understandings about our complete and unitary being. Following from such meanings, the use of the psychoanalytic concept of abjection clearly exposes the shades of emotions in play when nurses attempt to control defiling substances or work hard to 'civilize' disease (Douglas 1966). These emotions lie in wait to locate nurses as 'subject of or subject to abjection' (Kristeva 1982: 209). Using the psychoanalytical concept of abjection shows contradictory forces in play during the operations that nurses use to civilize, sanitize and order the various settings where they work. Its presence confirms how the silenced maternal function always already overwhelms scientific, technical or managerialist positionings.

To show this, I explore one instance of care for its positioning, for what it reveals about the multiple levels of containment in operation only discernible when we bring the emotional substance of what nurses and patients are doing into the analysis. Gendered interactions are revealed, for the way that these transgress nursing's ideologies of care and taken for granted understandings about nurses and patients in such situations. In the following section I present moments of containment and transgression in the work of the unit for what they have to say about nursing, emotions and their containment. In using the concept of abjection, the hope is to uncover how such containments have to work against the abject body that always already waits with its intransigent horrors. I show that the abject does not just relate to clearly visual horrors such as wounds, but to a wounded self, where practices that sustain identity are disordered.

---

4   Also other feminist authors (see Spivak 1981) have asserted that Kristeva's work essentializes gender and does not provide a way of exploring within and between group variations. We hope that this edited collection goes some way towards countering such a view.

Blood on the Floor: When it All Goes Awry

One of the major issues for care of people with severe burns is the control of the dressing process and the consequent pain of these dressings and skin loss. Skin has many nerve endings, and when burnt to middle levels some of these pain sensors are permanently activated unless covered sufficiently by dressings or analgesia (medication). The covering that occurs in the care of burns is not just the more recognizable forms such as dressings, but the prescribed acute pain relief as well as a carefully managed dressing technique which controls pain experienced by the patients. In the episode that forms the basis of this section I explore how a less than satisfactory dressing process can happen.

The observation which forms the basis of this chapter is difficult to recount. I found the circumstances difficult to observe, experience and to record objectively. The pain present in the observation is as much mine as the nurse's and patient's whose interaction it records. I had to do a lot or research of records around the incident for it to begin to make sense. Moreover, the effects I observed go wider than the actual dressing itself. They show how the dressing procedure, while a tightly bound space is not hermetically sealed by the technologies and sciences of wound management (Rudge 1998, 1999). The position of abjection always awaits nurses and patients, intruding into their 'boundedness' and the systems of wound management which technologize this space. In this observation, Nurse Irene was taking Phil for his second shower after the grafting of his legs. This dressing took place eight days after the surgery that took skin from his back to replace the skin on his legs. He had been in bed for five days after the surgery, and his progress from the bed to the dressing room had included a trip to the toilet. The incident which is the focus of this analysis occurred 25 minutes into an observation which lasted one hour and 25 minutes.

Observation: blood on the shower stall floor

Irene turns on the shower and tests the temperature of the water. She allows some of the water to fall onto Phil.

Irene: is it the right temperature?

Phil: yea it's alright
She gives him the shower nozzle and the sponge for him to wash of his cream and exudate from recently grafted and still burnt areas on his body. He is also washing unburnt and healed areas. He has grafted hands and is finding it a difficult task to hold the shower head and the washer to undertake the rinsing. He is sitting on a shower chair in the shower stall. Irene starts cutting and removing the paraffin gauze on the recently grafted skin on his legs. Some of it has stuck to the areas around the grafts and Phil flinches as this is removed. A piece of tulle is

hanging beneath the chair from the back of Phil's leg. She pulls at this gauze and it comes away. Phil shouts in pain and starts sobbing. The bottom of the shower is covered in bright blood from his leg. Phil is sobbing; Irene is apologising.

Irene: I'm sorry Phil. I thought that piece of gauze was just hanging there [which it was, researcher note], but it must have been over a raw area at the top of your leg. I'm really sorry.

Phil continues to sob. Colin appears in the bathroom, and puts a bolus through the IV line from the pump. [Phil is having an IV infusion of Morphine, 1mgm/hour.] He then moves out of the bathroom again, not saying anything to Phil, Irene or to me. Phil is shaking and moaning.

Irene: I'm sorry about this. I didn't know that you had some raw areas. I'll put a dressing on the area when we get out of the shower and that will help with the pain. Let's get clean quickly.

Irene continued on through the dressing process. She tried to calm him down by talking about how he could take deep breaths to relieve the pain. I asked them if they wanted me to leave, but Irene said for me to stay, and Phil was not talking. She continued to coach him with his breathing by getting him to follow her breathing calls of 'in and out'. Phil did try but as he was still crying and moaning made it impossible. Phil did gradually calm down, probably due to the effects of the bolus taking hold from the extra pain medication. Irene attempted to do his shave and face care, but it was clear that Phil had had about as much as he could take. She abandoned this after a few tries only. To get the shower and the dressing completed quickly she took over the removing of cream and washed his pubic area. Phil said that he hoped that the burn won't affect the action. Irene got flustered. All the way through the dressing, from getting up and down the hallway, into the shower and beyond the accident, Phil had been addressing Irene as 'dear' or 'dearie' and as the length of the dressing went on the term was increasingly imbued with a sarcastic tone.

Irene was not a young nurse, or inexperienced in burns care. She was however, small, petite even; Phil was a tall, now raw-boned, working class man from a country town. As I noted before this, he was determinedly 'hypermasculine', and very loud (Rudge 1998). After the mistake of pulling on the tulle gras that was over an area that had been debrided but not covered with donor skin, the emotional climate of the dressing disintegrated. Irene was unable to reassure Phil, indeed, he refused to be reassured. Further, he used ways of putting up boundaries to Irene's efforts through sexual innuendo about his penis, and by using diminutives to destroy any sense of authority Irene attempted to re-establish.

The next day when I arrived on the ward to observe Phil's dressing process again, Louise took me aside to ask what had happened. I said I couldn't say without the consent of Phil and Irene, but did say that it seemed to be an accident. Louise said that the tulle was located on an un-grafted section from theatre. She said that Irene had been on leave for three days before showering Phil and that it was likely she did not know of this, and that this information had not been passed on. Louise went on to confide that Phil had told the nurse who was caring for him in the afternoon what had happened during the morning shower. This nurse had said that he had the right to complain about the nurse to the patients' ombudsman, and now Louise had to defuse a very inflamed situation. As Louise noted at a later interview about the incident,

> The type of work we do here means we've got to support each other. I mean it's difficult enough without nurses supporting each other and seeing when someone might be having some difficulties and helping that nurse. It's not that we shouldn't listen to the patients – it's that we need to do that so that we can support each other, and deal with the patient's concerns at the same time.

As I had noted before, Phil was a patient who was skilled at pitting nurse against nurse; gender against gender. On the whole, he manipulated the situation so that the female nurses kept away from him. When Phil needed to return to the ward for extra work less that one month after his discharge, many of the nurses realized that they had let him get away with his splitting and distancing. They knew that this meant that he had not received the optimum care, or the skin care education that he needed as he was able to fob them off for much of this. In his attempt to contain his emotional and physical situation (that is post traumatic disorder (PTSD)[5], depression[6], infected grafts and contractures[7] for release only one month after initial discharge), Phil had become a treatment failure.

---

5   Post traumatic disorder is a mental health condition that is defined in specific ways in the diagnostic manual for mental health conditions. It is a syndrome that is considered a psychological reaction to stress or a group of stressors and characteristically occurs after experiencing an event with is outside of normal human experience. For example forms of these types of experience are: war, torture, violence or witnessing of it, trauma (in this case, burn trauma). Post-traumatic Stress Disorder (PTSD) is the most debilitating of these conditions, and is characterized as evidence of stress which is still present six months after the event (Yu and Dimsdale 1999).

6   Depression is a diagnosis characterized by depressed affect evident in: lack of activity; poor sleep pattern (sleeping all the time or difficulty with sleeping at night; feelings of guilt and worthlessness; feelings that life is not worth living; loss of appetite. This condition often co-occurs with PTSD (Yu and Dimsdale 1999).

7   Contractures occur over joints where a skin graft has constricted and does not allow normal range of movement of function and therefore requires surgical release of the skin, often with re-grafting of the area that needs to be released. With modern techniques of

Moreover, as I tried to understand what had happened I returned to his complete medical record which showed how the above accident occurred. The failure to harvest enough skin to cover his surgical debridement was recorded on his operation notes. It was not recorded in his progress notes, nor in his dressing notes beyond that day. On removal of the dressings from his grafts, tulle gras[8] only had covered this raw area rather than the dressing of choice (that is, silvered dressings[9] or duoderm D™[10]). The lack of dressing was not noted or handed down to anyone new doing his dressing, and over time the tulle fell away from a small section of the raw area. An inevitable accident was framed by several system failures or gaps in Phil's record and in the communication practices of the unit. Dressings were not recorded in full in the medical record but in a note book for nurses, where this lack of cover for Phil's grafted areas was not repeated – the abject escaped!

Hygienic Spaces of Nursing Practice? The Intransigent Personal

In this next section I identify how this event was almost impossible to avoid. There were other contextual issues which I believe complicated this event for Irene and Phil. Some weeks previously I had come upon Irene, in tears, in the tearoom. Irene had experienced a very traumatic event in her personal life and was often in tears, having difficulty focussing on her work and needing constantly to get away from the unit to get time to herself while she was on duty. Prior to this dressing she had had the maximum period of bereavement leave (three days) to get over what I will term the finale of her situation. Irene had felt that this amount of time was not sufficient and she had not received much support from anyone during this protracted situation and crisis. Indeed she acknowledged that her personal situation had made things more difficult for her, and to do the work. As I have suggested elsewhere (Rudge 2009), marking out the journey into 'burns nurse' identity as residing purely within the context of a specialized area of nursing practices denies the effects from sociocultural aspects of nursing identity formation. It is also possible that many nursing ideals do not take account of specificities, such as when a nurse and a patient experience difficulties with their interactions. Instead, such ideals suggest that these difficulties can be overcome by merely resorting to

---

grafting and with the use of pressure dressings such events are not so frequent as they used to be. In Phil's case he had not complied with exercise or other techniques.

8   Tulle gras is a form of dressing gauze that is impregnated with paraffin gel that keeps the wound soft and protected.

9   Silvered dressings is a particular technique of impregating a dressing cream into a fabric to place on the burns. Silver sulphadiazine was the cream of choice at this time, but other kinds of products are available now. This cream has silver nitrate (a debriding agent – takes off dead skin) and an antibiotic to protect from infection.

10   A trade mark or proprietary dressing product that provides a moist healing environment for optimal healing of wounds.

psychotherapeutic technologies (see Rose 1996) or communication techniques that put aside the sociocultural positions of either nurse or patients (see Wilkinson et al. 2008, Stein-Parbury 2009). Also unlike in other professions that experience such issues, there is no routine for supervision or counselling of a nurse to overcome any countertransferance or other emotional issues that arise in the care of the client [11] (Menzies Lyth 1959). Moreover, the abilities of the nurses on the unit did not lead to their structuring or setting limits of this patient who in this situation also required more support and therapy (Herman 1992). Moreover, the emotional politics of this are revealed in using a psychoanalytical approach.

As Moore (1988) alludes to in her analysis of masculinity, abjection is an emotional state potentially available to men, while their usual dominant positioning will mean a different entry point and experience from that of women. Also in the case of these burnt men, any sureties of positioning available through a straight forward masculine identity are difficult to sustain in the face of their experiences of being burnt. The point of this form of analysis is that given these particularities, how are nurses and patients positioned discursively? If males have fantasies about their dominance, certainty, and invulnerability, is it possible to analyse these for what they say when all of these are transformed (Theweleit 1989). These considerations of the construction of meanings in the spaces where burn trauma and trauma nursing take place have both conscious and unconscious effects (Pile 1996). This relates to the way in which taboos, rules, exclusions and the braided horrors of the wounded body, constantly challenge ideologies and knowledge systems put in place to control for its effects (Braidotti 1994).

As part of this analysis also, I want to emphasize that nursing idealizations of care, evident within its preferred texts and practices, are only one part of how nurse-patient relationships come to be constituted. Nursing texts such as procedure manuals, case notes and the myriad journal articles about wound care and wound management practices, consciously or unconsciously, are attempts by nurses to control the emotionality of the spaces of wound care (Rudge 2003). Nursing texts contain the hopes of how to nurse (see also McCabe, Roderick in this collection). They also present certainties such as scientific facts about how wound healing and skin integrity can be recovered. Moreover, it is the tendency in such texts to portray nursing practices as merely techniques, technical responses and outside of the culture and history which form them (Rudge 1999). Such a process is also evident in the way in which nurses seek to control the processes of wound care. Nursing ideals are evident in what counts as competent practice, technical skill as these relate to patient comfort as well as controlled techniques of the self. Patient ideals are readily discerned in their understandable need for their own comfort, surrendering to nursing expertise or working to obtain some control over their

---

11   It is clear that little has occurred with this except in some specializations that work alongside other professions that are mandated to have supervision, such as psychologists and psychiatrists. Mental health nurses have instituted such practices in some areas in Australia, but it is rare elsewhere.

skin or pain management. In the scenario above, the male patient and female nurse are abject: she, because of the failure to not hurt and not keep her reactions under complete control with a professional persona; he, because of his on-going emotional grief over the loss of certainty and masculine invulnerability.

Moreover, systems of meaning, nurse and patient identity and representations of nursing and patienthood leak into and colour this space (Pile 1996). However, in spite of the constraints set by such meanings and understandings, this space always has the potential to fail in containing or controlling transgressive emotions that go unrecognized or are not available for conscious thought. Moreover, the on-going horror that patient Phil was facing was not over his literally wounded body, but was about how his sureties about his identity as a male had been so easily lost – his feelings of puzzlement were very obvious in the tone of voice in his interviews – in the struggle to get through each day. Simple things like holding a cup, shaving his face, managing to wash himself were a constant struggle; the daily shower and dressing a thing of constant dread. It was clear in the trauma of the burn his masculine identity was deeply wounded. To contain this and in the face of a re-traumatizing in the shower that day, he re-asserted his control through verbal and other forms of attack left open to him. While his wounds were now significantly healed, what remained intransigently wounded was his identity as male. His refusal to listen, his lack of forbearance and inability to negotiate would bring about the less than favourable treatment outcomes for him.

Kristeva's discussion of transgressions is illuminating and allows an analysis where we, as analysts, can suspend judgement about either Irene or Phil as we explore how the dressing played out. Kristeva traces the effects of abjection and the abject body on the sociocultural practices around notions of transgression and defilement. Following Douglas (1966), Kristeva asserts such practices are apparent in various taboos, exclusion, ritual practices of tribal societies and around defilement and guilt in Judeo-Christian belief systems (see also Douglas 1966, 1994). Her analysis of the movement from locating transgression and guilt in specific locations, to one more akin with the internalized and unavoidable guilt in Christianity, is heuristic of the containment practices of nurses. There is no doubt that at least one other nurse believed that nurse Irene was entirely culpable for what happened. Many others did not want to know about what was troubling her as they could not empathize with her, but they did not entirely blame her for what happened. Others showed forbearance and quiet support. It is clear that Irene was positioned as abject by her personal life and grief; at the moment of the dressing disaster she carried the unit's communication disorder on her shoulders alone[12] (Douglas 1994, see also Cooke 2007). For patient Phil, the moment of the dressing

---

12   I have written elsewhere (Rudge 2003) about how the absence of a full report on each dressing change in the progress notes erases the nursing presence, and is a type of organizational forgetting (Bowker and Star 2000). It is clear from this incident that such an erasure counts in the continuity of care and has outcomes for both nurses and patients at the level of work on the unit.

experience was just a major example of what went on all the time and what he dreaded every day. When he told me what happened that afternoon, he expected that he would go through with the complaint. That he never actually went through with it, was testament to the senior nurses who drew together around Irene, who got her the psychological support she needed, and who took over the care of Phil until the episode calmed down.

Abjection and Re-containing Boundaries

The burns unit identifies itself as a purified space, yet abjection waits within its cleaned and contained walls. At times its inhabitants are governed by the way in which, as product and process, this space is sterilized of its corporeality: flesh, blood and power (Moore 1988). Moreover, positioned by the effects of the abject body (unclean and disowned), and by the discourses of abjection such interactions can, at any time, move outside of the dominant frames into the in-between, ambiguous and composite (Kristeva 1982: 4). Nurses and patients therefore position themselves dynamically within this seemingly never ending stasis of burn trauma. Analysis of these dynamics suggests how nurses' and patients' space and time is consumed in a logic of both stasis *and also* movement. In such an event then, the way in which nursing and nurses (and patients) are best represented is not by recourse to ideological discourses, but by the way in which such a process is imbued with those horrors of postmodernism Moore alluded to earlier – flesh, blood and power – and conveyed in the nurses' and patients' actions and speech.

However, if one considers her work on abjection as metaphorical, located in the imaginary and symbolic realm, Kristeva affords an explanation of how abjection positions individuals in common and divergent ways. Her discussion of identity, system and its orderings in the emotional realm are immensely productive for understanding how nurses and patients, in traumatic situations, are situated in the ways that they are. Abjection, as a concept, has real, imaginary and symbolic efficacy for understanding the effects of skin loss, and the affects on the individuals who witness such loss. Furthermore, unlike other forms of conceptualization, theorizing them through the identification of abjection's role does not decrease or minimize their impact. Rather, it takes seriously the ontological affects of trauma, accounting for disorder and chaos, while explaining how the system seeks to cover itself from the abject. I assert that Kristeva's psychoanalytic insights afford a view on nursing ideals, and their correlate ideologies, that provide both a position from which to resist and therefore critique nursing's normalizing and scientistic projects.

Finally, I want to return to the symbolic effects of the rupture of skin on patients and the nurses who witness this trauma. A great deal of research focuses on recovering skin, however, the effects of skin's rupture and its centrality to sociocultural integration through the beliefs about its complete and plastic attachment remain unexamined. While it could be said that my argument about skin is over-determined, the anxieties and containment practices present when it no longer contains, suggests how integral it is to the maintenance of systemic order. It is skin's imaginary and symbolic relevance that has an on-going affect on nurses and patients in such units. The diagnosis of PTSD goes only some way to explaining what happened to Phil, for many others were and are more disabled than him, yet they maintain a firmer hold on their sense of self. I consider that it is the significance of the accident, to both Irene and Phil that over-determines this incident. The science of wound healing and pain relief does not resolve all pain because resolution of such suffering takes time, acknowledgement and the provision of care based on this.

Yes, this accident was avoidable; but when it happened how it was resolved was completely avoidable. I think also that it is important that I do not over-dramatize these occurrences. Events like this happen everywhere where people try to work together, and where they seek to overcome with science, a human event. What such a re-telling can do is illustrate how humans can get hidden in the talk about costs, the science of care or cure and the need for health care to be effective and efficient. It is this that I want to disrupt. A few more days leave for Irene; an understanding that she was not the person to care for this hypermasculine man, and that was not her fault; a nurse is not a nurse is not a nurse. Male patients with a major burn are not the same as each other; each has their own relation with their bodies and with circumstances around their burn trauma. Little of this difference is accounted for in other forms of research. As Gatens (1996) stresses, a psychoanalytic approach allows for a view of the significance of imaginary bodies that other forms of analysis omit. To see this as merely interplay between masculine patient and feminine nurse disguises how the practices in the unit are subtly differentiated one from each other. This is not to go to an individualistic framing of self and practice but to see how patients and nurses are captured by the structures of science, rationalized health care and ideals about what a patient and nurse should be. Kristeva's analysis affords a different form of ethics; one acknowledging symbolic and imaginary pain, tempered with forbearance and patience, a counter to a singular focus on efficiencies and one size fits all mentality dominant in health care.

Conclusion

The concept of abjection makes sense of how medical scientific discourses have the power to seduce, contrasted as they are against death, disease and decay. This is not new. Rather, I believe such analyses allow nurses, patients and other health workers the freedom to acknowledge that we cannot make everything better. Rather, Kristeva's insights challenge us to imagine sitting in quiet contemplation, (rather than in frantic self-justificatory activity):

> As we lay bare, under the cunning, orderly surface of civilisation, the nurturing
> horror that is pushed aside by purifying, systematising, and thinking; the horror
> they seize on in order to build themselves up and function ... (1982: 210).

Contemplation of nursing wounds is presently more necessary than ever as we deny the nurturing contained in the recognition and acceptance of such horror. If we but allow such a situation, then nurses do not feel that they are working against a system where their work is hidden, but instead is central in how a patient recovers from such a traumatic event.

Containment is in operation at several levels, physical through dressings, social through the way gender is articulated in dressing process, and emotionally through the containment of pain and suffering for all involved through defence mechanisms such as disavowal, sublimation and denial. If abjection's processes are acknowledged, patients and nurses can discuss how this work proceeds. We then establish a process of potential healing through recognition of affective effects. The availability of abjection, as a position, allows nurses and patients to be healed and to recover through its nurturance and acceptance of the maternal function.

References

Anzieu, D. 1989. *The Skin Ego*. Translated by C. Turner. New Haven: Yale University Press.

Bland, R. 1996. More than just a bit of a nark. *Primary Intention: The Australian Journal of Wound Management*, 4(4), 17–19.

Bowker, G. and Star, S.L. 2000. *Sorting Things Out: Classification and Its Consequences*. Cambridge, Mass.: MIT Press.

Braidotti, R. 1994. *Nomadic Subjects: Embodiment and Sexual Difference in Contemporary Feminist Theory*. New York: Columbia University Press.

Cooke, H. 2007. Scapegoating the unpopular nurse. *Nurse Education Today*, 27, 177–184.

Douglas, M. 1966. *Purity and Danger*. London: Routledge and Kegan Paul.

Douglas, M. 1994. *Risk and Blame: Essays in Cultural Theory*. London: Routledge.

Evans, A., Pereira, D., and Parker, J. 2008. Discourses of anxiety in nursing practice: a psychoanalytic case study of the change-of-shift handover ritual. *Nursing Inquiry*, 15(1), 40–48.

Frosh, S. 1987. *The Politics of Psychoanalysis*. London: MacMillan.

Gardner, G. 1996. The walking wounded. *Primary Intention: The Australian Journal of Wound Management*, 4(4), 5–8.

Gatens, M. 1996. *Imaginary Bodies: Ethics, Power and Corporeality*. London: Routledge.

Herman, J. 1992. *Trauma and Recovery: From Domestic Abuse to Political Terror*. New York: Plenum Press.

Kristeva, J. 1982. *Powers of Horror: An Essay on Abjection*. Trans. L. Roudiez. New York: Columbia University Press.

Lacan, J. 1977. *Ecrits: A Selection*. Trans. A. Sheridan. London: Tavistock.

Lechte, J. 1990. *Kristeva*. London: Routledge.

Madjar, I. 1997. The body in health and illness, in *The Body in Nursing: A Collection of Views*, edited by J. Lawler. Melbourne: Churchill Livingstone, 53–74.

Menzies Lyth, I. 1959. The functioning of sound systems as a defence against anxiety: a report on a study of the nursing service of a general hospital. *Human Relations*, 13, 95–121.

Moore, S. 1988. Getting a bit of the other – the pimps of postmodernism, in *Male Order: Unwrapping Masculinity*, edited by R. Chapman and J. Rutherford. London: Lawrence & Wishart, 165–192.

Oliver, K. 1993. *Reading Kristeva: Unraveling the Double-bind*. Bloomington: Indiana University Press.

Parker, J. 2004. Nursing on a medical ward. *Nursing Inquiry*, 11(4), 210–217.

Pile, S. 1996. *The Body and the City: Psychoanalysis, Space and Subjectivity*. London: Routledge.

Rose, N. 1993. *Inventing Our Selves: Psychology, Power and Personhood*. Cambridge: Cambridge University Press.

Rudge, T. 1998. Skin as cover: the discursive effects of 'covering' metaphors on wound care practices. *Nursing Inquiry*, 5(4), 228–237.

Rudge, T. 1999. Situating wound management: technoscience, dressings and 'other' skins. *Nursing Inquiry*, 6(3), 167–177.

Rudge, T. 2003. Words are powerful tools: discourse analytic explanations of nursing practice, in *Advanced Qualitative Research for Nursing*, edited by J. Latimer. Oxford: Blackwell Science, 155–181.

Rudge, T. 2009. Beyond caring? Discounting the differently known body, in *Un/knowing Bodies*, edited by J. Latimer and M. Schillmeier. Oxford: Blackwell, 233–248.

Spivak, G. 1981. French feminism in an international frame. *Yale French Studies*, no. 62, 159–164.

Stein-Parbury, J. 2009. *Patient and Person: Interpersonal Skills in Nursing*. Chatswood, NSW: Churchill Livingstone Elsevier.

Theweleit, K. 1989. *Male Fantasies – Volume 2 Male Bodies: Psychoanalysing the White Terror*. Translated by E. Carter and C. Turner with S. Conway. Minneapolis: University of Minnesota.

Wiechman, S. and Patterson, D. 2004. Psychosocial aspects of burn injuries. *BMJ*, 329, 391–393. Online http://www.bmj.com [accessed 22 August 2007].

Wilkinson, S., Perry, R. and Blanchard, K. 2008. Effectiveness of a three-day communication skills course in changing nurses' communication skills with cancer/palliative care patients: a randomized controlled trial. *Palliative Medicine*, 22, 365–375.

Wynn, F. 2002. Nursing and the concept of life: towards an ethics of testimony. *Nursing Philosophy*, 3, 120–132.

Yu, B.H. and Dimsdale, J. 1999. Post-traumatic stress disorder in patients with burn injuries. *Journal of Burn Care and Rehabilitation*, 20(5), 426–433.

Conclusion

Defacing Horror, Realigning Nurses

Joanna Latimer

The abject 'disturbs identity, system, order. What does not respect borders, positions, rules (Kristeva, 1982: 4) [it] is [what is] radically excluded and draws me toward the place where meaning collapses' (Kristeva 1982: 2).

In this concluding chapter I think through some of the consequences of bringing together Kristeva's theory of abjection with ideas about the body, patienthood and nursing practice. In *Defacement* (Taussig 1999) asks:

> what happens when something precious is despoiled. [The book] begins with the notion that such activity is attractive in its very repulsion, and that it creates the sacred even in the most secular of societies and circumstances. In specifying the human face as the ideal type for thinking through such violation, the book raises the issue of secrecy as the depth that seems to surface with the tearing of surface. This surfacing is made all the more subtle and ingenious, not to mention everyday, by the deliberately partial exposures involved in 'the public secret' – defined as what is generally known but, for one reason or another, cannot easily be articulated (available at http://www.sup.org/book.cgi?id=432, accessed 16 August 2009).

It seems to me that the preceding chapters in this book in their various ways of 'thinking with' (Puig in press) Julia Kristeva's work 'lift the veil' that occludes the most threatening aspects of patient experience and nursing practice. The book tears the surface, to expose nurses' involvement in what can be thought of as one of the most sacred of modernity's public secrets: the ambivalence and fascination in our materiality and mortality. What is so important in the application of Kristeva's analysis in the context of patienthood and nursing care, is the association of the feminine with the ever-present threat of the dissolution of the self-other, object-subject duality that supports the figure of the individual as an *undivided being*. The abject is that space that most excites and disturbs because it instantiates the fragility of the integral, singular, sovereign subject (see also Latimer 2009b).

The book illuminates how nurses' participation in this occlusion[1] is deeply paradoxical. It is paradoxical because, while they work to contain and order the

---

1 Occlusion: the act of occluding: the state of being occluded: as the complete obstruction of the breath passage in the articulation of a speech sound (http://www.merriam-webster.com/dictionary/occlusion).

abject *in silence*, nurses maintain all that is most sacred to modern Euro-American culture, as at the same time the association between nurses' work and the abject despoils what is most precious. This paradox creates the need to deface the identities of those most associated with the abject: patients' *and* nurses'.

To start, I elaborate what I think the perspectives created by drawing together theories of abjection with analyses of health, illness and nursing care offered in this volume help accomplish. I go on to consider the consequences for ways to rethink patienthood, the meanings of particular aspects of health and illness, and the place of nursing and care. In this I emphasize nurses' dilemma in how to preserve the dignity of patients caught in the conditions that produce the abject. But I also show how the book suggests that nurses, by realigning themselves with different perspectives through which patients' troubles come into view, can help rewrite the conditions of possibility that produce the need for the abject as a realm of both patients' and nurses' experience.

Unveiling the Abject

In the first instance the book acts as a critique of the silencing of some of the most affective aspects of both patienthood and of mundane nursing care. As Rudge and Holmes (this volume) assert:

> Kristeva's theorisation of the psychical defence of abjection affords the possibility of voicing the incomprehensible in bodies that leak, in the chaos of illness and disease, and in the monstrosity of illnesses such as cancer, as well as much that is deemed 'out of place' in nursing and health care.

Each chapter offers ways to articulate and make visible the abject as what Scarry (1995) following Foucault refers to as the inexpressible and the invisible. But the book has a further interest here: that this unveiling brings some of the affective experience of patienthood, as well as the affective aspects of nursing practice, into the light of language. Here, the chapters in Part III, *Containment of Bodies,* focus on patients' and nurses' experience of containing abjection, while the chapters in Part II, *Abject Positioning,* focus on patients' experience of abjection. Each of the chapters reveals how aspects of health and illness, and their treatment and care, can transgress modernity's big stories.

This dimension of the book, through unsilencing those horrific and transgressive facets of illness and care, reinforces the need for processes and practices that can support attention to the affective in patients' and nurses' experience. I have in mind two studies here. First, Rudge's (2003, 2009, and this volume) ethnography of burns intensive care, in which the affective dimension of being burnt is not given attention, time or space, but is aggravated by how the burns unit is organized around a focus on the recovery of skin. By not attending to the affective and symbolic significance of skin, Rudge shows how it is skin alone, rather than personhood, that is recovered, while the psychical dimension is merely covered-up and repressed. Second, Parker and Wiltshire's analysis (2003) of the meaning of nursing handovers at the change of shift. Nursing handovers in this study emerge not as just functional moments for the passing on of information, as many hospital managers and nursing educationalists would assert, but as important occasions for story telling: through the exchange of stories about patients, nurses articulate and 'contain' their experience of the abject.

But the editors and some of the authors, in the current book have another, even more complex and perhaps even more profound mission in their unveiling of the abject. This second dimension is aimed at helping progress a way to expose *the apparatus*, and, to use Foucault's (1973) term, the 'conditions of possibility' that make aspects of being body-persons into abject objects.

Mundane Dividing Practices Performing Culture

For some time it has been understood that so much of what nurses do, and of what patients experience, has to be done, as Jocalyn Lawler (1991) puts it, 'behind the screens'. This need to hide the work that goes on between patients and nurses partly arises because nurses are preserving cultural notions of dignity and privacy: they are helping people to maintain their normality in the face of its potential dissolution. Nurses thus continually work to order and reorder bodies, persons and their parts, in order to help them keep face (Goffman 1955, 1963) and resume or maintain place.

But in conducting spaces of care in terms of what is public and what is private, what is potentially polluting and what is dangerous, also involves nurses and patients in 'categorical work' (Bowker and Star 2000) and 'dividing practices' (Foucault 1982). This mundane 'labour of division' (Munro 1997) helps, to borrow from Mary Douglas (1966), keep things, ideas and identities 'in place'. As it does so, the labour of division displaces possibilities for *other kinds*, of ideas and identities. It is this work of placing and displacing things that helps preserve the distinctions between the sacred and the profane. Indeed, working these distinctions is what constitutes the sacred. This is Foucault's (2006/1961) point over the antimony madness and reason: in marking and sequestrating the mad we continuously reconstitute what (and who) counts as reasonable. Ditto for what is normal and abnormal: we need the abnormal to help us (re)define and (re)member the normal. What is most threatening *and* most good to think, as Douglas emphasizes, is the in between, and that which, like dirt, defies or transgresses categories. Thus the work of sorting things out constitutes both identity-work and a form of alignment. In short, in the arranging of things, people and their significance, nurses and patients align with particular discourses and regimes of truth, or don't.

Let me exemplify what I mean here. I recently attended a workshop in London on Gender, Ageing and the Body organized by the British Sociological Associations Ageing, Body and Society Study Group. A paper by Angela Dickinson (2009) presented research on maintaining nutritional status in hospitalized older people. While the project focused on older people's experiences around food and eating, Angela also explored organizational practices. She showed a slide of a photograph she had taken during this project. The slide was of an elderly man, seated by his bed in front of a hospital table. He was eating his lunch. Next to his plate of food on the table, and amongst other bits and pieces belonging to the nurses, was a cardboard urine bottle. The juxtaposition of the urine bottle and the plate of food, as Dickinson pointed out, was deeply problematic because it contravened cultural norms. She emphasized how hospital practices around food contravened those taken for granted, implicit practices of division around the body, and which become embodied. It is these embodied practices of division that, as Mauss (1973) and Bourdieu (1984) have helped us to understand, perform us *as* 'civilized', and *as* full persons and members.

The difficulty for Dickinson, and the connection that she was making, is that the neglect of these kinds of critical dividing practices put patients in positions that mean it is not just difficult for them to eat, or that there is a risk of infection, as important as these things are. Rather she was stressing how the neglect of these kinds of mundane dividing practices are important aspects of older people's difficulties with eating in hospital *because* of their entanglement with the performance of identity. That is, the body, and how its materiality is ordered, for example in terms of dividing practices around consumption and excretion, is deeply social and cultural. So that the moral universe is without not within (Garfinkel 1967); and in the specifics their 'conduct of care' (Latimer 2000), nurses are, critically, at the centre of its ordering.

Questions arise then as to whether, in the context of the current focus on abjection, the everyday dividing practices, such as the separation of the consumption of food from processes of excretion, are mundane practices that in a sense help to obviate the need for abjection because of how matter, in this case the urine bottle, is made to mean and kept in place.

Rewriting Body-Persons

In some of the chapters in this book there is a suggestion that the abject, and the need for the abject as a defence mechanism, are *effects*. Effects signify processes and conditions of possibility. That is to say, some of the essays here seem to me to extend Kristeva's psychoanalytic emphasis, to suggest that abject objects are not necessarily horrifying or transgressive because of anything inherent: they question the assumption that phlegm, or vomit or faeces are *inherently* disgusting and transgressive. For example, Holmes and Federman (this volume) show how the quality of semen has been rewritten by the discursive apparatus of sexual health promotion, to despoil its association as a source of masculine power. Specifically, they show that public health institutions aimed at increasing people's awareness of HIV risk, in their alignment with popular associations between HIV and homosexuality, are reinscribing 'semen', in ways that afford its reconstitution as an abject object.

Where bodily parts and processes, or aspects of illness, become despoiled the conditions for the defacement, to use Taussig's terms, of persons becomes a necessary defence. Abjection as an *effect* can be reconsidered as the affects of complex social and cultural relations. With Surin (2001: 205), we are thus being invited to ask:

> What do the knotted feeling in the gut, the constriction in the throat, vomit, and faeces have to do with the orderly syntax of knowledge and truth? What do such visceral phenomena have to do with the flows of social power that are regimented by this syntax? How are we to think about those decisive moments of physical and affective communication that precede and exceed interpretation, the sensation that comes before and goes beyond logic but is somehow logic's operative basis, its *sine qua non?*

This complexity and entanglement of the particularities of what produces bodily parts and processes as abject objects with dominant Euro-American, masculinized ontologies is stressed by some of these chapters. Schmied and Lupton (this volume), for example, explore how and when breast milk and lactating breasts become abject objects. The analysis helps illuminate the complexity here: women who are breastfeeding become disgusted, and feel threatened, by breast milk at the point at which it is leaking from their breasts. Pregnancy and breast-feeding can be seen, from the perspective of the integrated, sovereign subject, as periods when in many ways the body becomes not just most animal like, but also when a woman as an individual self is most effaced: her boundaries are most obviously breached and she 'exists' for, and contains, 'an other'. During childbirth, for example, the mother's body labours to become a passage: the cervix literally effaces itself. In pregnancy and breastfeeding then a woman-self as an individual also becomes partially effaced. What Schmied and Lupton's chapter helps us to see is that the revulsion, and the abjection, is the effect of what I have called elsewhere a body-world relation (Latimer 2009a) that gives a particular perspective (Strathern 1991, 1992, 2007) in which the effacement of the woman is experienced as *defacement* of her self, and concomitant spoiling of identity. Only when sited within a particular perspective do lactating breasts become despoiled and despoiling of that most precious of Euro-American preoccupations: the integrated body-self or individual. Thus women who find themselves at times disgusted by having leaky, lactating breasts are deeply implicated in the construction of conceptions of personhood that revolve around the individual, and the singular, integral self. What I want to press therefore is how a shift in perspective (and relations) could rewrite the experience of leaking breasts to obviate a need for the abject as a defence against anxiety, because there would be no despoiling, no anxiety to defend against.

Public Secrets and the Sacred

Nurses are in a dilemma. As many chapters here show, nurses are, like Serres' (1995) angels, messengers who continuously work the border between order and chaos to hold and contain the horror 'behind the screens'. But at the same time they are in a sense contaminated by their knowledge of all that has the potential to rock the sacred, all that needs to be repressed in order for us to live:

> A wound with blood and pus, or the sickly, acrid smell of sweat, of decay, does not *signify* death. In the presence of signified death – a flat encephalograph, for instance – I would understand, react, or accept. No, as in true theater, without makeup or masks, refuse and corpses *show me* what I permanently thrust aside in order to live. These body fluids, this defilement, this shit are what life withstands, hardly and with difficulty, on the part of death. There, I am at the border of my condition as a living being ... (Kristeva 1982: 3).

But some of the chapters in this volume, I am suggesting, invite us to reconsider the very construction of what and when aspects of body-persons – semen, breast milk, mastectomy scars, blood, or burnt skin – are despoiling, and how those associated with these aspects need to be defaced. That is, the authors indicate the relationality of the abject. And as such, how such relations can be *unwritten*. In this latter mission, I think the book shows us the dilemma and offers us a way to a radical ethics of care: as at the same time as authors recognize the need to contain and support people placed in potentially abject positions, they help us keep in mind how the need for the abject is itself an effect of dominant ontologies that nurses can help unwrite. This is the balancing act that calls for a reflexivity that is a lot to ask: it requires awareness, sensitivity and carefulness over how to align and with what/whom, and at what moments.

Defacing Horror

Taussig (1999) suggests that knowing what not to know is the most powerful form of social knowledge. Nurses are continuously associated with the veiling of the greatest and most sacred public secret of them all: not just the vulnerability and materiality of mortality, but the perspective that maintains the figure of the sovereign individual and that allows us to hold the self as apart from, rather than as a part of, others (see Latimer 2009b). But nurses can also act in ways that help preserve yet another critically important secret: that the character of persons and their parts does not inhere, but is an effect of how people – patients, doctors, families, nurses – in their interactions *make worlds together*.

In summary then, what the book helps us to see is that the paradoxical and ambivalent place of nursing is in part due to the very location of care as helping to hold, contain, reorder and/or reconceal the problematic and defacing effects of all that reminds us of our mortal materiality, and of the fragility of our singularity and sovereignty. But some of the screening pertains to the silencing of aspects of what nurses and patients do and experience: a silencing that reinforces and reinstates the processes and conditions of possibility that produce the need for the abject. What the book is doing is both helping us to understand this silencing as a process through which the affective is covered in order to recover the status quo and the normal. So that the book gets at this as nurses' dilemma, and poses questions that point to the need for a radical ethics of care: when should nurses engage in moments in which they are confronted by and indeed are complicit in, the making of the abject, the defence mechanism through which all that is most threatening is made into an object of horror? And when, and how, can they rewrite those aspects of illness, and of persons, to obviate the need for the abject? Taking the perspective of the abject thus helps us to rethink the cultural and social meanings of particular bodily troubles as well as the experience of patienthood, and the construction of stigma, and the possibility that these can be unwritten, that horror itself can be defaced, through how nursing is done.

References

Bourdieu, P. 1984. *The Logic of Practice*. Oxford: Blackwell.

Bowker, G. and Star, L. 2000. *Sorting Things Out.* Massachusetts: MIT Press.

Dickinson, A. 2009. Maintaining the Older Body in Hospital: Patient experiences of hospital food provision. Paper presentation, *Gender, Ageing and the Body Conference.* BSA Ageing, Body and Society Study Group, British Library Conference Centre, London, 20 July.

Douglas, M. 1966. *Purity and Danger.* Harmondsworth, Middlesex: Penguin.

Foucault, M. 1973. *The Birth of the Clinic: An Archaeology of Medical Perception.* Trans. A.M. Sheridan. London: Tavistock Publications.

Foucault, M. 1982. The subject and power, in *Michel Foucault: Beyond Structuralism and Hermeneutics* (2nd edition), edited by H.L. Dreyfus and P. Rabinow. Chicago: University of Chicago Press, 208–226.

Foucault M. 2006/1961. *The History of Madness*. London: Routledge.

Goffman, E. 1955. On face-work: an analysis of ritual elements in social interaction. *Psychiatry: Journal of Interpersonal Relations*, 18(3), 213–231.

Goffman, E. 1966/1963. *Behaviour in Public Places.* New York: The Free Press.

Garfinkel, H. 1967. *Studies in Ethnomethodology*. Englewood Cliffs, New York: Prentice Hall.

Kristeva, J. 1982. *Powers of Horror: An Essay on Abjection*. New York: Columbia University Press.

Latimer, J. 2000. *The Conduct of Care: Understanding Nursing Practice.* Oxford: Blackwell.

Latimer, J. 2009a. Introduction: body, knowledge, world, in *Un/knowing Bodies*, edited by J. Latimer and M. Schillmeier. Socological Review Monographs. Oxford: Wiley-Blackwell, 1–22.

Latimer, J. 2009b. Unsettling bodies: Frida Kahlo's self-portraits and dividuality, in *Un/knowing Bodies*, edited by J. Latimer and M. Schillmeier. Oxford: Blackwell, 46–62.

Lawler, J. 1991. *Behind the Screen: Nursing, Somology, and the Problem of the Body.* Melbourne: Churchill Livingston.

Munro, R. 1997. Introduction – ideas of difference: stability, social spaces and the labour of division, in *Ideas of Difference,* edited by K. Hetherington and R. Munro. Oxford: Blackwell, 3–26.

Mauss, M. 1973/1936. Techniques of the body. *Economy and Society*, 2, 70–88.

Parker, J. and Wiltshire J. 2003. Researching story and narrative in nursing: an object-relations approach, in *Advanced Qualitative Research for Nursing,* edited by J. Latimer. Oxford: Blackwell Science, 97–114.

Puig, M. In press. Thinking with care. *The Sociological Review*.

Rudge, T. 2003. Words are powerful tools: discourse analytic explanations of nursing practice, in *Advanced Qualitative Research for Nursing*, edited by J. Latimer. Oxford: Blackwell, 155–182.

Rudge, T. 2009. Beyond caring? Discounting the differently known body, in *Un/knowing Bodies*, edited by J. Latimer and M. Schillmeier. Oxford: Blackwell, 233–248.

Scarry, E. 1985. *The Body in Pain.* Oxford: Oxford University Press.

Serres, M. 1995. *Angels: A Modern Myth.* Paris: Flammarion.

Strathern, M. 1991. *Partial Connections*. Savage, Maryland: Rowman & Littlefield.

Strathern, M. 1992. *After Nature: English Kinship in the Late Twentieth Century.* Cambridge: Cambridge University Press.

Strathern, M. 2007. Using Bodies to Communicate. Paper presented at *Social Bodies*, Department of Social Anthropology, University of Cambridge.

Surin, K. 2001. The sovereign individual and Michael Taussig's politics of defacement. *Nepantla: Views from South*, 2(1), 205–220.

Taussig, M. 1999. *Defacement: Public Secrecy and the Labor of the Negative.* Stanford: Stanford University Press.

Index